Sex

and

Health

SEX AND

Drawings
by Millicent Rader

HEALTH

A PRACTICAL GUIDE
TO SEXUAL MEDICINE

Armando DeMoya, M.D.
Dorothy DeMoya, R.N.,M.S.N. and
Martha E. & Howard R. Lewis

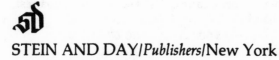

STEIN AND DAY/*Publishers*/New York

First published in 1983
Copyright © 1982 by Armando DeMoya, Dorothy DeMoya,
Martha E. Lewis, and Howard R. Lewis
All rights reserved
Designed by L. A. Ditizio
Printed in the United States of America
STEIN AND DAY/*Publishers*
Scarborough House
Briarcliff Manor, N.Y. 10510

Library of Congress Cataloging in Publication Data

Main entry under title:

Sex and health.

  Bibliography: p.
  Includes index.
  1. Generative organs—Diseases—Dictionaries.   2. Sex—Dictionaries.
3. Sexual disorders—Dictionaries.   4. Health—Dictionaries.
I. DeMoya, Armando.
RC881.S525   616.6′5′00321   80-5799
ISBN 0-8128-2794-5   AACR2

The DeMoyas:
For Marc, Andre, Lourdes,
Emily, and Harold

The Lewises:
For our brothers and sisters
Joyce and Sid, Hersh and Mary Anne, Vida and Erik

CONTENTS

A

B

R

S

T

How This Book Can Help You
A Note From The Authors

This book brings you practical information derived from the new, multidisciplinary branch of health care called sexual medicine.

The field of sexual medicine deals with how sexual activities can affect physical health and how medical conditions can influence sexual functioning. This new specialty draws on advances in gynecology, urology, pharmacology, endocrinology, psychiatry, and many other fields.

A major concern in this book is providing the reader with a better understanding of how diseases and physical conditions may interact with sexual health. Too often, physicians and other health professionals gloss over such information—or fail to discuss it at all.

Both patients and health professionals are widely misled by the stereotype that equates sexuality with vigor and thus decrees that the sexual urges of the aging, sick, or disabled are somehow inappropriate or nonexistent. This leads many patients to assume that an illness makes a satisfactory sex life impossible.

We are happy to help break down this misconception. A major part of this book offers information relevant to specific impairments. We also provide the reader with terminology that will be useful in describing sex-related concerns and asking pertinent questions that may otherwise be too difficult to express to the physician or other health professional.

Many people take medications without considering that drugs may influence their sexual functioning or reproductive capacity. We describe a wide variety of medications (and other drugs that are in common use) and how they may affect sexuality.

Also covered by this book are the health effects of sexual activities. We deal with a large number of sexually transmitted diseases. We also discuss other types of genitourinary conditions, including injuries and anatomical problems. In addition, you will find in these pages a guide to birth control methods, covering their relative effectiveness and risks.

The field of sexuality is rife with quackery. Myriad products are touted to restore potency, increase bust size, or whatever. We tell you which products are useless or possibly dangerous. We also dispel widespread sexual myths and misconceptions, and encourage people to explore a variety of choices in the expression of their sexuality.

This book is organized to lead you to information efficiently: The entries are in alphabetical order for quick, easy access.

The table of contents gives you a complete list of all the individual entries in the book. If you do not find the subject you are seeking in the table of contents, check to see if it is listed in the body of the book. That may refer you to an entry in which your topic is included. Also check the index at the back.

At the end of most entries, we refer you to related topics. In addition, general entries (e.g. VENEREAL DISEASE) will refer you to more specific ones (GONORRHEA, SYPHILIS, and so on). In general, we title entries with the terms most likely to be used by a layman, such as STROKE instead of "cerebrovascular accident."

Like anyone who works in the field of human sexuality, we are indebted to the outstanding pioneers, most particularly to Dr. William H. Masters and Virginia E. Johnson.

We hope our own efforts will bear healthy fruit by enlarging the public's understanding of the many ways in which sex and health are related. We hope also to help provide people suffering from disabilities or diseases a new hope for sexual fulfillment.

Armando and Dorothy DeMoya
Martha and Howard Lewis

ABORTION is the interruption of a pregnancy.

In a *spontaneous abortion* (miscarriage), the embryo or fetus is involuntarily expelled. Most miscarriages occur during the first twelve weeks of pregnancy.

Vaginal bleeding is typically the first sign of an impending miscarriage, suffered in about 1 in 10 pregnancies. Other symptoms include cramps, backache, and nausea.

Such symptoms should be reported to the doctor, who should preferably be a board-certified obstetrician-gynecologist (OBGYN), a physician who specializes in childbirth and female medical problems. His (or her) certification by the American Board of Obstetrics and Gynecology indicates a high degree of competence in the specialty.

Little can be done to avert a threatened miscarriage, especially if there are heavy bleeding and severe cramps. If the bleeding is slight, with little or no abdominal cramps, the doctor will most likely advise bed rest until twenty-four hours after the bleeding has stopped. Strenuous physical activity as well as sexual intercourse is usually forbidden until the bleeding has completely stopped for 24-48 hours. These measures may save the infant.

After a miscarriage, a woman needs a pelvic examination to be sure all the fetal and placental tissues have been expelled. If she experiences an *incomplete spontaneous abortion,* in which some of the material remains in the uterus, she must have the remaining material removed. This is done either by a D & C (dilation and curettage: stretching the cervix and scraping the uterus), or by the use of a drug that stimulates the uterus to contract and expel the remaining material.

The pregnancy that ends in miscarriage usually has an abnormal fetus. In other cases, the miscarriage may be due to the mother's malnutrition or to a medical condition such as genital infection, anemia, diabetes, hepatitis, or heart disease.

Spontaneous abortion can be a traumatic event. If the pregnancy was planned and a baby eagerly awaited, the loss to the couple can be particularly sharp.

This grief may be compounded by a woman's feeling inadequate or incompetent after a miscarriage. She may in addition blame herself for

1

doing something—or failing to do something—that she mistakenly believes caused the spontaneous abortion.

It's important for the couple to work through such feelings of guilt, mourning, and frustration, possibly with the help of a professional counselor.

A woman who has had a miscarriage may wish to become pregnant again as soon as possible. To avoid obstetric complications, she should wait about three months before trying to become pregnant. That is the average amount of time needed for the uterus to get back to normal and again be ready for egg implantation.

In *voluntary abortion,* a woman, with the concurrence of her doctor, chooses to interrupt the pregnancy. A *therapeutic voluntary abortion* is done when medical reasons dictate the necessity for the procedure. A woman who has a heart condition, for example, may not be able to safely bear a child.

No one should ever try to abort herself. Attempting to dislodge a fetus with knitting needles or coat hangers can be fatal.

So can an attempt at do-it-yourself suction with a vacuum cleaner. This could perforate the uterus and suck out part of the intestine. Other home remedies for abortion—drugs, herbal drinks, laxatives, violent exercise—range from useless to dangerous.

Just how safe are abortions? Early abortion is considered a minor and relatively safe surgical procedure. The more advanced the pregnancy is, the more dangerous the abortion becomes. But in the hands of a competent physician, abortion at any stage is no riskier than delivering a full-term baby.

The vast majority of women having legal abortions develop no complications of any kind. A study of 73,000 abortions by the Joint Program for the Study of Abortion shows that during the first twelve weeks of pregnancy a woman's chances of having abortion complications are about 5 percent. After twelve weeks, this percentage increases to 22 percent. Most complications are minor—such as a day of vomiting and fever. Other possible risks of abortion include damage to the cervix or to the uterus. There also may be infection, hemorrhage, and adverse reaction to anesthesia.

Death from abortion is extremely rare. In some years, the Center for Disease Control has reported only one death for every 100,000 legal abortions. The death rate increases as the pregnancy progresses. Out of

100,000 abortions done before the ninth week of pregnancy, there are 0.7 deaths; at twenty-one weeks or later, there are 22.9 deaths.

Does abortion affect future pregnancies? The answer to this question largely depends on whether there were any complications. A World Health Organization study—done at institutions in eight countries where abortion is legal—indicates an increased risk of spontaneous abortion in subsequent pregnancies. But this risk is probably related to the method used for the termination of pregnancy. The rate of spontaneous abortion was more than twice as high for women who had had an abortion by D & C (8.2 percent) as for women who had had an abortion by suction (3.3 percent).

The preliminary findings of a study funded by the National Institutes of Health (NIH) similarly show that women who had abortions— usually by D & C—tended to have more miscarriages and other problems in subsequent pregnancies. The study compared the experiences of more than 65,000 women in New York and Hawaii. Women who had had abortions had 35 percent more miscarriages, plus other pregnancy problems, such as low birth-weight and premature births (25 to 50 percent higher than in the non-abortion group).

On the other hand, studies of uncomplicated abortions done with current medical techniques find no correlation between abortion and any later pregnancy problems. An investigation of the pregnancy records of some 32,000 women at the Kaiser-Permanente Medical Center in Walnut Creek, California, detected a higher rate of miscarriages among women who had abortions before 1973, when D & Cs were common. Since 1974, the researchers found, suction removal of the fetus has been the norm. Now women who have abortions face "little or no risk," according to the Kaiser study, of suffering unusual numbers of miscarriages thereafter.

Dr. Janet R. Daling, an epidemiologist with the Washington State Department of Social and Health Services in Olympia, studied 590 women who had had an abortion, usually by suction. Dr. Daling found that abortions were in no way related to low birth-weight, premature delivery, stillbirth, infant death, miscarriage, or congenital malformations in subsequent pregnancies. Moreover, the abortion procedure itself and the length of pregnancy were not related to any occurrence of low-birth-weight babies or premature delivery.

Dr. Stephen C. Schoenbaum, director of medical services at the

Boston Hospital for Women, studied five thousand deliveries over a nine-month period. He compared three groups of women: those who had had no prior pregnancies, those who had had a pregnancy resulting in a live baby, and those who had had a previous pregnancy that was aborted. Dr. Schoenbaum found "few differences among the three groups." There was no excess of low-birth-weight babies among the women who had had previous abortions. Nor did those women experience a higher incidence of birth defects or infant deaths.

Abortions may be done at hospitals or clinics. Since the legalization of abortion, there has been a proliferation of freestanding abortion clinics. In 1973, hospitals accounted for 57 percent of abortions and clinics 40 percent. By 1976, that trend had been completely reversed; clinics accounted for 60 percent and hospitals only 37 percent.

Abortion clinics are usually the most commonly used facilities for low-cost abortions. They range from pleasant, competently operated facilities to the dregs of the medical world, with substandard equipment and rude personnel.

The cost of abortion may depend on when in the pregnancy it is performed, and whether it is done in a hospital or clinic. Some private health insurance policies pay some or all of abortion costs.

Several nonprofit agencies—such as Planned Parenthood and the National Clergy Consultation Service on Abortion—help women obtain safe, low-cost abortions. They charge no fee for referrals.

Private abortion referral services should be avoided. Such commercial enterprises have sprung up in the first states with legal abortion, like New York, and have victimized mainly out-of-state women seeking abortions. These referral services have charged women over $150 merely for abortion referral—the same information the nonprofit organizations offer free of charge.

Most abortion facilities provide counseling before—and sometimes after—the abortion.

It is the obligation of a counselor at an abortion facility to spell out for a woman who is considering abortion *all* the options open to her. A skilled counselor also provides an opportunity for the woman to ventilate any anxieties she has about the procedure.

Before the abortion, the woman should be firm in her belief that abortion is the best course for her to follow. If she is more than a little ambivalent—or if she is being pushed by someone else into having an abortion—she is much more likely to have a negative emotional reaction to the event.

The method of abortion is determined by the length of the woman's pregnancy. This is measured from the first day of her last menstrual period or estimated from the date of probable conception.

Up to twelve weeks, the most commonly used abortion procedure is suction, or vacuum aspiration, usually done under local anesthesia. The cervix (the opening of the uterus) is usually anesthetized, then dilated. A vacuum pump attached to a thin tube is inserted into the uterus. Gentle suction dislodges the fetus, and a curettage follows to ensure complete evacuation.

Dilation and curettage (D & C) was formerly the most common abortion procedure in the United States. It is now used in only a small percentage of abortions. For D & C the cervix is dilated more than for suction and the uterus is scraped with a curette, a surgical scraper.

Beyond the twelfth week, a woman's risks increase. After sixteen weeks, saline is used for most abortions. In this procedure, the physician applies a local anesthetic and inserts a hollow needle through the abdominal wall into the amniotic sac surrounding the fetus. He draws out some amniotic fluid and replaces it with a concentrated salt-water solution. The salt injection induces an abbreviated form of labor within three days.

Complications of the saline method include infection and retained placental tissue, often with bleeding and fever. Infection can generally be treated with the proper antibiotics. Retained placenta is usually treated by performing a D & C.

Hormonelike chemicals called prostaglandins have been approved by the Food and Drug Administration for use in inducing labor between the third and sixth months. Like saline, the prostaglandin technique involves an injection into the amniotic sac, but of a much smaller amount of fluid. Most women experience some degree of nausea and vomiting. Prostaglandins may also be prescribed in the form of vaginal suppositories.

A menstruallike flow of blood is normal after abortion. It may stop completely for a few days, then resume. The woman should wear sanitary pads, not tampons. She needs to report to her doctor any bleeding heavier than the heaviest menstrual flow she's experienced, and any passage of large clots.

ABSTINENCE

She should also report severe cramps which begin later than a day after the abortion. Other danger signs: fever, a greenish foul-smelling vaginal discharge, and burning or frequent urination. She should have a follow-up examination about two weeks after the abortion.

A woman can safely resume intercourse about 48 hours after the cessation of all bleeding. This usually occurs a week to ten days after the abortion.

If intercourse is resumed prematurely, bleeding may increase. Moreover, the cervix is still open. During intercourse, the penis can act like a plunger, pushing bacteria toward the uterus and causing pelvic inflammatory disease.

See also CONTRACEPTION; PELVIC INFLAMMATORY DISEASE; PREGNANCY.

ABSTINENCE. Voluntary refraining from sexual contact.

The reasons for abstinence are extremely varied. People often abstain from sex during periods of stress or illness. Some may find themselves so preoccupied with work or creative activity that they don't think about sex for months at a time. Others find that in the absence of a particular sex partner they are not interested in sex at all. Still others abstain from sex for a time following a series of unpleasant sexual relationships. They find a sexless period a comfortable respite from the dating game.

Some of the people who abstain may avoid sex altogether. Others refrain from sexual involvement with other people but achieve sexual release through masturbation.

Many people who give up sex for a time find the experience instructive and satisfying. They often have a sense of independence and freedom in not feeling compelled to engage in sexual activity simply because they have the opportunity.

For others, however, their lack of interest in sex is a cause for concern. People may become distressed if a period of abstinence stretches into years, and they feel no desire for sex. Such people may seek help from sex therapy clinics. Indeed, sex therapists find that a lack of sexual desire has become one of the most prevalent complaints in recent years. Often, physiological factors are found to account for diminished desire—illness, medication, depression.

Guilt over sexual impulses may account for abstinence. Emotional

6

conflicts about their sexuality can cause both men and women to avoid sexual encounters. A man who has an excessively strong attachment to his mother, for example, may be abstinent because no one can ever equal his mother in his mind; or he may associate all women with his mother, and sexually avoid them in order to escape unconscious incestuous guilt.

Similarly, young girls often focus their budding sexual feelings on their fathers. In some young women, the guilt of their forbidden sexual impulses becomes generalized to all men, and they can't overcome this guilt sufficiently to engage in sexual relations.

When such neurotic conflicts account for abstinence, psychotherapy or sex therapy may be helpful. Therapy may also be of help in the rare instances when people abstain because of an aversion to sex. Such people experience irrational, overwhelming anxiety at the thought of sexual contact.

Some people choose abstinence out of religious conviction, feeling that the finest way to pursue their religious beliefs is to forgo the sexual preoccupations of dating and family life. Some enter religious orders in which celibacy is prescribed.

Abstinence is not harmful. Lack of sex causes no organic illness or medical condition. However, people who repeatedly become sexually aroused without sexual release are likely to experience pelvic congestion and discomfort.

Nor does abstinence cause psychological disturbances. A popular notion holds that abstinence leads to frustration, which causes neurosis. There is no evidence for this belief.

See also EPIDIDYMO-ORCHITIS; MASTURBATION; PELVIC CONGESTION; SEX THERAPY.

ACROMEGALY. See HORMONE DISORDERS.

ADDISON'S DISEASE. See HORMONE DISORDERS.

ADRENOGENITAL SYNDROME. See HORMONE DISORDERS.

7

AFTERPLAY. See FOREPLAY.

AGING. Older people in reasonably good health can continue an active sex life into their eighties or nineties or beyond if they and their partners remain sexually interested.

In general, people who have had satisfying sex lives in youth and middle age are more likely to continue sex into old age.

Many older people, however, are victims of myths about sexuality and the elderly. There has been a prevailing notion that the elderly are no longer interested in sex—and that they no longer have the capacity even if they should be interested. Further, some say, sex is debilitating for the old and likely to be dangerous. Perhaps most important, there's a feeling that sex in old age is somehow unseemly, inappropriate.

Grown children with elderly parents may be particularly reluctant to view them as sexual beings. If the parents do express some interest in sex, they may get the feeling that their children see this as obscene or unnatural. What is considered normal sexual desire in a 25-year-old is considered lechery in a man of 50 years or older.

Many older people accept society's myths that sexuality ceases with aging. This expectation becomes a self-fulfilling prophecy. If people believe that sexual interest disappears with advancing age, they often find that it indeed does.

Institutions for the elderly perpetuate the myth of sexless older years by separating males and females—sometimes even if they are married to each other—and providing little or no privacy.

Some older people who find that they remain interested in sex may feel abnormal or sinful.

Recent research has dispelled the myths by showing that many older people retain an interest in sex and maintain active sex lives well into old age. In one study, 93 percent of the respondents said that they liked sex. An overwhelming majority of the participants—even those who were unmarried—said they continued to be sexually active.

Most people experience gradual changes in their sexual responses. Sexual processes slow down with advancing age, often beginning in the 40s, 50s, or 60s. In general, regular and frequent sexual activity seems to maintain sexual responsiveness.

Among women, aging need not decrease sexual desire or capacity for orgasm. After menopause (see entry), women cease ovulating and are no longer fertile. But their interest in sex and their capacity for sexual enjoyment needn't decline:

Aging does cause some changes in a woman's sexual response cycle. Her vagina is slower to lubricate with sexual arousal, and the amount of lubrication may be decreased. Her clitoris may become less prominent. There is likely to be less expansion of her vagina with sexual arousal.

She may be slower to reach orgasm, and her orgasmic phase may be shorter; she may experience fewer orgasmic contractions than she did when she was younger. Some older women may have a painful spasm of the uterus during and/or after orgasm because of decreased estrogen. Estrogen replacement therapy can bring relief. After orgasm, older women have a rapid return to the nonexcitement phase.

Some older women experience painful intercourse because of vaginal changes due to estrogen starvation (see MENOPAUSE). They should seek medical advice.

Among men, aging usually causes slower and less firm erections. An older man is less likely to experience spontaneous erections. He'll probably have an increased need for direct stimulation of his penis to attain an erection.

An older man also typically has an increased ability to maintain an erection for long periods before ejaculating. If he loses an erection before ejaculating, he may have some difficulty returning to a full erection.

With aging, a man has less need to ejaculate. Often, an older man can have very satisfactory intercourse without ejaculating at all. When he does ejaculate, an older man will have a decreased force and volume of ejaculate. There may be fewer expulsive contractions on ejaculating, and an increased interval between contractions.

After ejaculation, there is a rapid detumescence of the penis, and a longer refractory period before an erection can occur again.

Many men, unaware that these changes in sexual response with aging are common and expected, become anxious and/or depressed. Wrongly assuming that such changes herald the beginning of the end, such men may prematurely give up on sex. For others, performance anxiety may result in psychogenic impotence.

Men with such concerns can be reassured that, from a woman's point of view, sexual changes resulting from a man's aging are often welcomed. Since sexual arousal occurs more slowly in an older man, he's likely to engage in sexual play at a more leisurely pace before insertion. Many women find this slower pace more satisfying.

Furthermore, an older man's ability to maintain an erection for long periods allows the woman more opportunity to attain orgasm.

After a period of abstinence, older people may have a much harder time resuming intercourse than they would have had in earlier years. An aging woman who abstains from sexual intercourse may have a greater degree of shrinkage in the size of her vagina than a woman who has continued sexual activity. A man after prolonged abstinence often finds he is unable to have erections when he attempts to resume intercourse.

General poor health or chronic illness in one or both partners may lead to a cessation of sexual activity.

Other stresses in the lives of the elderly may contribute to the end of a sex life. The aging typically have to cope with the loss of role and status associated with employment; with relocation; with the end of parenting; with the deaths of friends and family. Lessened physical vigor and physical signs of aging may damage their self-esteem. The aging may thus feel less sexually desirable and may be loath to initiate sex.

Death of a spouse poses many sexual problems for the aging. Widows and widowers generally lose their sex drive during bereavement. This absence of sexual feeling is part of a painful, disruptive grief process that also disturbs sleep and appetite, worsens medical problems, and causes mood swings and depression.

But in healthy men and women, sexual appetite is only dulled by grief. As time passes, the sex drive reemerges, increasingly so as grief wanes.

Such reemergence of sexual feelings may disturb widows and widowers. They typically associate sexual feeling with pleasure shared with the spouse. Thus sexual feelings can be painful reminders of yet another way in which the loved one will be missed.

Reemerging sexual desires also may make the widowed feel guilty. A common reaction of the survivor is: "How selfish of me—to want sexual gratification when my husband (or wife) is dead."

Being deprived of a satisfying, intimate sexual relationship is a grave, but little-discussed, loss to the widow or widower. If sex was rich and fulfilling in marriage, the widowed will feel its absence all the more.

This sexual loss may be especially difficult to bear if they consider such feelings improper and are reluctant to discuss them. The elderly bereaved rarely get much encouragement from physicians and others who work with the widowed. Such professionals seldom initiate discussions of sexual needs, a silence that serves to reinforce a sense of shame.

In the absence of acceptable sexual partners, widows and widowers tend to masturbate. Sexual dreams are another sexual outlet among the elderly widowed. Older women as well as older men have frequent sexual dreams of orgasm.

Widows may have particular difficulties in finding sexual partners. Because men tend to die younger than women, there are nearly 5 widows for each widower: almost 10 million women for about 2 million men. Even if every widower were to marry a widow, nearly 8 million women would still be denied marital sex. Of course, many widowers never remarry. And, while widows generally marry men close to their own age, a substantial number of widowers seek out women considerably younger—reducing the pool of eligible widowers still further.

Some widows and widowers are lonely but cannot become sexually or emotionally involved with members of the opposite sex, even years after the death of a spouse. Widows may find a practical problem in a lack of suitable partners. Organizations such as the "Widow to Widow Program" or local social service organizations can be helpful.

Many elderly widows and widowers live together without formal marriage. If they legally married, their total social security income would be reduced. Despite the common belief that aging makes people more puritanical, a substantial subculture of older people share housing for social, sexual, and economic reasons.

See also MALE CLIMACTERIC; MENOPAUSE.

ALCOHOL. As Shakespeare's porter in Macbeth observes of drink, "It provokes the desire but it takes away the performance."

Many people find that a small amount of alcohol (possibly one or two drinks) allows them to feel more relaxed. Anxieties about sex may be overcome, and their sexual response may be enhanced. Some people are able to use just enough alcohol to overcome some sexual inhibitions—yet not enough to impede their performance.

But the difference can be critical. Alcohol is a central nervous system depressant. In men, it evidently depresses the pudendal nerves and erection reflex. Alcohol consumption is one of the most common causes of impotence (after fatigue, both physical and psychic). That one drink too many explains why couples coming home from a party are often disappointed when they try to make love.

The effect depends on the man's tolerance to alcohol and may be subtle. A man may have a martini for lunch, another after work, wine with dinner, then a cognac with his coffee. He doesn't feel drunk—he may not even think of himself as drinking. But the level of alcohol in his blood may make an erection impossible.

A man's tolerance may be even lower if he smokes, is under stress, overeats or eats poorly, or suffers poor health. In women, alcohol may similarly diminish sexual response.

ALCOHOLISM often leads to sexual dysfunction in both men and women. It is estimated that 50 percent of alcoholic men and 25 percent of alcoholic women suffer impaired sexual functioning.

In men, alcoholism typically results in decreased sexual desire. Impotence is common. Some men have problems ejaculating.

Alcoholic women often experience difficulty in becoming sexually aroused. Some report that they are able to have orgasms much less frequently, less intensely, or not at all.

Chronic abuse of alcohol can directly interfere with a man's sexual functioning by causing male hormone disruptions. Testosterone production may decrease or testosterone may in other ways become unavailable. Sperm production may decline. Nutritional deficiencies—common in alcoholics—may contribute to hormonal difficulties.

With prolonged alcohol abuse, the testicles may atrophy.

Relief of the sexual dysfunction depends on how well the tissues repair. In men—even after abstention from alcohol for months or years—sexual functioning returns to normal in only about half of the cases. Little is known about the long-term effects in women.

Psychological factors may also be involved. Recovering alcoholics typically suffer low self-esteem, guilt, or depression—any of which can contribute to sexual difficulties. What's more, the psychic pain of such feelings can lead to a return to drinking.

Marital discord is common when one partner is an alcoholic. Typically, such marriages are characterized by distrust, hostility, and poor communication. The sexual relationship may have been physically abusive. Such feelings and patterns may persist, even after the alcoholic has stopped drinking, and contribute to sexual problems.

So, too, recovering alcoholics who have experienced sexual difficulties often become anxious about their sexual performance. They watch themselves carefully, monitoring their sexual responsiveness. Such anxious watchfulness typically causes sexual difficulties to persist.

A recovering alcoholic would be wise to engage in intimate sexual activity—but with no goal in mind such as orgasm, full erection, or ejaculatory competence—for 3 to 6 months after drying out. This period of time allows for the alcoholic to resolve any medical, drug-related or nutritional problems associated with the alcoholism. Personal and marital difficulties may also be sorted out during this time.

If sexual difficulties persist beyond 6 to 12 months, sex counseling or psychotherapy may be helpful.

See also ALCOHOL; IMPOTENCE; SEX THERAPY.

AMEBIASIS is an intestinal infection caused by one-celled protozoa called *Entamoeba histolytica*. In the United States, about 4,000 cases are reported each year, and the incidence seems to be rising.

The parasite usually causes intermittent diarrhea and constipation, flatulence, and abdominal cramps. Appetite is typically diminished, and there may be nausea. Children may further suffer pallor, mild fever, and growth retardation.

Amebic dysentery, a virulent form of amebiasis, is marked by crampy abdominal pain and diarrhea with blood and pus, sometimes with a slight fever. The patient may become anemic and lose a great deal of weight.

Infection is transmitted through exposure to contaminated feces. This may be by hand-to-mouth contact, drinking contaminated water, or eating raw fruits and vegetables. In places where human feces are exposed in the absence of sanitary latrines, the infection can also be carried to foods by roaches and house flies.

The parasite can also be sexually transmitted as a result of anolingual contact, or anal intercourse followed by oral-penile contact.

Amebiasis is treated with either dilanoxide furoate (Furamide) for mild cases or metronidazole (Flagyl) for mild to severe. Treatment usually lasts 10 days. Metronidazole is not recommended for pregnant women, particularly in the first trimester.

See also ANAL SEX.

AMNIOCENTESIS is the procedure for withdrawing and analyzing amniotic fluid during pregnancy. It is used mainly to determine whether the fetus is suffering from a wide variety of fetal disorders or genetic defects such as Tay-Sachs disease or Down's syndrome. It can also determine a fetus's stage of development.

Amniocentesis is performed in a doctor's office, genetic laboratory, or hospital between a woman's 14th and 16th weeks of pregnancy. A local anesthetic is applied to the woman's abdomen. The physician then inserts a hollow needle into the woman's lower abdomen. The needle withdraws some fluid from the sac that surrounds and protects the fetus.

Amniocentesis is done in conjunction with a sonogram: by means of ultrasound, the fetus's image is projected on a screen, aiding the physician in determining where to insert the needle.

The amniotic fluid contains fetal cells that can be cultured in the laboratory. After 2 to 4 weeks, chromosome studies and biochemical analysis can uncover any of about 300 defects. If the fetus is found to be afflicted with a serious disorder, the couple can decide whether to continue or terminate the pregnancy.

Amniocentesis should not be routinely performed before age 36. The procedure is done on younger women when there is a strong family history of birth defects.

See also ABORTION.

AMPHETAMINES are commonly prescribed to decrease appetite and promote weight loss. There is also a substantial illicit amphetamine trade.

Little research has been done on the effects of amphetamine use on sexuality. In small oral doses, little effect on sexuality is observed— although some men report impotence or changes in sexual desire.

Women who are chronic amphetamine users may experience sexual disturbances and dissatisfaction with sexual activity. Some are promiscuous. But these sexual problems are not thought to be caused by their use of amphetamines. Rather, the drug abuse and sexual difficulties are both thought to be the result of personality factors.

Men usually report more positive sexual experiences with amphetamine use. Particularly in men, large intravenous doses appear to enhance sexuality. The initial "rush" produces a numbness and tingling that is often described as a diffuse orgasm. Some men report prolonged erections, delayed ejaculation, and increased capacity for repeat orgasm.

See also MEDICATIONS.

AMPUTATION is the surgical removal of an arm or leg.

For most people, losing a body part and function alters their sense of themselves. Amputees frequently experience distortions of body image. Phantom sensations in the missing limb may trouble them. Anxiety and depression are common after amputation surgery.

Amputation often leaves people feeling helpless and diminished. Loss of control and an inability to do ordinary tasks at will contribute to feelings of worthlessness and vulnerability.

Amputees typically worry about sexual rejection. A man or woman with an amputated limb commonly believes that the surgery is a liability in attracting, or keeping, a sexual partner. This may or may not be true. It is possible that the amputation may indeed repel a potential sexual partner or a spouse. More commonly, however, this feeling is an unrealistic fear based on loss of self-esteem.

Amputees find that the surgery initially limits their sexual expressiveness and physical maneuvering. A person with a missing arm is unable to stroke the partner in the same manner. Loss of a leg means less control of the body during intercourse. If the person is accustomed to taking a more active role in sexual activity, the role changes necessitated by surgery may be very threatening. The sexual partner may have equal problems adapting to changed roles and techniques.

Amputees should experiment with various new coital positions if the loss of the limb makes usual positions uncomfortable or impossible. Pillows can be used to maintain a level pelvis when a leg is missing.

Sexual dysfunction after amputation may result from particular feelings some people bring to amputation surgery. Impotence may develop if a man equates the amputation with castration. Others may suffer sexual problems if they experience the surgery as punishment for past sexual indulgences or indiscretions.

Most hospitals have rehabilitation programs for amputees. Ideally, such a program should include not only physical, but also emotional, rehabilitation. An amputee should expect that a new adjustment to spouse, friends, family, work, society—and sexuality—will take several weeks or months. It is usually beneficial for the spouse to be involved in the rehabilitation program.

A prosthesis—an artificial limb—often aids in the adjustment process and helps the amputee become more self-reliant and mobile. Anything that increases the amputee's self-esteem is likely to enhance feelings of sexual desirability and improve sexual functioning.

In general, the nature of the problem requiring amputation determines the ease and degree of sexual rehabilitation. Those amputated for traumatic injury usually have the easiest course of readjustment. They tend to be young, healthy, and in good physical condition, and usually soon find that their sexual functioning is unimpaired.

If the amputation was for a tumor, the patient is likely to suffer a more profound psychological impact and to require more counseling.

Those people amputated for disease (primarily the effects of diabetes or arteriosclerosis) are likely to be older, ill, and to have had a higher incidence of sexual dysfunction before surgery.

See also MASTECTOMY.

AMYL NITRITE is a fast-acting smooth-muscle relaxant and coronary vasodilator, expanding blood vessels around the heart. Its medical use is to relieve attacks of angina pectoris, characterized by spasmodic chest pain and the feeling of suffocation.

Some people intensify their orgasms by popping an amyl nitrite vial and inhaling the vapor. The drug probably causes engorgement of the genitourinary blood vessels, which could cause a heightened rush during the decongestion accompanying organism. By abruptly lowering blood pressure, the drug also may produce feelings of dizziness and giddiness that add to the experience. The skin may become more sensitive, enhancing tactile pleasure.

While there have been no reports of serious complications among those who use the drug in this fashion, recreational use, particularly by heart disease or stroke patients, is best avoided. The drug may also briefly raise pressure in the eye, making its use questionable by patients with glaucoma and other eye diseases.

The most common side effect is a severe headache, usually short-lived and rarely dangerous. Fainting, especially after drinking alcohol, is another common occurrence.

A final precaution: amyl nitrite vapors are highly flammable, so they should not be used near a flame or intense heat that could cause them to ignite.

ANAL SEX revolts many people because they have grown up learning that the excretory system is "dirty." Sexual pleasure associated with the anorectal region may therefore be viewed by them as a "perversion."

Anal sex for many couples is an acceptable form of sexual expression, for heterosexual as well as homosexual partners. The anus is richly endowed with nerve endings. It can be experienced as an erogenous zone, suited to pleasurable stroking and penetration.

The receiving partner may feel satisfaction from deep penetration comparable to that from deep vaginal insertion. While stretching of the anal sphincter is uncomfortable to many, this same sensation is erotic to others. Some men prefer anal to vaginal coitus because of the tighter grip the sphincter offers the penis.

Some heterosexual couples enjoy digital stimulation of the anus—but are afraid to try anal intercourse because they erroneously believe it betrays a "homosexual" preference. In fact, sexual activity of any kind between a man and woman is, by definition, heterosexual. Homosexuality has to do with the matter of preference regarding the person with whom one shares a sexual experience—not with what is done. Anal sex thus is simply one of many options available to any sex partners.

Injury can result. Tissue damage from anal intercourse is much more likely when the practice is forced or violent. The anus and rectum are capable of tremendous dilation without injury. But cuts and tears can lead to dysfunction of the sphincter, muscles that control bowel release.

Thus, couples should engage in anal intercourse only if the receiving partner is willing. When the recipient enjoys it, the sphincter dilates fairly easily—and the insertion is essentially painless. But if the recipient submits only to please the partner, there is likely to be sphincter tightening, difficult penetration, and considerable pain.

Couples should use a lubricant. Petroleum or surgical jelly will help the penis glide into the anal canal. Natural lubrication is too scanty to promote insertion, even though there is a slight moistening of the skin around the anus during sexual excitement.

Penetration should be gentle. It eases insertion if a bowel movement has emptied the receiving partner's rectum. Along with adequate lubrication, slow insertion helps avoid fissures (cuts in the membrane), the most common injury resulting from anal intercourse. If tears in the anus are irritated by repeated anal friction, there may be severe pain, bleeding, and pus-laden discharge. Having bowel movements may be agonizing. Doctors usually prescribe pain relievers, antibiotics, and stool softeners.

Several times a day, receiving partners need to tighten their sphincter muscles, as if holding back a bowel movement. Otherwise, the stretching of this ring of muscle may cause problems in holding in gas, with possible leakage and soiling of undergarments. If anal intercourse is discontinued, there is generally some recovery of muscle tone.

No large objects. Perhaps the most extreme injuries associated with anal sex arise from the insertion of the hand into the rectum. The rare practice commonly causes severe rectal lacerations, sphincter injuries, and varying degrees of incontinence. Proctologists widely consider it tantamount to mayhem.

Foreign bodies inserted into the rectum—vibrators, artificial penises, cucumbers, candles—can likewise cause severe tissue damage. The rectum joins the sigmoid colon at a right angle. Objects can thus slip out of reach into the colon. They may cause perforation and potentially fatal peritonitis.

If an object is lost in the rectum, no attempt should be made to retrieve it. The victim should go to a hospital emergency room. Anesthesia and special instruments may be needed.

Safeguards against infection. Feces may harbor many germs. Urethritis (inflammation of the urinary passage) may result from fecal contamination of the penis—another reason for the receiving partner's defecating beforehand. Also, a contaminated penis may transfer rectal bacteria to the vagina and female urinary tract. The major danger is from Escherichia coli. Salmonella and Shigella organisms also may be transferred this way.

The inserting partner should wear a condom for anal penetration, then dispose of it before entering the vagina. As an alternative, a couple might have the vaginal intercourse before the anal—there is little danger of vaginal organisms infecting the rectum. At the minimum, the penis should be washed with soap and water as soon as possible after anal penetration, certainly before entering the vagina.

A physician should be consulted if there are such signs of infection as frequency of urination, urethral discharge, burning on urination, or cloudy urine. Infection may also cause a slightly elevated temperature, malaise, and chills.

A condom is essential if either partner has a venereal disease. Gonorrhea is the most common anorectal venereal disease. Rectal symptoms, if there are any, range from mild itching or burning to severe discomfort.

All other venereal infections—syphilis, anal warts, chancroid, granuloma inguinale, herpes simplex, lymphopathia venereum—can be transmitted through anal intercourse.

Recipient men often suffer prostatitis (inflammation of the prostate gland). Treatment usually calls for increased fluid intake, antibiotic therapy, and avoidance of anal intercourse.

Infection also may be spread by anal-oral contact (anilingus). The anal region should be washed to reduce the spread of disease if the area is licked and kissed in love play. Viral infections such as herpes simplex, infectious hepatitis, and viral diarrheas can be acquired in this fashion. So can parasitic infections such as amebiasis, giardiasis, and pinworm infections.

See also PROSTATITIS; VAGINAL INFECTION; VENEREAL DISEASE.

ANDROGENS. See HORMONE DISORDERS.

ANIMAL DISEASES (zoonoses) can be contracted through close contact with an animal.

Some people treat their animals, especially their pets, as intense love objects—cuddling, fondling, hugging, and kissing them. Others use their pets for masturbatory sex play. A small number of people have sexual intercourse with animals, a practice called bestiality or zoophilia.

The greater the amount of contact, the greater is the risk of contracting a disease from the animal. Such diseases include leptospirosis (from pigs, sheep, dogs), which can enter through the mucous membranes; anthrax, rare in this country, can be contracted from a wide variety of animals through touching and inhalation; and toxicariasis (roundworms), which can be contracted from cats and dogs through mouth contact or contact with contaminated feces.

Toxoplasmosis is a generally mild infection which often has no symptoms. Contracted from cats through mouth contact or feces, the infection can be dangerous during pregnancy. When a pregnant woman is infected, there is a 20-30 percent chance that the fetus will be affected, with consequences ranging from mild visual impairment to mental retardation and central nervous system disorders. Pregnant women should therefore avoid close contact with cats. Another family member should dispose of the kitty litter.

Venereal disease cannot be contracted from an animal. The organisms that cause herpes, syphilis, gonorrhea, and other venereal diseases do not grow on nonhuman animal tissue.

ANOREXIA NERVOSA (Greek, "psychic loss of appetite") is a disorder in which the victim virtually stops eating.

While males and people of all ages may suffer from this disorder, its typical victims are girls between 12 and 18. They become emaciated. Some literally starve themselves to death.

Parents should be alert to symptoms in their children. Anorectics have the best chance of cure if they receive treatment at the onset of the illness. Here are the syndrome's characteristic symptoms:

● *Extreme weight loss.* It is not uncommon for anorectics to lose 40 percent of their body weight. One youngster dropped from 128 to 71 pounds.

● *Cessation of menstruation.* As a young woman's level of nutrition falls, her endocrine balance goes awry. She stops ovulation and can suffer long-term damage to her reproductive cycle.

The majority of women with anorexia nervosa stop menstruating when they have lost about 15 percent of their body weight. Many do not resume menstruating for months or years after regaining their normal weight. In fact, the menstrual cycle may never become regulated.

● *Lack of sex drive.* Anorectics commonly have little interest in sex. They usually have negative attitudes toward sex and masturbation and lack orgasmic responsiveness.

● *Refusal to eat*—or insistence on tiny meals, usually once a day. Such compulsiveness is usually hard to miss. One young woman had her daily meal at 9 P.M. She calculated it to consist of exactly 776½ calories: dried cottage cheese, low-calorie rice patties, eggplant, and one apple—all carefully measured and weighed.

● *Distorted body image.* An anorectic may be told that she looks like a concentration-camp victim, but she will insist that she is still too fat. Anorectics seem unable to perceive their deteriorated physical condition. Standing before a mirror, they contend they are just beginning to become pretty and healthy-looking.

● *Excessive exercise.* Although she runs herself ragged, an anorectic may show no sign of fatigue. Anorectics seem sustained by some miracle of energy.

● *Denial of hunger.* An anorexia nervosa sufferer may actually be very hungry but has developed a morbid aversion to food. She is likely to feel that food will make her sick or in some other way harm her. She may associate eating with sinfulness; starvation, with virtue.

● *Wasting of muscle tissue.* In the later stages of the syndrome, the body begins to eat away at itself in a desperate search for protein. Heart, lungs, and other vital organs may be damaged.

What causes anorexia nervosa? Psychiatrists speculate that the disease is a rejection of adulthood, a refusal to accept the inevitability of becoming sexually mature. An adolescent may try to defy the course of natural physical development in a dramatic effort to control her body. And, indeed, her self-starvation has the effect she desires: her curves recede, her breasts nearly disappear, and her menstruation stops.

Refusal to eat also may represent a power play. Food provides weaponry in the struggle between an anorectic and her parents. The reaction of a starving youngster's family is naturally, "EAT! EAT! EAT!" Parents often become desperate and try to force their anorectic child to take food. The child is almost always successful at frustrating their efforts.

Anorexia may reflect a teenager's mixed feelings about growing up.

21

Adolescents commonly crave both independence and dependence. A child's not eating may represent her giving up her dependence on her parents. At the same time, parents inevitably become concerned with the child's health. She thus has it both ways. She can act independent of her parents, yet she also has them hovering over her.

While anorexia nervosa often begins when a youngster goes on a diet, the disease is always associated with significant emotional disturbance.

Some girls stop eating, it is thought, because of fantasies of oral impregnation: they imagine they can become pregnant through eating. A girl may unconsciously have the impression that obesity and pregnancy are the same thing.

Most treatment for anorexia combines a medical regimen with some form of psychotherapy. At the Stanford University Medical Center and University of Pennsylvania hospitals, for example, patients are hospitalized and, through contractual arrangements, agree to gain specified amounts of weight while undergoing psychological therapy. Intravenous feeding is used as a last resort to save the youngster's life.

Parents whose child suffers from anorexia nervosa may receive valuable assistance from an organization called Anorexia Nervosa and Associated Disorders, Inc. (550 Frontage Road, Northfield, Illinois 60093). ANAD offers free services—including counseling, information, and referrals; self-help groups for both victims and parents; educational programs; and a listing of therapists, hospitals, and clinics treating anorectics.

APHRODISIACS are foods, herbs, ointments, powders, perfumes, potions, lotions, and drugs that have been thought to increase sexual desire, to improve sexual performance, and to cure infertility. The term is derived from Aphrodite, the Greek goddess of love and beauty.

Some examples:

● In Ancient Greece, lentils were believed to stimulate desire.

● Pliny the Elder, the Roman encyclopedist of the first century, reports that the root of the mallow in goat's milk excites the sexual urge. He also had great faith in white beets, carrots, and turnips.

● In the Middle Ages, eating the mandrake root, which is shaped like a man, was believed to aid conception.

● In seventeenth-century France, some dishes and pastries made with chocolate were considered aphrodisiacs. Monks were reportedly forbidden to drink chocolate.

● Now, in the twentieth century, the search goes on, but a true aphrodisiac remains undiscovered. However—just as a sugar-pill placebo can cure illness—spurious aphrodisiacs often work simply because people believe in them so fervently.

Ginseng has recently been revived as a supposed aphrodisiac. This plant was first used as a sexual stimulant in ancient India. In contemporary oriental medicine it is considered a remedy for all kinds of sexual inadequacy. Some claim that it restores fertility. Among some American Indians, ginseng is reported to improve sexual desire, attractiveness, and performance.

A recent study of ginseng users in the United States found that only 7 percent felt it enhanced sexual performance. Many users reported a general feeling of well-being, reduced fatigue, and stimulation. As with other stimulants, such effects can sometimes reduce sexual anxiety and lower inhibitions. But claims of increased sex drive and restored fertility remain unproved.

Ginseng interacts with the endocrine system in ways not completely understood. Disruption of the menstrual cycle has been documented.

While most aphrodisiacs are ineffectual but harmless, some are extremely dangerous. "Spanish fly" (cantharides) has been in use as a sexual stimulant since the Greek and Roman era. Actually, Spanish fly is a powerful poison. The active ingredient of the beetle Cantharis vesicatoria is an irritating substance that passes unchanged into the urine. It irritates the urinary tract, causing urinary frequency and sometimes erection. In women, the clitoris may become engorged.

Spanish fly can be fatal. Symptoms of poisoning include cramping abdominal pain and frequent urination that may contain blood and bits of sloughed off bladder lining. Priapism, an abnormally sustained erection, may occur just before death. The only antidote is to dilute the poison with a large amount of fluid.

The current search for aphrodisiacs has centered on drugs. Claims have been made for the aphrodisiac qualities of a wide variety of prescription and recreational drugs.

Alcohol and other drugs in moderate doses may temporarily reduce anxiety about sex, lower inhibitions, and free sexual desire. But excessive use of drugs is usually accompanied by diminished sexual interest and performance.

Further, drug effects are highly subjective and vary considerably from person to person, and even for the same person at different times. Psychological factors, such as expectations and setting, are thought to play a large part in the subjective experience of sex during drug use. Perceptions about sexual performance may be distorted under the influence of drugs and therefore unreliable. Thus no particular drug can be said to consistently stimulate sexual desire or functioning in all people.

Ironically, the most reliable aphrodisiac is androgen—male sex hormone—taken by women. In high doses, androgen causes markedly increased sexual desire. But it has a major drawback that precludes its use as an aphrodisiac: it has masculinizing effects—hairiness, acne, and overgrowth of the clitoris.

See also ALCOHOL; AMPHETAMINES; AMYL NITRITE; COCAINE; HALLUCINOGENS; HEROIN; MARIJUANA.

ARTERIOSCLEROSIS

ARTERIOSCLEROSIS is a condition in which degenerative changes in the arteries—the large blood vessels that convey blood from the heart—result in thickening of the arterial walls and loss of their elasticity. The condition predisposes to heart disease and stroke.

Arteriosclerosis is associated with certain risk factors which increase the likelihood of suffering from the condition or its complications.

The major risk factors are hypertension, elevated cholesterol and triglyceride levels, cigarette smoking, diabetes mellitus, and obesity. Other factors believed to increase the risk include physical inactivity, certain types of personality and patterns of behavior, and a family history of premature arteriosclerosis. Eliminating or modifying some or all of these risk factors is thought to decrease the incidence of arteriosclerosis complications such as heart disease.

The risk of arteriosclerosis increases with age. It affects many more men than women. The condition usually has no symptoms until serious complications develop. In many cases, arteriosclerosis has no effect on sexual functioning.

Some men with arteriosclerosis suffer from impotence. This is especially likely when the condition occurs in the artery of the lower abdomen or in the pelvic arteries. Decreased blood flow in this area may prevent adequate blood supply for erection. A symptom of arteriosclerosis in these arteries may be an aching muscular cramp in the hip, thigh, or buttocks. It is usually brought on by walking, and relieved by several moments of rest.

Surgical correction of the arteriosclerosis can restore some patients to full sexual potency. However, others remain impotent even after successful surgery. In such cases, help may be attained by a penile prosthesis. Some men after surgery suffer from ejaculatory problems, such as failure to ejaculate or retrograde ejaculation.

See also EJACULATION, RETROGRADE; HEART DISEASE; HYPERTENSION; PENILE PROSTHESES; STROKE.

ARTHRITIS (chronic joint inflammation) patients may be hampered during sexual activity by joint and back pains.

To help avert pain, chronic arthritics can plan intercourse for the time of day when pain is usually least severe. They can prepare by taking analgesic and anti-inflammatory medications. They can also take a warm bath or shower beforehand and apply hot packs to afflicted areas. Loosening up exercises may further help to ward off pain.

Patients can experiment with a variety of positions to discover which are the most comfortable. One problem is likely to be keeping weight off the hip and spine. When a woman has hip contractures and cannot stretch her legs, her partner may have some trouble accommodating to her.

The female-superior (on top) position usually puts the least amount of strain on an arthritic woman. The couple may also enjoy positions that permit vaginal entry from the rear, or allow both partners to lie on their sides.

Some arthritis patients suffer severe joint limitations or an inability to perform repetitive movements. Water beds and massage oils can help reduce friction and fatigue.

Counseling can also prove valuable. A sex partner may interpret an arthritic's expression of pain as rejection—or might withdraw sexually out of fear of causing injury. Actually, sex can have a painkilling effect that sometimes lasts for hours.

A patient who suffers persistent sexual dysfunction from a hip disability may benefit from a prosthetic hip replacement. But patients with such prostheses are cautioned against coital movements that can produce forceful or extreme motions of the hip—lest the prosthesis become dislocated.

ARTIFICIAL INSEMINATION. See INFERTILITY.

ASTHMA (bronchial asthma) attacks are characterized by labored breathing, wheezing, and coughing.

Airways become narrow as a result of inflammation, muscle spasm, and edema (excessive fluid retention). Mucus production further reduces air flow.

Attacks range from very mild to life-threatening. The underlying mechanism responsible for asthma attacks is unknown.

In susceptible people, asthma attacks may be precipitated by a variety of stresses. These include viral respiratory infections, exercise, and the exposure to specific allergens (agents responsible for allergic reactions). Inhalation of cold air may bring on attacks, as may the inhalation of such irritants as gasoline fumes, fresh paints, and cigarette smoke.

Emotional stresses may contribute to the onset of an asthmatic episode. This is usually true even when the asthma is caused by allergy. The emotional and physical demands of sexual activity may aggravate or precipitate an asthma attack. Indeed, some asthmatics find that sexual activity is nearly always accompanied by distressing asthmatic symptoms. Such experiences naturally make a person approach sex cautiously—or avoid it altogether.

Personality traits common to many asthmatics may contribute to sex-related asthma attacks. Many asthmatics are found to have attacks when their sense of security is threatened. This may be true of some sexual situations such as sex with a new partner.

Some asthmatics tend to be dependent on other people and have difficulty in assuming responsibility for themselves. This attitude can lead to their assumption that the sex partner ought to take the initiative and know what is sexually satisfying without having to be told. This assumption can result in the asthma patient's feeling angry, frustrated, and sexually inadequate, emotions that can trigger an episode.

Some asthmatics tend to be conscientious and task-oriented. They may set certain sexual goals, and then observe themselves to see if their sexual activity is adequate. Such an orientation often leads to sexual performance anxiety, which may be related to asthma symptoms.

Various drugs may improve sexual functioning. Some asthmatics find that tranquilizers lessen their anxiety and may avert asthmatic symptoms associated with sex. In others, the treatment of depression with an antidepressant will significantly increase sexual functioning.

Some asthmatics are helped by the use of antihistamines such as Intal (chomolyn sodium). Taken about 30 minutes before sexual activity, such drugs may abort an asthmatic attack in some people. For a large number of asthmatics, the use of bronchodilator medications prior to sexual activity significantly increases their ability to function. Treating the asthma sufferer's general health problems is also likely to improve sexual functioning.

In some asthmatics, attacks may be caused primarily by allergic hypersensitivity. Sometimes, the allergen may be closely related to sexual activity—for example, an allergy to the goose down in a pillow or quilt can precipitate an asthmatic attack. In such cases, the allergen can be identified and removed. The patient may wish to receive desensitization treatment.

Counseling often aids sexual functioning. Patients who experience asthmatic episodes in relation to sexual activity are often helped by discussions with a physician, social worker, psychologist, or other trained professional. In counseling sessions, patients can explore emotions that may be contributing to sex-related asthma attacks. Early parental prohibitions against sexual activity, for example, may help account for the patient's guilt or anxiety.

Joint sessions with the sex partner can attempt to deal with the couple's relationship and how it may affect the asthmatic. In some couples, for example, the *partner* may feel guilt, anxiety, lack of self-esteem, or insecurity. These emotions may be triggering an emotional reaction in the patient that is causing asthmatic episodes.

Standard sex therapy techniques may be used in treating specific sexual dysfunctions. This requires treatment of the couple as a unit. Help can be obtained from an experienced sex therapy team or clinic.

Asthma sufferers who experience severe guilt, lack of self-esteem or severe depression should consider psychiatric counseling.

An asthma sufferer with gonorrhea should ordinarily not receive penicillin injections, for there is an increased risk of anaphylactic shock from the drug. Other drugs, such as oral tetracyclines, can be substituted.

See also SEX THERAPY.

BACKACHE has a wide variety of causes. A physician should be consulted about any back pain that limits activity and lasts more than two or three days.

Backache most commonly results from placing too much stress on the back—as in lifting a heavy object, bending and digging for many hours, or sitting, standing, or sleeping in incorrect positions.

The spinal column is made up of bones called vertebrae. Each has a number of bony projections to which are attached ligaments and muscles. Between the vertebrae are discs of a firm but cushiony substance that serve as shock absorbers.

Excessive pressure or strain on the back may result in strains or sprains. A ligament stretched beyond its limit will flash pain signals. A muscle given too difficult or unnatural a job will respond with a severe tearing pain. It and nearby muscles may go into a temporary contraction—or spasm—to discourage continual use. The pain may make the sufferer tense, which tightens muscles and causes more pain, and go on to cause a chronic problem.

Discs may also be damaged. They can be forced out of position, become ruptured or "slipped," and often dig or press into a hypersensitive nerve.

Backache can be a symptom of serious illness such as cancer or arthritis. Low-back pain is often one of the earliest signs of osteoporosis. Pain may also come from an infection or congenital defect in the bones of the back.

Sometimes, back pain signals that something is wrong in another part of the body: kidney disease, heart disease, endocrine problems, prostate trouble, problems in the pancreas, stomach, or liver—all may have backache as a symptom.

During the last months of pregnancy, women often suffer from low-back pain. The weight of the child may cause "swayback" that cannot be compensated for by a change in posture.

Emotional problems often contribute to backache. This seems particularly true of a type of low-back pain which is accompanied by stiffness, difficulty in bending and moving, and shooting pains in the buttocks and legs.

Much psychogenic backache is due to the failure of the back muscles to balance correctly because of abnormal tension. With the pain, further muscular contraction occurs, intensifying the pain. Anxiety and depression can cause muscle spasm.

The stresses of sexual tensions and conflicts often contribute to backache. Uncomfortable intercourse positions may cause strain on the back. A woman who is repeatedly sexually aroused without reaching orgasm may develop pelvic congestion, which often has backache as a symptom. Both men and women often use back pain as an excuse for avoiding sex.

Many types of therapy are used to treat back pain—among them, massage, heat and cold therapy, bed rest, exercise, medication, surgery, and psychotherapy.

Sexual activity may ease back pain. During acute attacks of back pain with muscle spasm, patients are often concerned that sexual activity will cause permanent damage. In fact, sexual intercourse may relax muscle spasm and tension contributing to the pain.

It's advisable for the patient to take a hot bath or apply heat to the back before engaging in intercourse. An analgesic may be taken about an hour prior to intercourse. A massage as part of lovemaking is also recommended: it eases the pain and may create feelings of emotional warmth and sexual arousal in both partners. A massage after lovemaking may also be helpful.

The backache sufferer is usually most comfortable lying on the back with a pillow under the buttocks.

When people suffer from chronic backache, a common fear is that sexual intercourse will cause injury and pain. Even during periods of remission, when there is little or no back pain, the sufferer may worry that sex will cause a flare-up. Such anxieties may make a man impotent; a woman may have difficulty achieving orgasm.

Most chronic back pain sufferers have weak and inelastic muscles. The primary treatment is exercise to increase muscle strength, endurance, and elasticity. The pelvic thrusting of sexual intercourse is an excellent exercise. It improves back, lower abdominal, buttock, and thigh muscles, which may help combat chronic back pain. For the best

exercise results with the least chance of exacerbating pain, intercourse should be performed slowly, carefully, and frequently.
See also PELVIC CONGESTION.

BALANITIS. See PENIS INFLAMMATION.

BARBITURATES sometimes lower sexual inhibitions, thereby enhancing sexual enjoyment.

More commonly, however, chronic barbiturate users report that the drug interferes with sexual functioning. Used as hypnotics, sedatives, and anticonvulsive medication, barbiturates cause central nervous system depression. They also depress the activity of peripheral nerves and skeletal and smooth muscles.

Barbiturates can interfere with the release of sex hormones. Frequently, women who abuse barbiturates have menstrual abnormalities. Some users report diminished sexual desire, impotence, and difficulties in attaining orgasm.

Many people, however, who use barbiturates for long-term therapy experience no change in sexual functioning.
See also MEDICATIONS.

BESTIALITY. See ANIMAL DISEASES.

BIRTH CONTROL. See CONTRACEPTION.

BIRTH CONTROL PILL. See PILL, CONTRACEPTIVE.

BITING during lovemaking can be dangerous if the skin is broken. Human bites are often highly infectious—even more so than most animal bites.

To help guard against infection, a person who has been bitten should wash the bite with soap and water, then go to a physician or a hospital emergency room. The physician should thoroughly clean the bite with an antiseptic solution, then apply an antibacterial ointment and a bandage. A tetanus shot is necessary since the mouth may sometimes harbor tetanus bacteria.

If the bite does not heal within a week to 10 days—or if it becomes swollen, reddened, or pus-laden—a physician should be consulted.

There is no danger of rabies from human bites.

BLADDER REMOVAL. See CYSTECTOMY.

BLINDNESS deprives people of visual stimuli to sexual feelings and sexual behavior.

People with sight usually first react to each other's physical attributes. (A man may be attracted by the way a woman moves, by a light in her eyes, by the way she smiles; a woman may find a man's moustache appealing, or his clothes, or the gap between his teeth.) This initial attraction makes them want to get to know each other better.

Blind people miss the visual cues that ordinarily help people assess each other and act as a spur to sexual interest.

While a majority of blind adults achieve satisfying social and sexual relationships, they must do so by relying on their other senses—senses that may be more difficult to interpret and less informative than sight.

Children blind from birth require special sex education. A blind child may know what his own body is like. But he may have little or no conception of the anatomy of the opposite sex and no way of finding out. Blind children come up against strong social taboos against touching the bodies of other people, particularly other people of the opposite sex. They are likely to be completely ignorant about adult bodies of either sex. It is important for a blind child to be informed about the great variety of sizes and shapes people come in. The child needs to know how male and female bodies change at puberty, how a woman's body changes during pregnancy, and how people's bodies alter as they age.

In sex education classes for blind youngsters, realistic three-dimensional anatomical models are being used. These plastic models, often life-size, allow blind children to explore the shapes of breasts, testicles, and penises. Still, the children are deprived of the warmth, skin textures, and hair of real human beings. Some educators of the blind believe that live models should be substituted for the plastic replicas. This is the practice in some Scandinavian countries.

Blind teenagers typically have fewer opportunities for social encounters. They are often overprotected by their parents. Because mobility is a problem, dating is difficult.

Masturbating may also prove difficult for blind youngsters. Some may be inhibited in exploring their bodies for fear of being observed. Others may heedlessly masturbate in full view of other people and be perplexed at the negative reactions they elicit.

Parents can help a blind adolescent acquire a positive attitude toward sexuality and social and verbal skills that will help in coping with the sighted world. The child's privacy should be respected; at the same time, it should be made clear to the child that masturbating is considered a solitary activity, and that observing it may offend other people's sensibilities.

Blind children should be encouraged to accept as much independence and responsibility as they can manage. By restricting a blind child's freedom, overprotective parents may be reducing the short-term risk of physical injury; but they increase the long-term risk of psychological injury and social ostracism.

The blind adolescent needs a sympathetic adult who will answer sexual questions accurately and completely. This person may be a parent or an adult friend or relative.

Many adolescents are victims of sexual myths and misconceptions ("You can't get pregnant if you have sex standing up"). But a blind adolescent's misconceptions may involve gross physical distortions. The adult must be an unusually sensitive listener who can correct misconceptions without ridicule. Blind children are often gifted verbally and may use words appropriately to describe functions they do not fully understand. One blind youngster accurately described sexual intercourse but, on further questioning, reported that "the vagina is located beneath the right breast."

Blind people are at a social disadvantage. They cannot look around at a party to see who might be interesting to meet. Other people may be unsure of how to approach them. Eye contact and other visual cues to the other person's interest are absent. Subtle body-language messages, that sighted people take for granted, are meaningless to the blind.

What is more, the blind person's inadvertent gestures or mannerisms may be misinterpreted by other people. Some blind people may rock or move their heads in ways that people may take to mean "no." People blind from birth may be unaware of how sighted people react to dirty clothing or sloppy grooming.

For blind people, sexual attraction is usually rooted in friendship first. Personality is obviously more important than looks. Attraction is likely to arise through shared feelings and experiences.

When blindness occurs in adulthood, its impact is considerable. Particularly if it occurs suddenly because of injury, reactions commonly include impaired self-esteem, feelings of helplessness, social withdrawal, and depression—states of mind that frequently contribute to sexual problems.

In some instances, the cause of the loss of vision may produce sexual dysfunction—as in diabetes, multiple sclerosis, or brain tumors.

In treating sexual difficulties in blind people, it is important to distinguish between organic and psychogenic problems. Depression can be treated with drugs and supportive counseling. The patient's need to grieve for lost sight should be recognized; at the same time, the patient should be encouraged to return to work and social activity as soon as possible.

The newly blind may miss the visual stimulation of looking at a sex partner or reading erotic material. The partner can use methods of nonvisual arousal such as voice modulation, perfumes, textures of clothing, and sexual conversation.

Blind people may encounter stereotypes of the blind as uninterested in sex or sexually inadequate. Group sessions can help them gain perspective and counter such negative concepts.

See also DEPRESSION.

"BLUE BALLS." See EPIDIDYMO-ORCHITIS.

BREAST CANCER occurs more often (90,000 cases a year) and causes more deaths (34,000) than any other form of cancer among women. The 5-year survival rate is 65 percent.

Cancer of the breast is extremely rare in children and occurs only occasionally in men. Most cases are found in women after age 45, when numerous changes taking place in the body affect the breast.

Breast cancer is occurring more and more frequently among younger

American women. An explanation might be that girls tend to develop sexually at a younger age than formerly. With ovaries beginning to function earlier, these young women may be exposed to hormones that may promote the development of breast cancer. They thus may be at a higher risk than were their mothers at the same age.

There is evidence that daughters or sisters of breast cancer patients run a somewhat greater risk of developing the disease than women in whose families there is no history of this malignancy. Statistical studies also suggest that the risk of developing breast cancer is lower for married women than for single women and lower still for married women who have borne children.

There is no known preventive against developing breast cancer. Brassieres marketed with cancer-prevention claims are outright frauds.

By the time they are discovered, about 65 percent of all breast cancers have already spread to the axillary lymph nodes. When this happens, roughly 1 out of 2 women can be expected to survive for 5 tears. By contrast, of the women whose cancer has not yet metastasized, 8 out of 10 will survive 5 years or more, many of them with little more chance of death throughout their lifetimes than normal women.

Metastasis (spreading of the cancer) is twice as likely to be present when the tumor is the average size at which tumors are discovered—about the size of a golf ball—as when it is only a third the diameter. Thus, it is vital to discover the tumor at the earliest possible stage.

Immediate medical attention is needed by anyone who notices a breast lump or any change in the breast, such as nipple discharge, dimpling of the skin, inverted nipple, or enlargement of the pores to resemble an orange skin.

Since breast cancer usually is first apparent as a lump, the most common method of detection is by a fingertip exploration for lumps or areas of thickening. Many women have discovered breast cancer at a curable stage by giving themselves a monthly breast examination. The best time for this examination is three days after the end of each menstrual period.

Most breast lumps are not cancerous but rather are symptoms of chronic cystic mastitis, or fibrocystic breast disease. One in 20 women have cystic disease of the breast during their menstrual life. Treatment is rarely required, but women with the condition should have their breasts checked regularly—since they are almost 3 times as likely to develop breast cancer as women without the condition.

By the time a breast tumor can be felt it may already be out of control. Under ordinary circumstances, even the most astute examiner is unlikely to detect a cancer three-eighths of an inch in diameter.

One method to detect breast cancer while it is still of minute, curable size is mammography, a process of X-raying the breast's soft tissue to reveal cancerous lesions. So revealing is mammography that some tumors only one-quarter of an inch in diameter, which could not be felt, show up on the film. A Health Insurance Plan of Greater New York study shows that the breast cancer death rate was one-third lower in patients who received both examination and mammography than in the control group who received only routine medical care.

Immediate mammography is recommended for any woman with a breast mass or thickening, or persistent breast complaints. Women with nipple discharge or nipple erosion should also be considered for mammography. The National Cancer Institute recommends that women over 50 have mammography routinely.

Thermography is another diagnostic tool in breast cancer. Temperature changes in the breast may sometimes indicate cancerous tumors. Any suspicion should be confirmed by a mammogram.

Definitive diagnosis of breast cancer is made by doing a biopsy—excising the suspicious tissue and examining it under a microscope. Until recently, if the tissue was found to be malignant, the breast would be removed immediately.

Now, more and more women are demanding a two-stage procedure. If breast cancer is diagnosed, women may want the option of adjusting to the idea over a week or so. They may wish to have the diagnosis confirmed by another laboratory test. Above all, they may wish to discuss with their doctors the specific type of surgery that is recommended—for several different types of mastectomy (see entry) are in current use.

The two-stage procedure remains controversial. Some surgeons discourage the procedure on the ground that it is safer to be anesthetized once rather than twice.

In premenopausal women with metastatic breast cancer, the ovaries may be removed in an attempt to check the spreading of the disease.

Chemotherapy and radiation therapy are also used in treating breast cancer. In older women whose breast cancer has spread, the male sex hormone testosterone is sometimes used, either alone or in combination with other chemotherapeutic agents. This treatment causes the metastases to regress in about 15 percent of cases. But it may have unpleasant side effects. Women may experience signs of masculinization: they may develop undesirable hair growth and tend to overweight. They may begin to lose scalp hair and develop acne. The clitoris may enlarge. In many cases, these signs may be minimal and may be acceptable if symptoms of the disease are relieved. Hair removal by shaving or the use of depilatories may help alleviate embarrassment.

The use of testosterone also increases sexual desire. This is usually not a serious problem. But it may be a problem to women who are single or widowed—or to women whose elderly husbands are unable to meet their increased sexual needs. Many such women find relief in masturbation.

See also CANCER; MASTECTOMY; MASTURBATION.

BREAST DISCHARGE may be caused by a serious medical condition. The discharge may be pussy, blood-tinged, or a thin translucent yellow.

Among the conditions that may account for breast discharge are infection or a benign tumor in the breast duct system.

In some cases, however, breast discharge indicates cancerous changes. Careful breast examination, including a mammogram and thermogram, is recommended for women with breast discharge.

After vigorous sexual activity, some women discharge breast milk. Particularly when orgasm has occurred, a few women have brief episodes of galactorrhea, inappropriate breast milk discharge. This may be due to elevations in circulating prolactin (the hormone that stimulates milk secretion) that occur as a result of breast manipulation and are associated with orgasm. This type of galactorrhea is unlikely to be the result of disease. The woman should consult a physician if the milk discharge becomes more persistent or if it is associated with symptoms that might indicate intracranial tumor (headaches, visual changes, and changes in the sense of smell).

Inappropriate lactation may indicate other serious medical conditions. Among the wide variety of causes are head trauma, hypothyroidism, precocious puberty, and chest wall lesions. Many drugs, including oral contraceptives, may induce galactorrhea.

Some women experience the amenorrhea-galactorrhea syndrome, in which the breast milk discharge is accompanied by failure to menstruate. Elevated secretion of prolactin is often associated with this syndrome. Treatment with such drugs as L-dopa and bromocriptine (Parlodel) often restores ovation function and controls the galactorrhea.

Lactation may occur in men. Several cases are on record of males who give breast milk after repeated suckling. Galactorrhea in men may also occur as a result of endocrine disorders such as acromegaly and after extensive therapy with phenothiazines. These drugs are used in the treatment of many medical conditions. Thorazine, a phenothiazine derivative, is used to control psychotic disorders.

See also BREAST CANCER.

BREAST FEEDING (nursing). Breast milk is a more complete food for babies than cow's milk. A baby nursed at its mother's breast is less likely to suffer from diarrhea and other intestinal upsets and is less prone to food allergy.

Breast feeding is also more convenient than bottle feeding. All themother need do is accompany the baby—and the source of supply is available, clean, and free.

Many women report that the nursing experience is intensely pleasurable and satisfying. Breast feeding causes the uterus to return to its pre-pregnancy size faster.

Women may sometimes experience sexual arousal, even orgasm, during suckling. Some women feel guilty and anxious about this experience and may stop nursing their babies. They can be reassured that their breasts are simply responding normally to the tactile stimulation of the child's sucking.

If a woman plans to breast feed her baby, she should discuss it with her doctor during her pregnancy. It is also important for her to discuss her intention of nursing with her husband and to gain his support. Some husbands feel that their wives' breasts are their exclusive property and may be jealous of the infant's suckling. Open communication is needed to resolve such conflicts, preferably before the child is born.

It is a good idea to contact a local La Leche League, an organization that provides information and support to nursing mothers.

Milk supply has nothing to do with breast size. A woman can have extremely small breasts and still breast feed her baby. Nor does nursing infants cause breast sagging.

Women often do not begin menstruating for many months while they are breast feeding. But breast feeding is not considered a method of birth control. A woman may ovulate before her periods resume.

After childbirth a nursing mother should drink about 1½ quarts of milk or eat its equivalent in cheese or yogurt daily. She should get as much rest as possible.

Nursing mothers should avoid drugs. Almost every drug a woman takes passes to her baby through breast milk, with possibly harmful effects. If a nursing mother must take an aspirin she should do so just after nursing. Women who are taking anticancer drugs, steroids, or therapeutic doses of radioactive iodine should not breast feed. Ordinarily, a woman can have a drink or two of alcohol without its adversely affecting the child.

Some breast feeding mothers complain of painful intercourse months after delivery. During the postpartum period, there is a relative steroid starvation, causing dryness and thinning of the vaginal mucosa. Breast feeding can contribute to such a steroid deficiency. A water-soluble lubricant (such as K-Y jelly) or a contraceptive cream or jelly will make penetration more comfortable. While an estrogen vaginal cream will quickly relieve the condition, there is some concern that the amount of estrogen absorbed into the breast milk can be harmful to the infant.

See also CONTRACEPTION; POSTPARTUM PROBLEMS.

BREAST HAIR is common and normal. Many women have a few hairs growing around the areola, the darkened ring around the nipple.

In some women, breast hair is part of a generalized hairiness that may be hereditary or may be associated with endocrine abnormalities or other medical conditions.

If a woman is troubled by breast hairs, the best way of removing them is tweezing.

See also HIRSUTISM.

BREAST SAGGING may develop following pregnancy, most

likely because the breasts' elastic tissues are repeatedly stretched by increases in size during pregnancies. A great weight loss can also cause breasts to sag and flatten.

Surgery can temporarily relieve severely sagging breasts. The first stage raises the breasts by cutting out excess skin and tissue and ordinarily takes 2 to 3 hours and requires several days in the hospital. After 2 or 3 months' healing time, implants are inserted to augment the size of the breasts if needed for small breasts. Within 3 to 5 years, however, the sag may return to some extent.

To help avoid breast sag, it is advisable to wear a bra. Some physicians feel that the current fashion of bralessness may contribute to breast sag. While some degree of flattening is part of the normal aging process, the problem may be accelerated in women who habitually go braless.

This is particularly true of large-breasted women, and those who have had several pregnancies or large weight losses. Without the added support of a bra, the fragile breast ligaments may gradually weaken, giving the breasts a flat, pendulous appearance.

To properly support the breasts, bras should be selected carefully. A woman should try on each bra individually, since different styles and brands may require different sizes. A bra should not restrict a woman's movements—indeed, she should be barely aware of wearing it.

There should be no bulge of skin above the bra or at the underarm. The bra should permit a woman to take a deep breath without feeling constricted. A final check of whether the bra fits is the strap test: The woman drops one strap; if support is lost on that side, the bra does not fit. A wireless bra is preferable.

See also BREAST SMALLNESS.

BREAST SMALLNESS is a problem for some women. Women with unusually small breasts often report feeling self-conscious and sexually inadequate.

Often, a woman can increase her breast size merely by gaining some weight. Otherwise, there is no known preparation, system of exercise, or mechanical device which can affect breast size.

Small breasts do not prevent a woman from breastfeeding.

If a woman wants her breasts enlarged she should see a plastic surgeon. An operation called breast augmentation is the only way to increase breast size to any significant degree. It takes about one hour, and usually requires no hospital stay. Recuperation takes about one week.

Breast augmentation is usually done by cutting an incision at the underfold of the breast and inserting a silicone-rubber bag filled with silicone gel. The bag, which closely duplicates the shape and consistency of breast tissue, is harmless.

Purely for psychological reasons, many women who have had their breasts surgically enlarged report feelings of increased adequacy and a greater interest in sex. Many take greater pride in their general appearance, and are pleased to find that clothes fit better.

Breast enlargement results in fairly small and inconspicuous permanent scars beneath the breasts. A woman will have some degree of discomfort and pain during the two-to-four-week healing process. Sometimes, implants may sag or migrate, causing an awkward, asymmetrical look.

Some women experience discomfort and drainage from the surgical incision that may persist for many months. In such cases, the implants may have to be removed.

Implanted breasts may feel firmer than normal breasts, especially if a woman has little breast tissue of her own. The more tissue over the implant, the more natural it feels.

The same procedure is used in part of the relief for breast sagging.

Breast augmentation should not interfere with breastfeeding; nor should breast sensitivity be impaired.

The injection of liquid silicone for increasing breast size is prohibited by the Food and Drug Administration. A woman should not believe any doctor who tells her it is safe. Liquid silicone should not be confused with the silicone gel implants used in augmentation surgery.

The results of injectable silicone are unpredictable. Deaths have occurred. Some women have had to have both breasts removed to save their lives.

Injected silicone may mask malignancy. When silicone is injected into tissue, globules of the plastic are formed, each one surrounded by a layer of cells. These "pseudocysts" may make detection of breast malignancy by physical examination or X rays more difficult.

By contrast, in accepted plastic surgery procedure, the material is inserted under the woman's own breast tissue, and thus does not interfere with the detection of malignancy.

For women who have had silicone injections, it is often possible to remove the injected silicone and replace it with a silicone-gel implant.

Products which are said to increase breast size are frauds. Some mail-order operations advertise exercise plans for breast development. Such plans are almost entirely worthless.

Since the breast has no muscles, exercises can merely tone up the chest-wall muscles beneath them. This may contribute to the overall prominence of the breasts, but it may also give a woman a barrel-chested appearance. It cannot improve her breast contour.

Often, these come-ons are accompanied by impressive before-and-after photographs: on the left, a small-breasted woman; on the right, the same woman presumably after the exercise plan, with huge breasts. The difference may be merely a change in posture. Or it may be a matter of trick photography. Sometimes women who resemble each other are used in the before-and-after pictures.

Other mail frauds for breast enlargements may pose an actual threat to health. One manufacturer offered a gadget which claimed the ability to "transform a flat-chested girl into a girl with a lovely bosom, free from fears of inferiority and confident in her femininity." The product was a suction device which forced temporary swelling of the breast tissue. Users were encouraged to believe that, if they persevered, some of the temporary swelling would become permanent. At Post Office hearings the government's medical witness testified that the device was not only worthless but possibly dangerous. Using it might cause unknown cancer to spread more rapidly.

Other dangerous breast-enlargement products may contain female hormones like estrogen. These products can upset the body's own hormone balance, possibly disrupting menstruation and accelerating unsuspected cancer of the breast.

Some women suffer from the opposite problem: Extremely large breasts. There is no known cause for this disorder, nor is there any drug, hormone, or other medical treatment for reducing the size of the breasts.

Most women with overlarge breasts can live with this condition by using special brassieres. A surgical supply company can give advice on where to find such bras.

For women who suffer physical and/or psychological discomfort from huge breasts, surgery is available. Heavy breasts may cause severe upper back and neck pains. There may be deeply incised, painful grooves where bra straps cut into the shoulders. Surgery to reduce overlarge breasts is a major operation which may take as long as 4 to 5 hours. It involves not only excising tissue, but also moving the nipples upward.

The surgery leaves scars, and there may be decreased or lost nipple sensation. Women may lose their ability to breastfeed. Breast reduction surgery should not be performed during pregnancy, or in women with heart disease, chronic lung disease, or other serious medical conditions.

See also BREAST CANCER; BREASTFEEDING; BREAST SAGGING.

BREAST STIMULATION. Women vary considerably in their response to breast stimulation. Some women find it unpleasant or irritating. Some derive no particular pleasure from having their breasts caressed or sucked. Others experience intense sexual pleasure.

Kinsey and his associates found that about half the female population responds with enjoyment to breast fondling. A small number of women have such sensitive breasts that they achieve orgasm through breast stimulation alone. The size of a woman's breasts do not determine their sensitivity.

During sexual arousal, a woman's breasts respond—even if the breasts are not directly stimulated. Breast changes are more marked in women who have not nursed.

During the excitement stage of sexual response, breast size increases and the nipple becomes erect. The breast becomes engorged with blood.

In the plateau and orgasm stages, the breasts further increase in size and become more engorged. The areola becomes engorged, causing the nipple to appear less erect. A rash-like "sex flush" may appear on the breast and upper abdomen.

During the resolution stage, the breast slowly returns to normal size over 5 to 10 minutes. The sex flush rapidly disappears. The areola engorgement subsides, then the nipple returns to its nonerect state.

A woman's response to breast stimulation may depend to a great extent on the quality of her relationship with her sex partner. Some women report arousal by one partner but not another.

Arousal from breast stimulation may be inhibited by a woman's excessive modesty or shame about her body, or by negative feelings about her breasts. Fear, guilt, or anger regarding sex may also interfere with response to breast fondling.

Technique in breast stimulation likewise has a lot to do with a woman's reaction. Most women respond negatively to rough handling or too-vigorous sucking. Women often report greater enjoyment when both hand and mouth are employed simultaneously. And, while the most sensitive area of the breast is usually the nipple, many women enjoy stimulation of the entire breast.

Breast sensitivity varies according to the time of the menstrual cycle. In general, a woman's breasts may be receptive to stimulation during midcycle, when she is ovulating. Another peak of sensitivity may occur during menstruation.

On the other hand, some women find that their breasts are oversensitive and tender during midcycle and before and during menstruation. They may experience breast stimulation at these times as extremely irritating.

Some women have been reluctant to communicate this to their partners for fear of appearing to reject them. They should realize that there is no way for a man to know when a woman's breasts are receptive to stimulation. Breast sensitivity and receptivity are individual—and it is up to the woman to let her partner know when she finds breast stimulation pleasurable.

Many couples use breast fondling as a prelude to sexual intercourse. Nipple stimulation often triggers clitoral distention and vaginal lubrication.

Many men have sensitive breasts. Most heterosexual males have little experience with breast eroticism. But Kinsey found that among homosexual males breast stimulation is common, and many males are known to have highly sensitive breasts. As many males—both heterosexual and homosexual—may be sensitive to breast stimulation as females. "A few males may even reach orgasm as a result of breast stimulation," Kinsey found.

Some cautions: Intense biting of the breasts can cause bruising and infection. Trauma to the breast may hasten the spread of breast cancer. In experiments with mice, massage of the tumor caused rapid dissemination of cancer.

Breast stimulation may trigger uterine contractions, and may induce premature labor in a woman prone to premature delivery.

BREAST TISSUE MISPLACEMENT affects about 1 to 3 percent of men and woman.

Misplaced (or ectopic or aberrant) breast tissue is a congenital condition. In the embryo, breast tissue develops from the ectoderm at about 6 weeks. Two ectodermal bandlike structures extend from the underarms to the groin, and are called milk lines or mammary ridges.

Soon, most of the ridge disappears, leaving breast tissue on the chest alone. Ectopic breast tissue occurs when other areas of the mammary ridge remain. Only very rarely does breast tissue occur in areas outside the mammary ridge, such as face, arms, legs, or buttocks.

Most ectopic breast tissue is located in the underarms, or between the breasts and the navel. With no nipple to help identify it, misplaced breast tissue often goes undetected, or is mistaken for other kinds of growth.

Ectopic breast tissue is affected by hormones—during menstruation, pregnancy, and the postpartum period. Women with ectopic breast tissue often report a sense of fullness or pain premenstrually.

In one unusual case, a 29-year-old woman, pregnant for the first time, noticed a swelling on her vulva. The enlargement persisted through pregnancy, increased in size during labor and delivery, then subsided only slightly over the next several weeks. When the swelling was surgically removed and examined, it was found to be normal breast tissue.

Misplaced breast tissue is subject to the maladies of normally placed breast tissue: infection, abscess, and fibrocystic breast disease. But such breast tissue is not usually capable of erotic sensations.

There is no general agreement about the risk of cancer in misplaced breast tissue. Some researchers believe that aberrant breast tissue is more subject to malignancy, particularly if it occurs in the underarms or vulva. There may also be a greater tendency for cancer of ectopic breast tissue to spread.

It is wise for misplaced breast tissue to be removed if it begins to grow or causes pain. Vulvar tissue is probably best removed in any case. Underarm tissue should be removed at the first suspicion of a lump or abnormality. Many patients elect to have misplaced breast tissue removed for cosmetic reasons.

Some people have extra (supernumerary) breasts. Most often, they consist of a small nipple and areola. They have no physiological function and do not respond to erotic stimulation.

In rare cases, a supernumerary breast will have underlying breast tissue as well as a nipple and areola. Such a breast usually occurs just below a normal breast. It looks as if two small breasts have been incorporated into one larger one with two nipples. Such complete breasts are likely to be erotically responsive. As with misplaced breast tissue, supernumerary breasts respond to hormonal changes.

Most people with supernumerary breasts choose to have them surgically removed. Underarm breasts can be removed so as to leave the scar hidden. Extra nipples may sometimes be small enough to resemble moles, and may not trouble the person. But when they are as large as a normal nipple, they are likely to be a source of great embarrassment. Surgical removal leaves a small scar, which most people consider a reasonable trade-off.

BREASTS, OVERLARGE. See BREAST SMALLNESS.

BRONCHIAL ASTHMA. See ASTHMA.

BRONCHITIS. See RESPIRATORY DISEASE.

CANCER is not a single disease, but a group of over 200 diseases that have in common an abnormal, unrestricted growth of body cells.

Perhaps more than any major disease, cancer requires prompt treatment for the patient's survival. While a malignant cancerous growth still is limited to one area, it often can be destroyed or removed. If undetected, or ignored because it is small, it will almost surely spread and cause death.

More than 1,500,000 Americans alive today have been cured of cancer. By "cured" it is meant they are without evidence of the disease at least five years after diagnosis and treatment. The cure rate is now about 1 in 3—up from 1 in 4 in 1950 and 1 in 5 in 1930. If all patients received adequate diagnosis and treatment, it is widely estimated that the cure rate would jump to 1 in 2. The false notion that cancer is incurable is so ingrained in our culture that some patients refuse surgery or other treatment that might have provided a cure.

Some people are so terrified by the thought of having cancer that they simply cannot accept the doctor's diagnosis and therefore disregard his instructions. Others shut their eyes and pretend the problem will vanish if they wilfully ignore it for a time. In a California survey, four patients in ten waited more than three months to seek medical help after noticing the symptoms of cancer. One in every five waited longer than a year—during which time the cancer spread. In such cases, fear itself may be the biggest obstacle to cure.

An annual physical exam can save more lives from cancer than any other preventive measure, says the American Cancer Society. Quitting smoking is another smart move. Cigarette smoking is the major cause of lung cancer and an important factor in other diseases.

The American Cancer Society emphasizes the Seven Warning Signals—which don't mean that cancer is necessarily present, but nonetheless call for medical attention. A doctor should be consulted if any of the following lasts longer than 2 weeks:

1. Change in bowel or bladder habits.
2. A sore that does not heal.
3. Unusual bleeding or discharge.
4. Thickening or lump in breast or elsewhere.
5. Indigestion or difficulty in swallowing.
6. Obvious change in wart or mole.
7. Nagging cough or horseness.

Have any blood in the urine checked immediately. *Pain is seldom an early cancer signal.*

What is cancer? Cancer cells seem to be runaway cells that multiply rapidly and without purpose. The cancer growth takes nourishment needed by the normal cells. It compresses and invades healthy tissues.

Cancer cells may break from the original cancerous mass and move, via the bloodstream or lymphatic system, to other parts of the body. There they form secondary sites (metastases). If vital centers or important organs such as the liver or kidneys are affected by the metastases, life expectancy will be shortened drastically. Because the ancient Greeks thought that spreading cancerous growths resembled the claws of a crab, they called it the crablike disease, *karkinos.* The Latin translation of the word was *cancer.* The zodiac sign of cancer is a crab.

Different kinds of cancer have different characteristics. Some cancers are slow to grow and spread to neighboring tissues. Others grow rapidly and spread swiftly to distant sites. What cures one type of tumor (growth) may be ineffective for another. Moreover, one part of the body may give rise to several different types of cancer, each following its own course and requiring different treatment.

Not all tumors are malignant. Benign tumors are clumps of cells that grow in a limited area and do not spread. They are harmful only when they press against other organs and disturb their normal functions.

Cancer is the second most common cause of death in the United States. Only heart disease surpasses it. Of the more than 200 million people in the United States, during one year approximately 635,000 develop cancer and approximately 280,000 die of it. At the present rate about 1 in 4 persons will eventually have cancer, and about 1 out of every 6 deaths in the United States will be caused by cancer.

Cancer in children 2 to 14 years old is a major cause of death, second only to accidents. The most common form is leukemia, followed by cancer of the brain and other parts of the nervous system.

For men and women, the risk of cancer increases steadily from childhood to the end of life. The death rate rises sharply after age 45. Between the ages of 20 and 60, more women than men develop cancer because of the high incidence of breast cancer and cancer of the uterus and other parts of the reproductive system. After age 60, overall cancer incidence is higher for men.

More men than women die of cancer by a ratio of 55-45. Responsible for the most cancer deaths in men are cancer of the lungs, cancer of the stomach, and cancer of the prostate. In women, cancer deaths are most often caused by cancer of the colon and rectum and of the breast and uterus.

The mere diagnosis of cancer can cause sexual problems. For some people, the shock of discovering they have this dread disease plunges them into depression, with consequent loss of sexual interest. Many people become so preoccupied with seeking confirming medical opinions, deciding upon treatment, and resolving when, how, or if to tell other people about the illness that there is little time or energy left to devote to sexual activity.

Moreover, cancer patients have to grapple with fears of pain, mutilation, weakness, and death. Most feel a combination of anxiety, anger, and a sense of despair. It is common for cancer patients to feel a sense of betrayal by their bodies. All these emotions may interfere with sexual functioning.

A large part of the psychological impact of cancer is the notion that the disease is somehow a shameful one. While other diseases—such as heart disease or diabetes—may elicit concern and sympathy, cancer may be greeted with such discomfort and dread that the patient feels in some way culpable, guilty, and shamed.

When the cancer involves the genitals or breasts, its impact on sexual functioning is likely to be even greater.

Not only is much sexual self-esteem focused on the genitals and breasts, but some people view cancer of these organs as punishment for real or imagined sexual sins such as masturbation, voluntary abortion, or sex with an illicit partner. They may vow to give up sexual activity forever in exchange for surviving.

Besides the psychological effects, certain physical effects of cancer—such as anemia, loss of appetite, and muscle atrophy—are likely to produce severe weakness and may thus make sexual functioning difficult or impossible.

Treatment for cancer may also impair sexual functioning. The most common treatment methods are surgery, radiation, and chemotherapy. Radiation and chemotherapy may cause nausea and vomiting, provoking strong feelings of revulsion and a sense of loss of control of the body. The hair loss that often results from some types of chemotherapy may further decrease self-esteem and feelings of sexual desirability. Surgery or radiation of the genitals may impede sexual functioning. A woman's reaction to mastectomy—or her sex partner's—may similarly affect sexual activity.

After treatment, a wide variety of psychological and interpersonal problems may affect sexual functioning. Guilt, poor self-esteem, and altered body-image may decrease the patient's interest in sex. Fear of recurrence may make a person chronically anxious and preoccupied. The patient—or the partner—may believe that sex is no longer appropriate.

Shame and embarrassment may affect sexual intimacy. A cancer patient may fear sexual rejection because of mutilating surgery. Feelings of self-disgust may be projected onto the partner. These feelings may interfere with the resumption of sexual activity after cancer therapy.

There has been little research on the impact of cancer on marital relationships. Some evidence shows that cancer patients of both sexes have an increased desire for physical closeness—but a lowered interest in sexual intercourse.

Despite many possible impediments to sexual activity, many cancer patients retain a keen interest in sex and wish to resume sexual relations. They should seek information from the doctor or nurse about how the illness or its treatment may affect sexuality.

Counseling may be needed to help resolve psychological or interpersonal problems that may be responsible for sexual difficulties. Ideally, sex partners should be included in counseling.

See also BREAST CANCER; CERVICAL CANCER; MASTECTOMY; PENILE CANCER; PROSTATE CANCER; TERMINAL ILLNESS; VAGINAL CANCER.

CANCER OF THE CERVIX. See CERVICAL CANCER.

CANCER OF THE UTERUS. See CERVICAL CANCER.

CANDIDIASIS. See YEAST INFECTION.

CASTRATION. See TESTICLE REMOVAL.

CEREBRAL PALSY rarely impairs sexual desire or capacity—although there may be mechanical difficulties because of the victim's motor problems.

The term cerebral palsy refers to a number of motor disorders. It usually results from central nervous system damage to the fetus or newborn and is characterized by an impairment in voluntary movement.

Children with cerebral palsy are usually spastic and rigid. Their limbs may be weak and underdeveloped. Impairment ranges from very mild to extremely disabling.

Speech impediments are common, and about 25 percent experience convulsive seizures. While some types of cerebral palsy are associated with mental retardation, in many cases intelligence is normal.

Parents are usually concerned that their children develop maximal independence within the limits of their disability. Physical therapy, occupational therapy, bracing, orthopedic surgery, and speech training may all be required.

Sex education is usually neglected. Cerebral palsied people almost always report that they received no sex education as children or adolescents. Many perceived an attitude that they were asexual or too different to be interested in sex. Some recall being considered too vulnerable to sexual advances to be allowed to function freely in social situations.

Victims of cerebral palsy are at a great social disadvantage and have sharply reduced opportunities for forming social and sexual relationships. Many fail to learn effective social skills or a means of expressing closeness. Rejection by peers is common. Speech problems may add to a sense of isolation.

Establishing mature sexual relationships demands a significant degree of independence from parents. Yet cerebral palsied youngsters are often dependent on parents for many more years than normal people.

Cerebral palsied children raised in institutions are often segregated by sex. They have little privacy and few opportunities for social contact with people outside the institution. They are typically deprived of normal touching and physical closeness. Feelings of isolation and difference are thus accentuated.

Cerebral palsy victims often benefit from being taught appropriate social skills. They are then frequently able to behave more assertively in establishing relationships and initiating sexual activity. Basic sex education and birth control counseling are usually required as well.

See also SEX THERAPY.

CEREBROVASCULAR ACCIDENT. See STROKE

CERVICAL CANCER is potentially one of the most curable forms of cancer, yet is commonly fatal.

Cancer of the cervix—the narrow part where the pear-shaped uterus opens into the vagina—can easily be detected by the simple, painless Pap test.

Named for Dr. George N. Papanicolaou who developed it, the test requires only the microscopic examination of cervical cells.

Sloughed-off cancer cells may be present even though the woman has no symptoms. If their presence is detected before the cancer invades surrounding tissue, the disease can be cured in almost every case. Cancer of the body of the uterus can also be detected by the same test.

Yet among women in this country some 85,000 cases of cervical and uterine cancer occur each year, with about 11,000 deaths. This happens mainly because so many women avoid routine gynecological examinations.

Every woman who is sexually active should have a periodic Pap test. The disease is most common during the reproductive years, but it can occur at any age.

Cervical cancer is associated with early sexual intercourse. Women who have begun intercourse in their teenage years, particularly if they had had several sex partners, are at greater risk of cervical cancer. It is postulated that a certain type of cell which is present in the cervix of teenagers and absent in women past 18 or 20 may be the target cell. Early childbearing also puts a woman at greater risk. The disease is very rare among virgins.

Exposure to herpes virus type 2 is associated with cancer of the cervix. Women who suffer from cervical cancer show a very high incidence—70 to 100 percent in a variety of studies—of antibodies to herpes, showing they have been exposed to this virus.

The first visible sign of the disease is irregular bleeding or unusual vaginal discharge. There is usually spotting of blood after intercourse or douching. These warning signals are the same as those of other, less urgent conditions, such as cervical erosion. But they should be reported promptly to a physician since the possibility of cancer poses too great a risk to ignore.

Cervical cancer and cancer of the body of the uterus usually develop slowly, and patients may live for years in rather good general condition. Irregularities in menstrual cycle, profuse periods, and the recurrence of a period after several months without periods are symptoms that call for checking with a physician. Only rarely does cervical or uterine cancer result in painful intercourse.

Cervical cancer is treated by surgery or radiation or both.

Sexual difficulties may follow treatment. Women often report decreases in the frequency of intercourse, loss of interest in sex, and less orgasmic responsiveness.

Psychological problems may be a large factor. Anxiety and depression are common after cervical cancer treatment. Women are often plagued by the unfounded fear that sexual intercourse will cause a recurrence of the cancer. Men may refrain from sex out of fear of injuring their sex partners. Sometimes, a man may fear that the cancer is contagious.

A woman may feel she developed cervical cancer as a punishment for forbidden sexual fantasies or practices. Such irrational guilt and shame typically result in sexual difficulty. Or a woman may harbor angry feelings toward men for having caused her cancer through intercourse. Counseling can help such people resolve their emotional problems.

Treatment also causes physical problems that may impair sexual functioning. In surgery, all of the cancerous tissue is removed. This often involves removing the uterus (hysterectomy). Hysterectomy usually has no physical effect on sexual desire or functioning.

However, when the surgery is very extensive—involving parts of the vagina, bladder, rectum, or pelvic structures—sexual intercourse may be very difficult or painful. Other sexual options remain available to the couple, including oral and manual genital stimulation.

When radiation treatment is used for cervical cancer, it may be beamed to the cancerous tissue from a source outside the body, such as an X-ray or cobalt therapy machine; or it may be placed directly in the body, in the form of radium. Often, radium is enclosed in a capsule which is inserted through the vagina to the cancerous site.

When the vagina is foreshortened after surgery or radiation, intercourse may be painful. The following intercourse position will limit penile thrusting and alleviate pain resulting from deep penetration: The woman lies on her back, then lowers her legs and brings them together so that the man's knees are outside her thighs. The female-superior position also gives a woman better control.

After radiation therapy, a common problem is narrowing and constriction of the vagina because of scarring. Sexual intercourse itself may help prevent such narrowing. Orgasm by any means helps maintain flexibility and good blood supply in the vaginal walls. Vaginal exercise—contracting the muscles around the vagina—will promote blood flow to the pelvic area and may also decrease any developing scarring. Women are usually also instructed in stretching their vaginas by daily using vaginal dilating instruments.

A lubricant such as K-Y jelly may be required for intercourse since vaginal lubrication may be impaired. Vaginitis caused by radiation may require antibiotic and hormone-containing creams. Women and their sex partners can be reassured that the radioactivity cannot be sexually transmitted.

See also CANCER; CERVICAL EROSION; HERPES GENITALIS; HYSTERECTOMY.

CERVICAL EROSION is a gynecological condition that affects perhaps 1 out of every 4 American women.

The cervix is the narrow tip, or neck, of the uterus, at the top of the vagina. An erosion is a sore—a worn-away grainy-looking area of redness—on the cervix.

Erosion of the cervix is almost always present after childbirth. Uterine contractions repeatedly force the baby's head against the cervix, causing it to bear a great deal of pressure. In some cases, the cervix is unavoidably injured during the delivery. Erosion that develops after childbirth usually heals itself within a few months.

Cervical erosion may also be caused by a vaginal infection. Changes in the acid-alkaline ratio of the vagina may destroy cervical tissue, leading to inflammation and subsequently erosion. During intercourse, the normal acidity of the cervix becomes more alkaline due to semen. Bacteria may also be introduced into the vagina and the cervix during intercourse.

Cervical erosion is often painless and does not interfere with the enjoyment of intercourse. The chief symptom is a whitish, odorous discharge. The discharge may be bloody if the erosion is deep. Inflammation around the erosion can cause pelvic pain or backache. Generally, the symptoms are so unspecific that women are unaware of the erosion.

Women should have semiannual gynecological examinations to detect the presence of erosion and other abnormal conditions. An erosion is usually benign, but many gynecologists consider neglected erosion a potential forerunner of cervical cancer.

Treating erosion. Vaginal douching is often recommended as treatment of mild erosion. One tablespoon of white vinegar in one quart of water will help maintain the normal acid contents of the vagina.

Common methods for treating cervical erosion include electric cautery with a fine-tipped needle, the application of silver nitrate to the erosion, the application of creams, and electrocoagulation. These office procedures cause little or no discomfort and require no anesthetic. For a few hours after treatment, some women note cramping like that of menstruation, which can be relieved with aspirin.

The newest method of treatment is cryosurgery—freezing of the cervix. It is as painless as other treatments and generally more effective.

See also CERVICAL CANCER; VAGINAL INFECTION.

CERVIX. See CERVICAL CANCER; CERVICAL EROSION; FEMALE SEXUAL ANATOMY.

CHANCROID (soft chancre) is a venereal disease caused by the bacteria *Hemophilus ducreyi*. It is characterized by soft, painful, ragged ulcers with grayish pus and a red border. Lymph glands in the groin often swell and may develop abscesses. Symptoms usually appear within a week after intercourse.

In men, the most common sites of infection are the foreskin, frenulum, and other parts of the penis. Sometimes the infection also involves the anus, thigh, scrotum, or lower abdomen.

In women, the infection commonly appears on the labia, clitoris, or perineum. Both men and women occasionally develop chancroid ulcers on the lip, tongue, or fingers.

Secondary bacterial infection is common and may produce a characteristic foul odor.

Chancroid usually responds well to sulfonamides. The physician may also recommend hot salt compresses to reduce pain and swelling. Topical antibiotic creams applied after the compresses will help reduce secondary infection. While this treatment will cure the infection, tissues already damaged or destroyed cannot be restored.

See also VENEREAL DISEASE.

CHLAMYDIA. See NONGONOCOCCAL URETHRITIS.

CIRCUMCISION has recently become a subject of medical controversy.

Removing the prepuce (foreskin) of the penis has been practiced as part of religious ritual among Jews and other groups for thousands of years. With parents' consent many United States obstetricians routinely circumcise newborn boys within a few days after birth. Recently some doctors have begun questioning the wisdom of the operation.

Circumcision is clearly needed when there is a decidedly abnormal overgrowth of the foreskin, fully hiding the tip of the penis. Contrariwise, when a child is of indeterminate sex, doctors recommend against circumcision, at least until the child's problems are resolved.

When the child's penis and general health are normal, the decision about circumcising rests with the parents. Some arguments on both sides of the question:

● There is a possible link between a lowered incidence of cancer of the penis and circumcision at birth. Smegma, an odorous, irritating cheeselike secretion that accumulates under the foreskin, may be implicated.

On the other hand, good genital hygiene may also prevent penis cancer. Studies do not confirm a widespread belief that circumcision prevents cancer of the cervix in the female sex partner.

● Circumcision tends to prevent repeated penis infections. Urologists in military service find that uncircumcised men have substantially more infections, particularly in hot climates. But good personal hygiene also cuts down the incidence of infection.

● There is no evidence that the circumcised man is deprived of any sexual pleasure. Nor is it necessarily true that intercourse is more prolonged for him than for the uncircumcised male. It is sometimes argued, without basis in fact, that the tip of a circumcised penis becomes less sensitive because of rubbing by underwear, pants, etc.

● Circumcision is a relatively simple surgical procedure, but it requires skill and careful aftercare. There may be complications, such as infection. The most serious complication, death from hemorrhage, is extremely rare.

In general, doctors feel that babies should be circumcised if it is consistent with the family's religious and esthetic values. The procedure seems especially warranted if busy parents feel circumcision will spare them—and their sons—the effort required to keep the area under the foreskin clean. Circumcision should be avoided in premature infants and newborns with any congenital abnormality of the penis, illness, infection, bleeding, or a family history of hemophilia.

When a child is not circumcised, high standards of personal hygiene are needed. About once a week, starting when a child is about 3, the parent should gently push against the foreskin with a washcloth, pulling the foreskin gradually back over the penis. It should not be forced or tugged, since this can cause tearing, with bleeding and possible scarring.

The parent should wash the exposed tip of the penis with soap and water and then rinse. Then the foreskin should be returned to normal position. If it does not go back down easily, the parent should try squeezing the rounded tip of the penis. If the foreskin still does not go down, a physician should be called immediately, before painful swelling occurs.

Psychiatrists urge fathers to supervise the bathing of a son until he can do it for himself. From about age 10 the boy needs to retract his foreskin daily and wash with soap and water.

Circumcision is sometimes needed by older boys and adults. Among the reasons for circumcising are repeated infection and difficulty in retracting the foreskin. Psychiatrists recommend against circumcising a child between 4 and 7 years of age, a crucial stage of psychosexual development.

Adults need to abstain from intercourse for 10 days after the circumcision. Doctors often provide patients with a drug to avoid erections.

After a baby is circumcised, the area should be kept clean and dry so that it will heal well.

Diapers should be changed often, or the child can be left undiapered. The doctor may prescribe a dressing or ointment. The doctor should be notified if the baby has a fever over 101° F, bright red bleeding, or a rash, swelling, or inflammation.

CLIMACTERIC. See AGING; MALE CLIMACTERIC; MENOPAUSE.

CLITORAL PROBLEMS. The clitoris is a small knob of tissue located above the opening of the urethra, the passage to the urinary bladder. It is surrounded by a fold of tissue, the clitoral hood. The hood is attached to the labia minora, the liplike structures at the entrance to the vagina.

In the embryo, a group of specialized cells becomes the clitoris. If the fetus is male, the same tissue becomes part of a penis. Unlike the penis, the clitoris has only one known purpose—as a focus of erotic sensitivity in women. In the entire human anatomy, it is the only structure whose sole function is sexual pleasure. The clitoris is much smaller than the penis but has an equal number of sensory nerve endings. Hence it is potentially far more sensitive than the penis. Structurally, the clitoris is like a penis in miniature: It has a shaft, a glans, and a hood.

Clitorises vary greatly in size and shape. Such factors have no bearing on sexual responsiveness.

Clitoral pain is unusual. Although the clitoris is richly supplied with nerve endings and is sensitive to touch, it is rarely a source of pain. Any irritation from sexual activity usually soon passes. A physician should be consulted for any persistent clitoral discomfort.

Clitoral pain may result because of an allergic reaction to a medication applied to the area, such as an anesthetic or antibiotic ointment. Some women have allergic reactions to clothes, deodorant sprays, or detergents (including bubble bath products). The clitoris may become irritated by a buildup of perspiration, urine, and smegma.

Almost all dermatological conditions can affect the clitoral area. The clitoris is subject to ulcers, abscesses, and tumors. Clitoral pain may result from vaginal infections. Urological conditions such as urethritis can cause referred pain to the clitoris. Scarring may result from severe infection, burns, or injury. Injudicious use of a vibrator may cause clitoral injury.

Some venereal diseases, such as chancroid and granuloma venereum, can cause painful ulcers, sometimes on or around the clitoris. Venereal warts, transmitted through intercourse, are sometimes painful. Herpes on or around the clitoris may also be painful.

Conversely, the clitoris may develop a lack of sensation. This may result from such physiological conditions as nerve injury, diabetes, or multiple sclerosis. Alcoholism and vitamin deficiency also may dull clitoral feeling. Lack of sensation may be psychological; if so, psychotherapy may be required.

The clitoris can be damaged by objects used in masturbation. One young girl was treated for a painfully enlarged clitoris—caused by a hair she had tightly wrapped around it. Another patient as a child would rub her clitoris on the branches of trees as she climbed. This damaged the nerve endings beyond recovery.

Also liable to cause clitoral irritation are some gadgets—sold in sex shops or through catalogs—that are advertised as clitoral stimulators.

One such device is a plastic penis-shaped mold that fits over a man's penis (the man presumably requires such a device because he has potency problems). At its base is a small protuberance. When the device is inserted into the woman's vagina, the protuberance supposedly stimulates her clitoris. But, since the man has little control over the degree of pressure exerted, the sensation is much more likely to be irritating than pleasurable.

Some women are born with, or acquire, clitoral abnormalities, most frequently clitoral enlargement. Pathological enlargement may be due to endocrine disorders. Sometimes, for example, abnormally high androgen production by the adrenal glands in females causes marked masculinization with enlargement of the clitoris. In rare cases, tumors of the ovary can have the same effect. Treating the cause of clitoral enlargement can often reverse it.

Testosterone treatment for breast cancer typically causes clitoral enlargement. Sometimes, the enlargement is due to inflammation, infection, or injury.

In baby girls, hormone disorders can result in an enlarged clitoris (sometimes it looks like a small penis) and other genital abnormalities.

Surgical removal of the clitoris (clitoridectomy) is rarely necessary. When it is done, as in cases of cancer or congenital deformity, the surgery does not seem to impair sexual functioning, erotic sensations, or orgasm. Evidently the nerve supply for sexual sensations is so lavish that a woman can lose large amounts of tissue without destroying her sexual gratification.

Claims have been made that surgically freeing up or removing the hood of the clitoris (clitoral circumcision) enhances clitoral sensations and sexual arousal. Research does not substantiate such claims.

Clitoris and orgasm. It is clitoral more than vaginal stimulation that produces orgasm. The clitoris is an organ with a dense concentration of nerve endings that transmit erotic sensations. By contrast, the vaginal walls are largely devoid of such nerves.

During excitement, the first stage of sexual response, the clitoris swells because of increased blood flow. But clitoral erection is not a good indicator of whether a woman is adequately stimulated. For about half the women studied by Masters and Johnson the enlargement was not sufficient to be noted by the naked eye.

These clitoral changes may be caused by direct stimulation of the genitals or of another sexually sensitive part of the body, such as the breasts. Erotic fantasies, too, may cause the clitoris to swell.

During the second (plateau) phase of sexual response the clitoris retracts. It draws away from the vaginal entrance and is covered by the clitoral hood. At this stage, the clitoris continues to respond to direct (manual) stimulation.

Intercourse generally provides only indirect stimulation. The shaft of the penis generally does not remain in contact with the clitoris. Rather, the thrusting of the penis exerts pressure on the labia minora. This rhythmic pulling is transmitted to the clitoral hood and then the clitoris itself.

For some women, this indirect stimulation can bring orgasm. But most women require more direct stimulation than the penis alone provides.

Physiologically, orgasm—the third stage of sexual response—is a release of the sexual tension and engorgement of blood vessels built up by sexual stimulation. It is accompanied by many physical changes other than clitoral, for orgasm is a total body response.

The clitoris returns to its normal position 5 to 10 seconds after orgasmic contractions stop. Its swelling subsides during the final (resolution) phase of sexual response. This can take from 5 to 30 minutes.

See also HORMONE DISORDERS.

CLITORIS. See CLITORAL PROBLEMS; FEMALE SEXUAL ANATOMY.

COCAINE use is reputed to enhance sexual enjoyment.

Some cocaine users have described intensified orgasms, increased desire, and increased firmness and durability of erections.

At the same time, negative sexual effects have also been reported, including priapism and loss of erection. Chronic, sustained use may result in decreased sexual interest and performance.

Objective research is scanty, and no conclusions can be drawn at this time. Further, all drug effects are highly variable and subjective and difficult for researchers to assess.

See also APHRODISIACS; PRIAPISM.

COITUS. Another term for sexual intercourse.

COITUS INTERRUPTUS. See WITHDRAWAL.

CONDOMS (rubbers, prophylactics, trojans, safes, sheaths, scumbags) offer high protection against both pregnancy and disease. Used properly, they are 90-97 percent effective.

If used correctly with foam or a diaphragm, the condom is practically foolproof. It has virtually no side effects. Moreover, it is inexpensive, widely sold, requires no prescription, and is easily carried in a pocket or purse.

Condoms are about eight inches long and generally come prerolled and powdered. Some have a nipple-shaped reservoir at the tip to catch the semen and help prevent the condom from bursting. If a condom does not have a reservoir, the man should leave half an inch loose at the end when putting it on.

The condom must be fitted over an erect penis. This can be made part of the sex play, the woman helping the man put it on. With practice, this can be done in the dark in a few seconds, avoiding needless interruption of lovemaking and possible loss of the erection. To add to the sensuousness of condoms, they are manufactured in a variety of designs and colors. Textured condoms, including "French ticklers," are advertised to provide a range of sensations.

The condom may slip off inside the vagina as the penis shrinks after ejaculation. The man should therefore remove his penis before it becomes soft. While doing this, he needs to hold his fingers around the base of the condom so that it does not slip off. He should then move away from the woman while he unrolls the condom, since sperm will now be on his penis. A new condom must be used each time intercourse occurs. If there is any chance that semen has leaked into the vagina, the woman should immediately insert an application of spermicidal jelly, cream, or foam.

In rare cases a man or woman may suffer an allergy to rubber, causing a rash on the genitals. Switching to a condom made from lambskin (a "skin") generally solves the problem.

To avoid breakage, condoms should not be subject to heat. They may deteriorate quickly if carried in a pocket or wallet, or stored in a glove compartment. Condoms should be bought from a store, not a machine—which may have overage merchandise. It is best to avoid foreign-brand condoms, which are not uniformly subjected to the testing given American condoms and may be defective more often.

A condom should be examined, but not tested, before use. It is likely to be damaged by needless stretching or inflating. Condoms that are lubricated in their packages are least likely to break from dryness. For do-it-yourself lubrication, spermicidal jelly or cream is recommended. Petroleum jelly or oils should not be used—they can cause the condom to deteriorate and they have no spermicidal properties. If there is any question whatever about the safety of condoms, they should be discarded.

Condoms come in packets of three or twelve. They are thin but tough. Manufacturing defects are extremely rare—condoms are made under the jurisdiction of the Food and Drug Administration and have to meet strict standards. In an unopened box they ordinarily last about a year.

Most men who complain of loss of sensitivity with regular condoms have found those made from lambskin more satisfactory. Indeed, by decreasing penis sensitivity, condoms may delay ejaculation, prolonging intercourse and enhancing pleasure for both partners. Condoms may benefit a man who has trouble maintaining an erection—the condom exerts a slight tourniquet effect on the veins of the penis.

It is unwise to improvise condoms from plastic sandwich bags or wrappings, an attempt that is uncomfortable and carries a high risk of pregnancy.

See also CONTRACEPTION; DIAPHRAGM; SPERMICIDES; VENEREAL DISEASE.

CONTRACEPTION (birth control). Any choice of contraceptive should take into consideration the protection the method affords, the risk of adverse reactions, and the method's suitability to an individual's preferences and frequency of sexual activity.

The accompanying table compares the effectiveness of birth control methods.

Birth control: How well does it work?

	Effectiveness if used perfectly all the time	Effectiveness based on surveys of actual couples who use the method
Pills (combined estrogen and progestogen)	99.66%	90-96%
Mini-pills.(progestogen only)	98.5-99%	90-95%
IUD	97-99%	95%
Condom *and* Foam or Diaphragm*	99+%	95%
Condom	97%	90%
Diaphragm	97%	90%
Foam	97%	84%
Withdrawal	91%	75-80%
Rhythm	87%	79%
Douching	?	60%
No method	10%	10%

These figures are for *fertile* couples, based on the *first year* of using a method. "90% effective" means 90 out of 100 couples using the method for one year *will not* have an unplanned pregnancy.

Source: *Contraceptive Technology*; adapted from the National Clearinghouse for Family Planning Information Health Education Bulletin.

For both safety and effectiveness, condom with foam is a good combination. Contraceptive foams and condoms are readily available in pharmacies at relatively low prices. The method requires little advance preparation, and may be best suited for women who have intercourse infrequently.

The condom with diaphragm, which is even more effective with as few adverse reactions, is suited to women who have intercourse more frequently and who can plan ahead reliably. The diaphragm requires a

---

*Figures are for foam. With diaphram, effectiveness is greater.

gynecological examination, a physician's prescription, and careful instruction in its use.

Women who have frequent sexual intercourse may choose to use IUDs, which require no preparation just before intercourse. This method—like the birth control pill—may be preferred by women who are loath to touch their genitals.

Birth control pills appeal to many women because they provide peak protection and allow for sexual spontaneity. On the other hand, the Pill requires perfect daily compliance, and there is the possibility of worrisome—and sometimes fatal—side effects.

Women who follow the precepts of the Roman Catholic church need to learn the natural family planning methods of birth control and should seek instruction in their use.

Some birth control methods are just marginally better than no method at all. Vaginal douching after intercourse is risky protection. Nor can withdrawal be considered reliable contraception. While breastfeeding may reduce a woman's chances of conceiving, it is not considered a method of birth control.

It is also unwise to rely on frequent ejaculations, through intercourse or masturbation, as a form of birth control. Frequent ejaculation does tend to decrease a man's semen volume and sperm concentration, possibly reducing the chances of pregnancy. But pregnancies occur even with very low sperm concentrations and poor semen quality. Furthermore, as soon as the man cuts down on the frequency of his ejaculations, his sperm count and semen quality quickly return to high enough levels to greatly increase the chances of pregnancy.

Abortion is a hazardous and expensive means of birth control. Sterilization is a birth control option for people who are sure they want no more children.

See also ABORTION; CONDOM; DES; DIAPHRAGM; IUDs; NATURAL FAMILY PLANNING; SPERMICIDES; TUBAL STERILIZATION; VASECTOMY; WITHDRAWAL.

CORPORA CAVERNOSA. See MALE SEXUAL ANATOMY.

CORPUS SPONGIOSUM. See MALE SEXUAL ANATOMY.

CORTICOSTEROIDS. See STEROIDS.

CRAB LICE. See LICE.

CROSS-DRESSING. See TRANSVESTISM.

CRYPTORCHIDISM. See TESTICLE, UNDESCENDED.

CUNNILINGUS. See ORAL SEX.

CUSHING'S SYNDROME. See HORMONE DISORDERS.

CVA. See STROKE.

CYSTECTOMY is removal of the bladder and the creation of an artificial urinary outlet. This surgery is most often performed as cancer treatment.

After a radical cystectomy, a man will be unable to have an erection because the peripheral branches of the pelvic nerves are interrupted. He will be unable to ejaculate because the prostate and seminal vesicles are also removed in this surgery.

He can still experience orgasm, however, through manual or oral stimulation of his flaccid penis. His testicles remain active, producing hormones and sperm that is reabsorbed. He will not experience any feminization.

A cystectomy patient is usually an excellent candidate for surgical implantation of a penile prosthesis. He is likely to be suited to either of the two types: the semirigid silicone rubber prosthesis, which results in a permanent erection; or the inflatable device, which allows him to control the presence or absence of an erection.

Even without a penile prosthesis, the patient can enjoy lovemaking and can provide his partner with physical and emotional gratification.

Women often retain complete sexual functioning. After cystectomy—if only the bladder and urethra are removed—a woman can be fully responsive sexually, and she retains her ability to have children. Often, however, a portion of a woman's internal reproductive organs also requires surgical removal.

Since cystectomy patients have an abdominal urinary stoma—an opening for urine in the abdomen—and must wear a urinary appliance, they are almost certainly bound to be embarrassed about lovemaking at first, but most people can learn to overcome this.

Patients almost always benefit from the services of an enterostomal therapist, a nurse specially trained to help such patients learn to adjust to their condition, both physically and psychologically. Membership in an Ostomy Club can be invaluable. Here patients who have to cope with urine and feces appliances can share their feelings and exchange practical information.

See also CANCER; HYSTERECTOMY; OSTOMIES; PENILE PROSTHESES.

CYSTITIS. See URINARY TRACT INFECTION.

DEAFNESS. Over 90 percent of deaf children are born to hearing parents, who have no idea what it means to be deaf or how to communicate with their deaf children. Although the very best lip-readers understand only one quarter of what is said, most parents communicate orally with their deaf children, expecting them to lip-read.

Thus, acquiring knowledge is a difficult process for a deaf child. To add just one word to the vocabulary is a major accomplishment. Sexual words and concepts are particularly hard to come by.

Deaf children are handicapped by not overhearing other children or adults discuss sexual matters. This is how hearing children pick up information about relationships, taboos, body parts, and their functions. When deaf children are taught sign language, they typically learn very few signs relating to sex.

Deaf children who point to their genitals to ask questions or make observations soon learn that adults consider such gestures inappropriate; this lesson erects further barriers to sexual communication.

65

Abstract ideas are particularly difficult to communicate to deaf children. Concepts such as maleness, femaleness, parenting, and reproduction are hard to convey.

Further, many deaf adolescents and adults have low levels of verbal and reading achievement—so they are handicapped in acquiring sexual information through books or pamphlets.

In residential schools for the deaf, administrators may assume that parents have provided their children with sex education. In any case, most residential schools ignore the sexual needs of deaf children. Even in schools where sex education is formally taught, few teachers are well equipped to assume the role of sex educator.

Moreover, residential schools are often segregated by sex. They provide few opportunities for social interaction between the sexes or for privacy. When sexual activity does occur in such residential settings, it is more likely to be homosexual than heterosexual.

Deaf children who live at home are likely to be overprotected, and their opportunities for social interaction may be severely limited. Parents of hearing children have a hard-enough time conveying sexual information; when the children are deaf, parents may be even more at a loss.

Deaf children require special sex education to overcome the limitations on their acquisition of sexual knowledge. Sex education for the deaf requires highly visual materials supported by clear, simple language. Pictures, films, photographs, and role-playing are important tools for enhancing sexual understanding and the development of sex-related concepts.

Conveying even a simple idea such as "Girls become women" requires making sure that the child understands each of the three words and has clear photographs or diagrams representing the concept.

Deaf adolescents frequently benefit from peer counseling sessions. Here they can share feelings, values, and attitudes relating to their social lives and sexuality. Parents groups can help parents of deaf youngsters deal with their children's sexuality and the problems of conveying sexual information and values.

Deafness does not impair sexual desire or responsiveness. But sexual ignorance and deficiencies in social skills may predispose a deaf person to marital and sexual problems. Deafness may have a negative impact on self-esteem and body image which may impair sexuality.

Deaf people who seek sexual counseling can best be helped by professionals experienced in communicating with the deaf.

When deafness first occurs in adolescence or adulthood, common reactions are depression, social isolation, and a sense of helplessness. Sexual problems caused by such states of mind are usually temporary.

DELAYED EJACULATION. See AGING.

DEPRESSION is a mental disorder in which melancholy and dejection are unrealistic and out of proportion to any known cause.

There is often a very thin line between a normal emotional reaction to negative events and a clinical depression. Most people experience a state of transient depression after an emotional trauma such as a divorce or a job loss. Illness or surgery may result in depression. Loss of a loved one almost always causes a depression for many weeks or months.

For most people, such depressive states disappear fairly quickly, and they are able to resume normal activity.

For others, however, the depression is unduly persistent or severe. Such people may be suffering from *exogenous* depression, a sort of depression triggered by a specific event or series of events.

Other people may suffer from *endogenous* depression, which appears independently of environmental triggering mechanisms. This sort of depression is more commonly psychotic. It is characterized by recurrent depressive episodes. Manic-depressive illness is a type of endogenous depression in which depressive bouts alternate with pathologic euphoria.

The cause of depression is not known. Some investigators suspect that an underlying biochemical abnormality or predisposition may trigger the disorder.

People don't always know when they're depressed. Some people may conceal their feelings even from themselves, or not be able to identify what is bothering them.

Symptoms typically associated with depression may help identify it. Depressed people often suffer from insomnia or irregular sleeping patterns. Loss of appetite and weight loss are common as are fatigue and agitation. Psychosomatic symptoms—such as headache, backache, hypochondria—affect many depressed people.

There is usually a diminished enjoyment in work, leisure activities, and other people. The capacity for intimacy diminishes. The depressed person may be less physically active and show less initiative and assertiveness. Feelings of despair and utter hopelessness afflict some depressed people. Some become unable to function at work or home. Suicidal thoughts are common.

Some people attempt to counter the joylessness of depression with impulsive pleasure-seeking. They may overeat, drink a lot, or take extreme physical risks.

Decreased interest in sex is a common symptom of depression. The depressed person often loses the capacity for sexual fantasy that for many people is an important prelude to sexual arousal.

The mechanism for decreased sexual desire in depression is not known. In some people, a purely psychogenic reaction may be involved. A person in the midst of an emotional crisis may be directing all energies toward mastering difficulties and may have little time or energy left for sex.

Physiologic and endocrine changes that accompany severe depression may interfere with sexual desire. Men under chronic stress show lowered blood testosterone levels. Menstrual disturbances—particularly failure to menstruate—frequently occur in depressed women. Stress may influence the hypothalamus, which may signal the pituitary to decrease the output of sex hormones.

Some people react to decreased sexual desire by increasing sexual activity. In an attempt to boost self-esteem and compensate for the lack of sexual desire, it is not unusual for depressed people to engage in impulsive sexual behavior. Promiscuous behavior in both men and women may occur as an attempt to escape loneliness and depression. It often results in mechanical and pleasureless sexual encounters. Some depressed people engage in homosexual experimentation. Compulsive masturbation may occur in a restless, agitated depressed person, often in an attempt to seek relaxation and attain sleep.

For a few people, sexual escape from depression may take the form of exhibitionism, pedophilia, incest, or sexual delusions.

All such impulsive sexual acts may cause the person to suffer agonies of guilt—which may deepen the depression, and in turn lead to more sexual acting-out.

Most depressed people, however, report *a decline* in the frequency of sexual intercourse. This may occur partly because of decreased sexual interest and partly because a depressed person withdraws from social interactions with others, thereby lessening opportunities for emotional intimacy and sexual activity.

For most depressed people, sexual functioning is not altered. While they may be less interested in sex and engage in intercourse infrequently, their bodies will respond normally on the occasions when they do have sex.

But others suffer sexual dysfunctions such as trouble reaching orgasm, ejaculation problems, or impotence.

Such problems may arise because of lowered sexual desire. A depressed man, for example, may feel little or no sexual desire. He may be upset when he realizes that his wife is frequently initiating intercourse. When he tries to have intercourse, he may have partial erections which he is unable to sustain. This causes him a great deal of anxiety. He is even more anxious before the next sexual act. Psychogenic impotence results as the man becomes more and more fearful of sexual failure and tries to force himself to have an erection.

In a few people, depression is *caused* by sexual problems. Typically, this is a mild depression that disappears dramatically with the resolution of the sexual difficulty. These cases of depression are unlikely to respond to drug therapy. Psychotherapy or sex therapy are recommended.

Depression is much more common in women than in men. The reason for this is unknown. While depression can occur in any type of personality, it is much more frequent in people who are rigid, constricted, and compulsive. A person who is characteristically intense, serious, hardworking, and humorless is more depression-prone than a more casual person.

Treatment for depression typically results in increased sexual desire and greater sexual enjoyment. Most depressed patients respond to a combination of antidepressant medication and psychotherapy. Electroshock therapy is recommended for some.

A thorough physical examination is necessary since some illnesses have depression as a symptom. Medications taken for a variety of illnesses may also cause depression.

Sex therapy is indicated for patients who continue to experience sexual difficulties after the depression is relieved.

DERMATITIS. See SKIN DISORDERS.

DES should be used as emergency contraception only.

This controversial "morning-after" contraceptive has been approved by the Food and Drug Administration for use in emergency situations such as rape. The pill, a large dose of a synthetic estrogen compound called diethylstilbestrol or DES, is over 90 percent effective in preventing pregnancy when administered within seventy-two hours after intercourse.

The FDA emphasizes that DES should not be considered as a routine means of contraception because of possibly severe side effects. It generally causes violent nausea and vomiting. Other common side effects include extreme breast tenderness, headaches, dizziness, and menstrual irregularities. If DES treatment is taken once, it should not be taken a second time. The contraceptive dose is equivalent to about ten months of birth control pills.

A controversy over DES concerns its possible cancer-causing potential. It was banned as a growth hormone for cattle and other food animals after it was found capable of causing cancer in some animals. At one time DES was used to prevent miscarriages. Daughters of women who received DES during pregnancy suffer an unusually high incidence of a rare type of vaginal cancer. Sons have an unusual incidence of genital abnormalities.

There is no data to show that DES causes cancer in the woman who takes it. The FDA believes that DES, used as a contraceptive, does not pose a "significant threat to the patient."

On the other hand, the cancer-causing potential of DES has not been fully explored. Doctors Roy Hertz and Mort Lipsett, experts in hormonal cancer at the National Institutes of Health, have stated that "DES is such a powerful carcinogen that it is used as a model for producing artificial cancers in animals."

DES should not be taken if there is a family history of cancer of the breast or of the genitals. There may also be a risk if other estrogens, such as birth control pills, have been taken.

See also CONTRACEPTION; PILL, CONTRACEPTIVE; RAPE.

DIABETES, a chronic disease of insulin deficiency, often causes sexual problems. In general, several years after the diabetes is discovered, a diabetic man notices a decrease in the firmness of his erection. For the next 6 to 18 months, his erections become less and less firm and of shorter and shorter duration. His interest in sex is usually unimpaired, and he retains his ability to experience orgasms and ejaculate.

Such impotence—the inability to achieve or sustain an erection—results from diabetic neuropathy, a process of microscopic nerve damage throughout the body. It leads to sexual dysfunction in about half of men with clinically apparent diabetes.

Impotence may also be an *early* sign of diabetes, often appearing before the underlying condition is recognized. In such cases, the impotence has a rapid onset and is accompanied by loss of sex drive. It's typically accompanied by the classic diabetic symptoms of itching, weight loss, and excessive hunger, thirst, and urination.

When impotence is an early symptom of diabetes, it usually can be resolved with good control of the condition. Even late-onset impotence can often be slowed down or stopped with proper treatment. Actual tissue damage, however, cannot be reversed.

Diabetic impotence often comes and goes. So if a couple maintain regular sexual contact, they are likely to enjoy intercourse during remissions. They can also explore ways of sexually gratifying each other besides penile intromission.

A penile implant is a possibility. Diabetic men may be suited to either of two types: the semirigid silicone rubber prosthesis, which results in a permanent erection; or the inflatable device, which allows the man to control the erection. One major caution: because of problems with wound-healing and infection, diabetics are often at increased risk of surgical complications. A diabetic patient's impotence may be due to factors other than his diabetes. It may be psychogenic—diabetics are at least as subject as other men to emotional stress. Indeed, their illness may make them feel less virile, thus anxious over their sexual performance and subject to erectile failure. In such cases, diabetic men are as amenable as nondiabetic men to sex therapy.

So, too, a patient's medications may be interfering with his erections. Many drugs have impotence as a side effect. A diabetic is also at increased risk for other illnesses that may interfere with sexual functioning—heart disease, infection, endocrine disorders. Resolving such a concurrent condition may resolve the sexual problem.

Some diabetic women experience decreased libido and difficulty or

71

inability in achieving orgasm. The onset of the problem is usually gradual and progressive, beginning several years after a diagnosis is made.

Sexual dysfunction is thought to be the result of diabetic neuropathy and/or vascular disease. Careful control of the diabetes may restore sexual functioning.

Other diabetes-related factors may account for, or contribute to, sexual difficulties: a diabetic woman's fatigue and weakness from the disease may leave her uninterested in sex; diabetic women are predisposed to chronic vaginal infection, which may make intercourse uncomfortable.

Some diabetic women—fearful of the added risks of complications in pregnancy and congenital defects in their children—may suffer sexual difficulties of psychogenic origin. The stress of coping with a chronic life-threatening illness may similarly contribute to sexual impairment. So may marital or work problems, medications, and alcohol use. Other endocrine abnormalities may account for sexual dysfunction. Thus, thorough medical examination is necessary when a diabetic woman complains of orgasmic difficulties.

See also ALCOHOL; IMPOTENCE; PENILE PROSTHESES; VAGINAL INFECTION.

DIAPHRAGM, a soft rubber device with a spring rim, is but one part of a contraceptive system. Another essential part is a contraceptive jelly or cream that kills sperm before they can get into the uterus.

While the diaphragm system alone is 83-97 percent effective, used with the condom it is nearly foolproof (99+ percent).

To properly use her diaphragm, a woman spreads on its saucerlike surface a teaspoon of spermicidal cream or jelly—foam doesn't adhere well enough. She then places the diaphragm into her vagina so that it blocks her cervix, the entrance to her uterus. Without the spermicide, she would be at great risk of sperm getting around the diaphragm rim and making her pregnant. The diaphragm has no side effects.

For a while the diaphragm fell out of favor because it seemed less convenient and effective than the Pill or IUD. Now the diaphragm appears to be making a comeback among women who, fed up with side effects and worried about long-term safety, have abandoned the Pill and IUD.

There is no need to interrupt sex play to insert the diaphragm. In fact, sexual arousal changes the location of the cervix, raising the hazard of an improper fit. A better practice: if a woman thinks she might possibly have intercourse, she can insert her diaphragm hours in advance.

The spermicide is certainly effective for up to two hours. If she has intercourse more than two hours after insertion, she will be safest if she leaves the diaphragm in place but introduces into her vagina more spermicide (cream, jelly, suppository, or foam). Each application protects her against the sperm in one ejaculation. Before each additional intercourse, she needs another applicator full of spermicide.

After intercourse, she needs to leave the diaphragm in place for at least six hours. She similarly should wait six hours before douching. The diaphragm can remain in place for days without adverse effect, but this is not recommended. Removing it allows the vagina to cleanse itself. Taking it out also reduces the chance of irritation and infection.

Properly cared for, a diaphragm can last for about two years. After removing it, the woman should wash it with mild soap and warm water, then air dry it and dust it with cornstarch before putting it back in its container. She should check it after every use for weak spots and pinholes by pulling the rubber gently away from the rim as she looks at it in front of a light.

A woman is likely to be a good candidate for a diaphragm if she is well-motivated, responsible, and not averse to touching her genitals.

The diaphragm should be used every time a woman has intercourse, even during her menstrual period. No harm results if she starts menstruating with the diaphragm in place. Indeed, some women use it to hold back the blood if they have sex during their periods.

It is essential to go to a doctor or a birth-control clinic—both to have the diaphragm fitted and to learn how to insert it properly. A woman may not realize that the cervix is so far back in her vagina. A full finger-length in, she will feel a lump somewhat like the end of a nose. That is her cervix, what her diaphragm must cover. The rim will slip into the recess above the cervix, out of reach. The rubber will feel wrinkled—it will not lie flat over the cervix.

A woman should never borrow someone else's diaphragm or buy one without a prescription. If the diaphragm is improperly inserted or if it is too small, it can fail to protect her from pregnancy. It might also be displaced during intercourse.

It is wise for a woman to see her doctor a week or so after she begins using the diaphragm to make sure that she is using it correctly and has no problems. If she was a virgin or had had sex only a few times when the diaphragm was fitted, she is likely to need a new size after a few weeks because her vaginal muscles will expand with sexual experience. Until she returns at the end of that week for a check of the size and her technique, she should use a backup method of contraception, such as a condom or additional vaginal spermicide.

A woman using a diaphragm should return for checkups at least once a year. Even if she uses a diaphragm for years, she may grow careless about her insertion technique. She may need a change in size if she loses or gains more than twenty pounds, or if she has an abortion or a baby. She also needs to go for a check on the size or her technique of insertion if one of the following warning signals appears. 1) Her partner complains of feeling the rim. 2) She develops such discomfort that she must remove the diaphragm prematurely. 3) The diaphragm rim no longer remains snug, or she can place a finger easily between the rim of the diaphragm and the recess of her vaginal wall, suggesting that the diaphragm is too small. 4) At a time other than her period, there is blood on the diaphragm when it is removed. This may indicate undue pressure from the rim, improper placement, or an injury or illness.

Should she suffer itching or irritation, she may be allergic to rubber or the spermicide. She may overcome an allergy to the cream by switching brands.

See also CONDOM; CONTRACEPTION.

DRUGS. See MEDICATIONS.

DYSPAREUNIA. See INTERCOURSE, PAINFUL.

ECLAMPSIA. See PREGNANCY.

E. COLI. See ANAL SEX; URINARY TRACT INFECTION.

ECTOPIC PREGNANCY. In a small number of women, the embryo implants itself in the Fallopian tubes, cervix, ovary, or abdominal or pelvic cavity instead of in the uterus. This is called an ectopic (meaning "out of place" or "in an abnormal position") pregnancy.

Ectopic pregnancy is more common in women using IUDs. Of pregnancies occurring with the IUD in place, 1 in 20 are ectopic.

The most common type of ectopic pregnancy is tubal—one that occurs in a Fallopian tube. Other types are rare. In about half the cases of tubal pregnancy, implantation is caused by a previous infection in the tube.

First symptoms of tubal pregnancy are spotting and cramping pain in the abdomen. These usually begin shortly after the first missed menstrual period and mimic signs of a threatened miscarriage. A woman experiencing such symptoms should consult a physician.

If the tubal pregnancy is not discovered earlier, at about 6 to 8 weeks of pregnancy the woman may experience sudden severe lower abdominal pain, followed by fainting. This usually indicates that the tube has ruptured and is hemorrhaging into the abdominal cavity.

Whether the tubal pregnancy is diagnosed before or after rupture, the treatment is surgical removal of the tube, along with the embryo implanted in it. Sometimes the ovary on the involved side must also be removed.

See also PREGNANCY.

EJACULATION. See ORGASM.

EJACULATION, BLOODY (hematospermia). Men who find blood in their ejaculate are likely to be very upset by the experience. The color of the semen may be black, brown, rust, or red—depending on how long it has been since the bleeding occurred.

In most cases—particularly if there are no other symptoms—the condition is not serious. Usually, blood in the ejaculate is a sign of infection in the genitourinary tract, most often the prostate, seminal vesicles, or urethra. Antibiotics usually bring about a complete cure.

*Venereal diseases—especially trichomoniasis and gonorrhea—*may account for the symptom. Tuberculosis may be a cause, as may congestion of the prostate, bladder neck obstruction, or blood abnormalities. Only rarely is bloody ejaculate a sign of a cancerous tumor. In some men, vigorous, repeated, or prolonged masturbation is thought to be the cause.

See also MASTURBATION; VENEREAL DISEASE.

EJACULATION, PLEASURELESS. In this uncommon experience, a man ejaculates but without the pleasurable sensation of orgasm.

Occasionally, the problem is due to organic conditions such as diabetes or a neurological disorder.

Inflammation of the urethra or prostate disease may be the underlying cause. Urethral scars caused by gonorrhea may sometimes account for this difficulty.

Most men who suffer from pleasureless ejaculation (also called ejaculatory anhedonia or orgastic impotence) have a psychological rather than a physiological problem.

Often, the difficulty reflects an emotional dissatisfaction with the sexual relationship. Unconsciously, the man may want to separate the sense of pleasure from the sexual act. He may be feeling anxiety, fear, or hostility about sexuality. Such feelings may lead to his suppressing intense sexual excitement at the moment of ejaculation. Psychotherapy or sex therapy may be helpful.

See also SEX THERAPY.

EJACULATION, PREMATURE. Premature ejaculation involves the male's reaching his climax too soon—either before penetration or within a minute or so thereafter. It is the most common sexual problem among men.

Premature ejaculation is deemed a chronic problem if a man cannot maintain control long enough to satisfy his partner at least half the time, assuming that she can reach orgasm through sustained intercourse.

Female partners commonly complain they feel used and frustrated. Both partners, of course, miss out on the pleasures of slow, leisurely sex.

The greater a man's formal education the more likely he is to seek relief. Such men tend to be concerned with their partners' satisfaction.

Conversely, grade-school and early high-school dropouts rarely seek help. Among this group, the husband generally dominates a couple's sex life. He may in fact regard quick ejaculation not as a problem but as a sign of his masculinity.

Premature ejaculation is often caused by faulty conditioning. There is no known medical condition that can account for premature ejaculation. Most cases arise from the male's being introduced to sex in a way that emphasizes his ejaculation rather than satisfying his partner.

He may thus become conditioned to ejaculating rapidly. This physical response develops outside his conscious control, and he automatically ejaculates very soon after beginning foreplay or intercourse.

A young man may develop such a habit of "coming quickly" if he starts by having intercourse in situations that call for a hurried response: in the backseats of cars, in living rooms with parents nearby, etc. Under such pressures he is likely to be concerned with attaining sexual release as soon as he can, with little time to worry about relieving the sexual needs of his partner.

Similar conditioning may result from a form of heavy petting often called "humping." The couple simulates intercourse through their clothes, with no actual penetration. This too is generally a one-sided activity, with the male's focus on his ejaculation.

Early encounters with prostitutes lie behind many cases of premature ejaculation. If the prostitute wants to turn as many tricks as possible, she may encourage the young man to hurry—rewarding him with smiles and compliments if he finishes in record time. Thereby a habit can be launched.

Using withdrawal as a birth control technique can promote premature ejaculation. Both partners may be preoccupied with the male's pulling out in time. He may withdraw and ejaculate after a few thrusts of the pelvis, and his partner's sexual needs may be left unfulfilled.

In some men, ejaculating prematurely may express a sexual conflict or an underlying emotional problem. Sexual anxiety is thought to be at the root of some men's premature ejaculation. Likewise, men who are unconsciously hostile toward their sex partners may express their anger by ejaculating before the woman can be satisfied.

Psychotherapy may be required before the man can attain ejaculatory control. A competent sex therapist will help a couple resolve differences that may be contributing to sexual difficulties.

The condition responds well to sex therapy. With the help of a caring, supportive, and informed partner, premature ejaculation is almost completely reversible through the "squeeze technique" developed by urologist James H. Semans of the Duke University School of Medicine.

Just before the man has an urge to ejaculate, his partner presses his frenulum—the sensitive spot at the bottom edge of the crown of his penis—firmly with her thumb for 3-5 seconds. She holds the opposite side of the crown with 2 fingers.

The goal of the squeeze technique is to keep the man sexually excited at a level short of ejaculation. If a man is uncircumcised, a little practice may be necessary to locate his frenulum in the nonerect state. If the woman worries about how hard she can press without hurting, the man can show her by placing his fingers over hers.

The Squeeze Technique
Three different angles show
exact placement of fingers

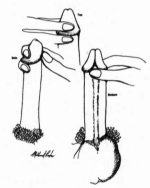

The man can expect to lose 10-15 percent of his erection after the squeeze is applied, but it's generally soon regained. Over several weeks the man is likely to become more and more able to bring his urge to ejaculate under his own control. Masters and Johnson report a 98 percent success rate applying the squeeze technique to the following regimen:

1. *Pleasuring.* "Pleasuring" (or "sensate focus") promotes a loving, sexually arousing relationship while freeing a couple from the pressure of performance.

The couple deliberately refrain from intercourse. Instead, on at least 4 days they set aside an hour or more a day for love play, indulging in sensations of touching and being touched.

They please each other by kissing, stroking, patting, massaging,

78

playing with each other's hair. They can take a bath together, washing one another. Vocalize pleasure. Share sexual fantasies.

They can tell each other what they like. And, short of actual intercourse, they can comply with each other's wishes.

2. *Training.* The woman sits up comfortably supported by a pillow against the headboard of the bed. The man lies so his genital area is between her legs:

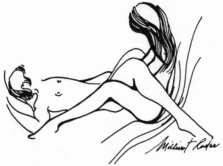

She masturbates him slowly, perhaps no faster than one stroke every 3 seconds or so. As soon as he feels an urge to ejaculate, he tells her. At once she applies the squeeze technique.

After 15-30 seconds, she resumes masturbating him. Perhaps 20 minutes of sex play may thus be experienced without the man's ejaculating. They repeat this for 3 or 4 days.

This training helps the man learn the level of sexual excitement he can sustain without ejaculating. It also helps the couple gain confidence that the problem can be relieved. And it encourages them to communicate openly about sex, thereby benefiting their relationship.

3. *Female-Superior Position.* The woman brings the man to a full erection and uses the squeeze technique 2-3 times. Then she assumes this position on top of him:

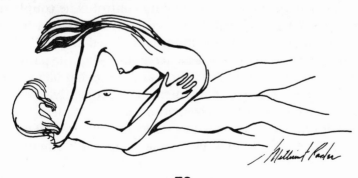

Her knees are as close to his nipple line as possible, above it if she's taller than he is. By leaning over him at a 45-degree angle, she can insert his penis into her vagina. Then she can move back onto it, rather than sit on the shaft.

She holds it in her vagina, and refrains from moving. As soon as he feels he is about to ejaculate, he tells her. She rises, exposing his penis—and applies the squeeze technique. Then she reinserts the penis. As before she remains motionless to avoid excessive stimulation.

After a few days of practice the man can provide just enough pelvic thrusting to maintain his erection. The woman does not thrust but applies the squeeze technique whenever needed. By the third day of this step, it is often possible to have intercourse for 15-20 minutes.

4. *Lateral Coital Position.* After control increases, they can try this position:

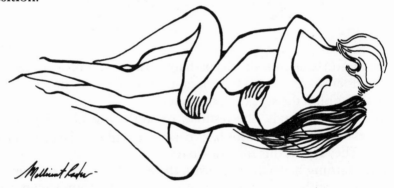

To get into it, they start with the female-superior position (preceded by the squeeze technique as in Step 3). The man rests one leg against the bed. The woman lies on the inner side of that thigh, straddling his other leg. For traction, both her knees can touch the bed.

5. *Subsequent Practice.* A man can expect to take between 6 and 12 months to achieve complete ejaculatory control. The couple should use the squeeze technique at least once a week for 6 months. Once a month, they may engage in the training outlined in Step 2.

It may be wise to use the squeeze technique after the partners have been apart from each other for a time, and sperm has had a chance to accumulate. It is helpful to have intercourse frequently.

After relieving premature ejaculation, many couples—flush with their newfound success—tend to overdo making love. This can so sexually satiate the man that he may be temporarily impotent. This problem almost always disappears as soon as he learns the frequency suited to him.

About Drugs and Distractions. Only as a last resort should a man ask his physician about prescribing tricyclic antidepressants such as Tofranil. Minute doses can slow down ejaculation without impairing erection.

In any case, premature ejaculators should avoid nonprescription drugs like anesthetic creams and jellies, which are supposed to prolong intercourse by reducing penis sensitivity. They are a waste of money and can trigger a drug allergy.

Masturbating before intercourse rarely delays ejaculation. Nor does wearing two condoms. Nor do attempts at distraction such as thinking about a job, counting backward from 100, etc. Physical distractions, like hair pulling or pinching, work no better.

See also SEX THERAPY.

EJACULATION, RETARDED. This relatively infrequent sexual dysfunction—also called ejaculatory incompetence or inhibited ejaculation—is the inability to ejaculate in the vagina.

Such men may be able to ejaculate through masturbation. Some may be able to ejaculate by manual or oral stimulation by a sex partner. In a small percentage of cases, a man may be able to ejaculate in the vagina of one partner but not another. Some men may not be able to ejaculate by any means. (Sex therapists have come across a significant number of men who have never masturbated.)

Typically, men suffering from retarded ejaculation have normal sexual desire and erections. They can usually maintain firm erections in intercourse for a long time.

In primary retarded ejaculation, the more common form, a male has never ejaculated in intercourse. The causes, most sex therapists currently believe, are usually psychological. Such men often have had a strict antisexual upbringing. They have feelings of guilt and shame about sexual activity. Some men with this condition have a great fear of impregnating their partners. Some fear the loss of control in ejaculation. Hostility toward the partner may contribute to the dysfunction. So may an unconscious fear of hurting the woman with the ejaculate— and possibly incurring her murderous retaliation.

In secondary retarded ejaculation, a man has been able to ejaculate in intercourse before developing the condition. In most such cases, retarded ejaculation is a symptom of problems in the relationship. Sometimes, a wife very much wants to become pregnant. Her husband may unconsciously fear fatherhood—thus withhold his ejaculate.

Some men can trace the development of the problem to a specific traumatic event: a man discovers his wife's adultery or finds out about a past rape.

While most cases of ejaculatory incompetence are psychogenic, organic problems sometimes inhibit ejaculation. Neurologic disorders may interfere with sympathetic nerves to the genitals. Some drugs may inhibit ejaculation. Chronic alcoholism may also cause retarded ejaculation.

Treatment for retarded ejaculation of psychogenic origin is a technique developed by Masters and Johnson. First, sensate focus exercises are employed, similar to those used in the treatment of impotence. The couple are encouraged to pleasure each other, taking turns caressing and stroking without touching the genitals or attempting to engage in intercourse.

The goals are to facilitate the man's awareness of his own physical sensations, to improve nonverbal communication between the partners, and to eliminate the pressure to perform.

The couple are encouraged to communicate their sexual preferences and aversions. Hostilities between them are explored. A woman may be angry at her husband if she believes he is willfully depriving her of children by not ejaculating.

When pleasuring progresses to genital touching, the woman is encouraged to manually stimulate the man's penis while he communicates to her what he finds most sexually pleasurable. She continues this stimulation until he ejaculates. This helps the man experience the woman as a source of pleasure. It may help if the ejaculation occurs near the woman's genitals, so that the man becomes more comfortable with an association between his ejaculate and his partner's vagina.

Next, the woman sits astride the man, facing him, or with her back to him (the reverse female-superior position), and stimulates his penis. When he is near the point of ejaculation, she inserts the penis into her vagina. If the man does not ejaculate after brief vigorous thrusting, the woman returns to manual stimulation until ejaculation becomes imminent. This procedure is continued until the man is able to ejaculate in the vagina.

A single successful ejaculation in the vagina may cure the dysfunction. If the man does not respond to sex therapy, psychotherapy may be necessary—or vice versa.

See also IMPOTENCE; MEDICATIONS.

EJACULATION, RETROGRADE. In this condition, semen is discharged into the bladder, rather than through the urethra. Normally, the bladder neck closes during ejaculation, and contractions compress the urethra to propel the semen outward through the urethra. When the bladder neck fails to close as a result of muscle or nerve damage, the semen flows backward into the bladder.

A man may discover—after intercourse or masturbation—that while he experiences orgasm there is no fluid ejaculate. The diagnosis is confirmed when sperm is found in the urine. Sexual performance is not affected by retrograde ejaculation.

The most common cause is prostate surgery. Scarring may prevent complete closing of the bladder neck, allowing semen to enter.

Other common causes include diabetes, spinal cord injury, and pelvic fractures, or other trauma to the pelvis.

Patients who receive ganglion-blocking drugs (usually for hypertension) may suffer from retrograde ejaculation. The condition usually reverses when the drug is discontinued.

Retrograde ejaculation may also occur after removal of the colon (colectomy) or after surgery for some tumors of the testicles. Patients who undergo lumbar sympathectomy—in which nerves in the groin are severed—may also experience retrograde ejaculation.

Men with retrograde ejaculation need not be sterile. While the condition is usually not correctable, sperm can be collected from the urine and used to inseminate the wife. In a small number of cases, surgery to the bladder neck can correct retrograde ejaculation.

See also DIABETES; INFERTILITY; PROSTATE ENLARGEMENT.

EJACULATORY DUCT. See MALE SEXUAL ANATOMY.

EJACULATORY INCOMPETENCE. See EJACULATION, RETARDED.

EMPHYSEMA. See RESPIRATORY DISEASE.

ENDOCRINE DISORDERS. See HORMONE DISORDERS.

ENDOMETRIOSIS may be the cause of severe pain during intercourse.

In this disorder, tissue from the lining of the uterus (the endometrium) is found in abnormal locations. Tissue fragments become embedded in sites with a rich blood supply, which provide nourishment for growth.

If endometrial tissue penetrates into the dense, muscular wall of the uterus itself, the condition is called adenomyosis. If the transplants are found elsewhere in the pelvic area, such as the ovaries, it's called pelvic endometriosis.

Endometriosis may result when tissue shed during menstruation is pushed up through the Fallopian tubes rather than out through the vagina. Why and how this happens is not known. In rare instances, the condition may result from previous pelvic surgery, and/or pelvic infections with scar formation.

A woman with adenomyosis commonly experiences aching pelvic discomfort. Her periods usually become progressively painful and heavy. Her uterus is enlarged and tender. Pelvic endometriosis likewise may cause painful, excessive menstruation. Periods may be irregular, and bleeding may occur between periods.

Pain during intercourse is usually the worst premenstrually, when the embedded fragments become engorged with blood and swollen. Particularly with pelvic endometriosis, the pain is usually felt deep in the vagina and may be excruciating.

A condition of women during their childbearing years, endometriosis is often associated with infertility. The exact relationship is unknown. In part, the cause may be decreased sexual desire and decreased sexual frequency as a result of pain.

Surgical removal of as many implants as practical often relieves symptoms and sometimes aids fertility. But the condition may recur, and women should be periodically checked.

Hysterectomy may be recommended for women with adenomyosis who have incapacitating symptoms or who have other gynecologic disease at the same time.

Removal of ovarian function by surgery or radiation often causes implants to shrink. Frequently women who become pregnant find that endometriosis symptoms are relieved.

Hormonal therapy—such as the use of a combination of norethindrone and mestranol—given daily for up to 9-12 months often relieves symptoms. Danazol (Danocrine) is a relatively new drug for the treatment of endometriosis. Because of many potential side effects, this drug should not be used without a definitive diagnosis of endometriosis made by laparoscopy.

In some women, the effects of the drugs persist for many months after withdrawal of therapy; in others, however, the implants quickly become active again. Endometriosis is often relieved with the onset of menopause.

See also HYSTERECTOMY; INFERTILITY; INTERCOURSE, PAINFUL.

ENEMAS are sometimes experienced as sexually pleasurable. Since the rectum is contiguous with the genitals in both sexes, it is not surprising that distention of the rectum may be sexually stimulating for some people.

Often, enemas are self-administered as a masturbatory act. In some cases, the enema is administered by another person. People who take enemas may have discovered their erotic potential while being given enemas as children. The practice in adulthood may be a secretive, "shameful" act—sometimes kept from a spouse for many years.

Use of enemas may be hazardous. The frequent use of enemas can result in enema-dependence: the person becomes unable to have a bowel movement without an enema. Improper use of enema equipment can cause rectal injury. Enemas may induce cramps and bowel spasms.

It is unwise to give children enemas for constipation. Not only is the practice medically unsound, but it can cause psychological problems as well.

Most children feel that the enema-giving mother attacks them and forces them into submission. When mothers give their sons enemas, any sexual excitation the boys feel may stir up uncomfortable incestuous feelings.

Occasionally, children may require enemas—before surgery or X ray, for example. They should be well prepared for the experience, told what the procedure will involve, what it will feel like, and just how long it will last.

See also ANAL SEX; MASTURBATION.

EPIDIDYMIS. See MALE SEXUAL ANATOMY.

EPIDIDYMO-ORCHITIS is inflammation of the testicles and the epididymis, an oblong organ attached to the testicles. Its slang term is "blue balls."

Blood vessel congestion from ungratified sexual excitement—such as petting without ejaculating—causes an ache in the testicles.

Teenagers are especially susceptible to it because of their dating patterns and because they are at a stage of heightened physical responsiveness.

Some boys fear they will suffer permanent damage. In fact, the condition is self-limiting. If intercourse does not take place, a boy often masturbates to bring relief.

Repeated episodes of sexual arousal without ejaculation may lead to a condition called congestive prostatitis (also called prostatosis or pelvic congestion syndrome). It is marked by an ache between the anus and the genitals, low-back pain, pelvic pressure, and frequent painful urination. There may be a clear discharge and bloody ejaculation. Rectal examination reveals a tender prostate. If prolonged, congestive prostatitis may produce partial obstruction of the bladder and bacterial prostatitis.

The condition often affects men who go through feast-or-famine sexual cycles: the prostate increases its secretion of prostatic fluid to meet higher demands, then becomes congested on sudden cessation of sexual activity.

The best treatment is ejaculation—by any form of sexual activity acceptable to the man. Prostatic massage is a poor and needlessly expensive substitute. Additional relief may be provided by sitz baths, and by avoiding coffee, alcohol, and spicy foods.

Bacterial infection should be ruled out by a physician.

See also AGING; MASTURBATION; PELVIC CONGESTION; PROSTATITIS.

EPILEPSY, a chronic disease of the central nervous system, is characterized by abnormal brain activity that may result in seizures (convulsions). These are often associated with altered consciousness or total loss of consciousness.

The disorder often begins early in life and commonly has no determined cause. Heredity is thought to play an important role. Epilepsy can also result from head injury, tumors, strokes, or other causes.

While epilepsy is not curable, the seizures can usually be controlled by lifelong drug therapy.

Epilepsy has for centuries been associated with sexual myths. In the middle ages, the disorder was thought to be caused by sexual excess. Masturbation was believed both to cause epilepsy and to result from it. Even as late as the turn of the century, castration and circumcision were often recommended to cure epilepsy presumed due to masturbation. Needless to say, this is all nonsense.

Some epileptics, advised by their physicians that any type of excitement can trigger a seizure and that they should avoid all emotional extremes, are fearful that sexual excitement or orgasm can bring on an attack. They can be reassured that it's extremely rare for sexual activity to precipitate seizures.

The sexual functioning of most epileptics is unaffected by their disorder. Reduced sexual desire seems to be the most widespread sexual effect of epilepsy. It may be a physiological feature of the disorder. It also may result from feelings—common among patients with epilepsy—of inferiority, social stigmatization, and anxiety and helplessness over their condition.

The reduction in seizure frequency that effective therapy provides may, in itself, increase sexual drive. On the other hand, the sedative side effects of such anticonvulsants as phenytoin (Dilantin) and phenobarbital may lower libido and interfere with the normal reflexes of sexual response.

Phenytoin may also cause excessive hair growth and overgrowth of gum tissue, which can lead to feelings of unattractiveness. The dosage of these drugs needs to be carefully regulated by a physician, with sexual and other side effects in mind.

EPISIOTOMY. See POSTPARTUM PROBLEMS.

ERECTILE DYSFUNCTION. See IMPOTENCE.

ERECTION. See IMPOTENCE; ORGASM.

EROSION OF THE CERVIX. See CERVICAL EROSION.

ESTROGEN. See HORMONE DISORDERS.

EUNUCHOIDISM. See TESTICLE REMOVAL.

EXERCISES, SEXUAL. Improved physical fitness is likely to result in enhanced sexual functioning and enjoyment.

For the best physical conditioning, an exercise regimen should combine:

• *Heart and lung fitness.* Increased heart-lung capacity may help protect against heart attack. What's more, the improved conditioning and breathing that result from heart-lung exercise often heighten sexual pleasure. Heart-lung training requires vigorous, sustained exercise at least 5 times a week. This can be accomplished by jogging, swimming, fast walking, jumping rope, etc.

• *Endurance.* Such exercises improve muscle strength and stamina. Pushups and swimming, for example, strengthen arm muscles. Walking and jogging strengthen leg muscles. Sit-ups tone back and abdomen muscles.

• *Flexibility.* Suppleness is important in lovemaking. Greater freedom of movement and pliability mean a greater range of intercourse positions are possible. Any stretching, bending, twisting, or range-of-motion exercises will improve flexibility. These include side bends and trunk bends, arm and leg swinging, toe touching, and back bends.

In addition to overall body conditioning, some groups of muscles are more directly involved in sexual activity. Sexual enjoyment may be enhanced by the following:

● *Buttocks and sphincter exercise.* At least 30 times a day the buttocks and sphincter muscles between the anus and the genitals are held for at least 5 seconds. These contractions can be done anytime, anywhere, in any position.

● *Stomach muscle exercises.* A simple exercise that can be done throughout the day in the course of other activities: Tighten stomach muscles, breathing normally. Hold for a count of 5. A more vigorous exercise involves lying on the back and raising legs slowly toward the ceiling, one at a time, then lowering them slowly. Next, raise both legs together and lower to a count of 20.

● *Pelvic exercises.* Gaining control of the pelvic area aids in sexual control. The basic pelvic exercise is standing erect with feet together and heels, buttocks, and back of head pressed against the wall. Pull in stomach, tilt pelvis forward and upward, trying to press the small of the back against the wall. Hold for 5 seconds, then reverse action, hollowing small of back and sliding buttocks up the wall as high as possible. Hold for 5 seconds. Then alternate, first thrusting pelvis forward, then backward, striving for the greatest possible range of motion. The same exercise can be performed with feet spread apart. If the exercise is done in a half-squat with feet apart, thigh muscles will also be strengthened.

● *Thigh exercises.* A simple exercise is sitting on the edge of a chair with an inflated ball between the knees. Squeeze knees together as hard as possible. Hold for 7 seconds, then relax and repeat 4 or 5 times.

Stand with feet about 10 inches apart. Pivoting on heels, force toes inward toward each other as far as they will go. Then force them outward, away from each other, as far as possible. Continue this thigh-rotating action 4 or 5 times. Rest briefly, then do the exercise 4 or 5 times again. Gradually add more repetitions.

See also VAGINAL EXERCISE.

EXHIBITIONISM is the deliberate exposure of the genitals in inappropriate settings. Exhibitionists are almost invariably males.

The typical exhibitionist is an otherwise responsible citizen: employed or in school, often married and a father, with an above-average education. He generally is passive and rigidly conventional. He is likely to be guilt-ridden over sex, suffering such problems as impotence and premature ejaculation. Often he is too frightened of women to make overtures to them in the normal way.

Even though the exhibitionist may have an erection and may be masturbating, his motivation is primarily nonsexual—typically an expression of anger stifled since childhood. He perceives his bodily sensations of rage as sexual urges; so in response to a situation he finds frustrating or provoking, he may have a compulsion to expose his penis rather than directly express his hostility. What he seeks is an expression of shock or fear—or admiration that reassures him of his masculinity.

The exhibitionist who admits to his condition generally has an excellent prognosis in psychotherapy. Once he understands the relationship between his act of exposure and his feelings of anger, he can usually be taught better ways of expressing his hostility. His impulse to expose himself may remain, but he will typically learn to control it.

A person who encounters an exhibitionist should pointedly ignore him. A small minority of men who expose themselves are potentially violent, so it is wise to do nothing that could be interpreted as humiliating. An exposer who makes threatening gestures or shouts obscenities should be avoided.

FAINTING with sexual excitement or after orgasm is an uncommon response. People who experience loss of consciousness associated with sex should have cardiovascular and neurological disorders ruled out.

Fainting in some may be due to the physical exertion of sexual activity. People who experience fainting after other physical exercise may have the same reaction after sexual exertion. Chronic or acute illness may account for the fatigue.

Fainting associated with sex may be due to emotional stress. The common faint is characterized by pallor, sweating, fast breathing, a drop in blood pressure, and loss of consciousness.

Some people may perceive the sense of loss of control preceding orgasm as fainting.

FALLOPIAN TUBES. See FEMALE SEXUAL ANATOMY.

FELLATIO. See ORAL SEX.

FEMALE SEXUAL ANATOMY. The female external genitals are collectively called the *vulva* and consist of the pubis, the labia majora, the labia minora, and the clitoris.

The *pubis* (or mons pubis or mons veneris) is a mound directly in front of the pubic bone; it is covered with pubic hair.

The *labia majora* (or large lips, or outer lips) are folds of skin that cover the labia minora, the vaginal opening, and the urethra, the tube through which urine is discharged.

The labia majora are covered with pubic hair on the outside and have sweat glands on the inside. During sexual excitement, the labia majora separate and flatten.

The *labia minora* (or small lips, or inner lips) are folds of skin within the labia majora. They possess many blood vessels, sweat and oil glands, and nerve endings. During sexual excitement, they turn from pink to bright red.

The *clitoris*, located at the point where the labia majora meet, just below the pubis, is a small knob of tissue richly endowed with nerve endings. Its only known function is as a source of sexual pleasure (see CLITORAL PROBLEMS).

A woman's internal sexual organs consist of the vagina, the uterus, two ovaries, and two Fallopian tubes.

The *vagina* is capable of considerable expansion in both length and width. It can accommodate penises of greatly varying sizes during sexual intercourse and expands enormously to allow the passage of the baby during childbirth.

In the sexually unstimulated state, the walls of the vagina are collapsed, touching each other. The vaginal walls are lined with a mucous surface that enables vaginal lubrication to pass through during sexual arousal.

The *uterus*, or womb, is a hollow pear-shaped muscular organ about 3 inches long. The *cervix*, the opening to the uterus, protrudes into the vagina.

The uterus is located in the pelvic cavity between the bladder (the sac

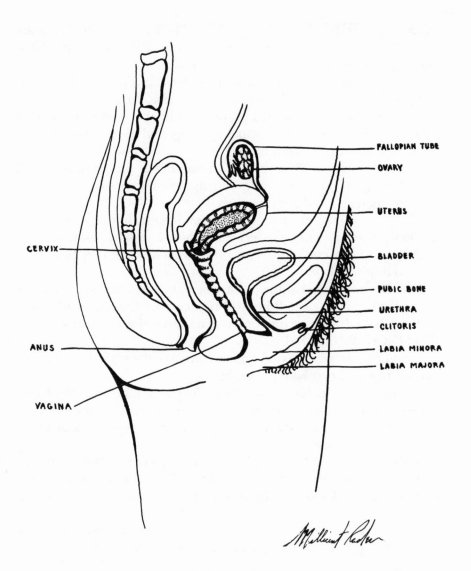

FALLOPIAN TUBE

OVARY

UTERUS

BLADDER

CERVIX

PUBIC BONE

URETHRA

CLITORIS

LABIA MINORA

ANUS

LABIA MAJORA

VAGINA

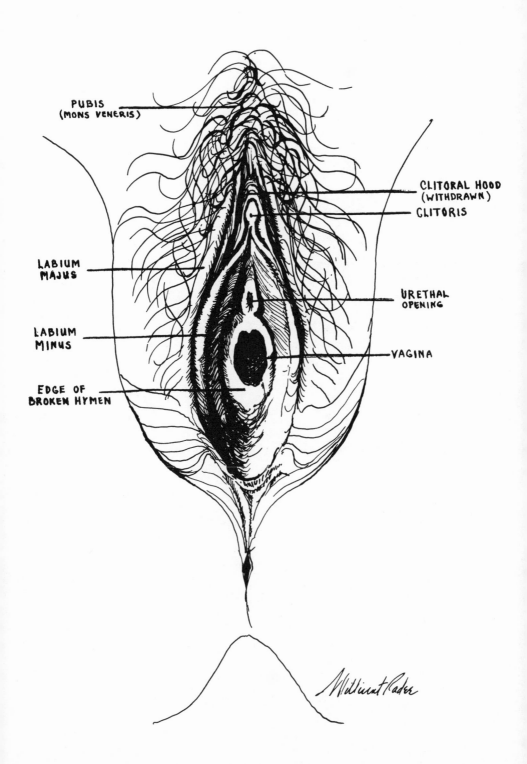

PUBIS
(MONS VENERIS)

CLITORAL HOOD
(WITHDRAWN)

CLITORIS

LABIUM
MAJUS

URETHAL
OPENING

LABIUM
MINUS

VAGINA

EDGE OF
BROKEN HYMEN

Millicent Rader

that holds urine) and the rectum (the lowest portion of the large intestine). It is the site for implantation of the fertilized egg and is capable of enormous expansion to accommodate the growing fetus.

The *two ovaries* are almond-shaped organs about 1 inch long. At birth, the ovaries contain a lifetime's supply of immature ova (eggs). At puberty, these eggs begin to ripen, and one is discharged each month during the reproductive years. If unfertilized, the egg is expelled during menstruation (see entry).

The *two Fallopian tubes* (or oviducts) originate at the uterus and open near the ovaries. The Fallopian tube is the usual site of fertilization of the egg by a sperm. The motion of the tube propels the fertilized egg into the uterus.

See also MALE SEXUAL ANATOMY; ORGASM.

FEMININE HYGIENE. See VAGINAL ODOR.

FERTILITY. See INFERTILITY; PREGNANCY.

FETISHISM is the attachment to an object (or sometimes to a part of the body) that is charged with special erotic interest.

The object (such as gloves, hair, shoes) becomes the primary source of sexual satisfaction. It may be used during masturbation. Or it may be incorporated into sexual activity with another person in order to produce sexual arousal.

For some fetishists, the object must be touched for the person to become sexually aroused and reach orgasm. For others, the object can be fantasized to produce the same effect. Some fetishists can become aroused and reach orgasm without the object—real or imagined; but the experience is considerably less intense.

The fetishist often has a collection of the particular type of object he or she requires to become sexually excited—spike-heeled shoes, for example, or rubber gloves. In some cases, the object has an association with early masturbatory experiences. Sometimes, it belonged to a particular person. The object starts out by representing and substituting for the person; in time, it becomes more important than the person, preferred as a source of sexual pleasure.

Fetishism requires no corrective therapy unless it causes the person concern.

FLASHING. See EXHIBITIONISM.

FOAM. See SPERMICIDES.

FOREPLAY is the sexual stimulation that takes place before intromission, the insertion of the penis into the vagina.

Couples often wonder how much foreplay is normal or adequate. The answer is, enough so that intromission is a pleasure, which usually means that both partners are sexually stimulated and the woman is adequately lubricated.

This varies from couple to couple and from occasion to occasion. There is no fixed amount of time for foreplay. The trick is to do whatever feels good for however long it is fun, treating lovemaking as a continuous episode of shared enjoyment.

"Foreplay" is therefore a misnomer. It implies that noncoital stages of lovemaking are but preliminaries building up to penetration, supposedly the main event. In fact, for women especially, sex play is often more productive of orgasm than is penile-vaginal thrusting. Indeed, containing the penis in the vagina may be merely one step in helping the woman become aroused and reach orgasm.

By the same token, afterplay, the fondling that may occur after intercourse, is also a misnomer. Like foreplay, it is best seen as part of the continuous process of lovemaking.

FREQUENCY. If sex partners are in general agreement about their frequency of intercourse—whether it is once a day or once a year—there is no cause for concern.

At one time or another, almost every couple differ over how often they should have sex. Couples are unlikely to share identical levels of sexual desire, just as they are not likely to respond in exactly the same manner to hunger, thirst, fatigue, joy, or frustration.

The imbalance is rarely crucial. Partners can usually adjust to each other's needs. Generally, partners are available to each other even if sometimes their interest is not strong.

Conflicts may develop if one partner wants sex significantly more than the other. Traditionally, it has been the husband who wants intercourse more frequently than his wife. He determines the minimum frequency, she the maximum.

Why do many happily married women want sex less often than their husbands? It may be because most men tend to rush foreplay, proceeding to intercourse too quickly. This leaves the wife too unstimulated to be within reach of orgasm.

Further, many men ejaculate within two minutes of insertion, and then terminate their lovemaking. As a result, many women become sexually excited but fail to achieve orgasm or to feel satisfied during or after intercourse. Recurrent dissatisfaction leads to less sexual interest for the woman.

This rarely occurs on a conscious level, so a husband is unlikely to realize that he contributes to the diminished frequency. The wife, too, may be aware only of wanting sex less. If she frequently finds herself excited but is left frustrated, then decline in level of desire becomes a defense.

To avoid frustration, a woman unconsciously avoids becoming sexually excited—which she may attribute to being too tired, too busy, etc. Her husband may resent her for being "cold" and "unresponsive."

Conversely, if the wife finds intercourse a pleasurable experience, frequency is likely to be satisfactory for both partners. One barometer of a couple's frequency is how the woman feels about her own sexuality. Is she comfortable in the nude? Does she communicate her sexual needs? The more positive her attitude, the more often she's likely to make love.

Family physicians are reporting more and more women complaining about insufficient frequency. Formerly, wives complained chiefly about lack of affection. This change is widely attributed to women's increasing awareness of their rights to sexual satisfaction. Now when wives are dissatisfied with the frequency of intercourse they are more likely than husbands to seek help.

Remaining sexually active develops the capacity for continued sexual expression in later life. It improves the functioning of the prostate gland. Intercourse is never physically harmful as long as it occurs between accepting partners and is not associated with injury or irritation.

Even so, it is important to keep sex in its proper perspective. The average married couple spends the equivalent in hours of one weekend a year having sexual intercourse. Therefore, it is unrealistic to suggest that sex is the major force sustaining the relationship. Many happily-married couples have what sex therapists consider serious sexual dysfunctions, such as potency problems or inability to reach orgasm.

Resolving conflicts. In any intimate relationship the key issue is not frequency of intercourse but the dovetailing of needs. Here are some suggestions to help a couple find a frequency suited to them both:

Communicate. It is important for partners to tell each other their needs and wishes. It is especially important for them to express their preferences if they avoid sex because they are chronically unsatisfied.

Partners may each be surprised at how the other perceives their sex life. In one study of couples married about 10 years, the typical wife reported having intercourse an average of some 8 times a month. This frequency matched her own desire. She estimated that her husband's preference would be 11 times a month, considerably more than her own.

The typical husband reported he had intercourse 7 times a month, about one time less than his wife's report. He estimated his wife would prefer some 6 times a month, less than she actually would. His own preference would be 9, less than she believed he wanted.

The couple can explore the desirability of alternate forms of sexual release. If they have a great disparity in sex drive, they can consider types of sexual activity besides intercourse, such as masturbation and oral sex. If a man has difficulty sustaining an erection, he can nevertheless give his partner considerable sexual pleasure by engaging in breast stroking, and clitoral and vaginal stimulation.

The couple can explore areas of marital discord. If a marriage is going through a bumpy period, there's likely to be less sex. Sexual interest may be restored if lingering resentment, anger, guilt, and frustration are resolved.

In a frank discussion, they may uncover conflicts arising from early sexual training. Many people are trained and educated during their developmental years to view sex as something evil, bad, and dirty. This may be the cause of impaired or late development of the usual or normal sexual feelings. This later may decrease frequency of sexual relations.

The same effect can be caused by being brought up in a home with too much permissiveness. In such homes, young people may have intercourse before they are ready or with partners who exploit them. These bad experiences can sour them on sex.

A couple can share concern over situations causing them anxiety. Job worries, financial problems, serious problems with a child—all can contribute to a decrease in sexual relations. So can lack of bedroom privacy, with the anxiety that small children may overhear or witness lovemaking.

Underlying marital discord or psychological problems that account for sexual disinterest may respond to professional therapy, either for one partner or for the couple.

Competent sex therapy may help alleviate the problem if avoidance of intercourse is the result of sexual dysfunction. Premature ejaculation, impotence, difficulty in achieving orgasm—all can lead to feelings of humiliation and anxiety over performance. A couple may prefer to avoid sex altogether rather than risk failure.

Schedule time for sex. Some couples have such cluttered, exhausting lives that a good sex life is a virtual impossibility. There is little opportunity or energy for sex when both partners are chronically overworked and preoccupied.

Therefore, it is important for a couple to set aside uninterrupted hours for making love. They can make an appointment, free of outside commitments and household worries, and work to improve the quality of such occasions. One good sexual experience a week can be more satisfying than three disappointing ones. When the quality of sex rises, the quantity usually will also. By contrast, boredom and routine are major reasons for sexual activity tapering off.

On which days of the week is intercourse most frequent? In a University of North Carolina Medical School study, married, middle-class women reported having intercourse most often on Sunday, with Saturday the next highest day. Unmarried women reported intercourse most often on Sunday, with Wednesday the next most popular day. Married black men reported the greatest sexual activity on Tuesday, with another peak on Friday or Saturday.

In temperate climates, birth statistics suggest that intercourse is most frequent in summer. In tropical climates it occurs most often in the cool season. In places where summers are very hot and winters very cold, intercourse rates are highest in spring and fall.

Check for physical causes. A thorough examination by a doctor can rule out physical problems that may be responsible for a lowered sex drive.

Aging may cause a natural decline troubling to a man. In general, men reach a peak of sexual feelings in early adulthood, with a gradual falling off thereafter. A man's rate often increases once he is convinced that he can enjoy a high level of sexual activity well into old age.

Women generally reach a peak in their 30s. Their sexual interest then remains relatively stable into the 60s or beyond.

Reliable birth control can help alleviate fear of pregnancy, which may be causing lowered sexual interest.

Improved personal hygiene can result in greater sexual frequency. Body or breath odors that are undesirable or offensive decrease desire and thus sexual frequency. The couple can shower together and apply fragrances and oils to each other.

Forget yardsticks. Couples are advised to have intercourse no more or less often than is comfortable for them, without trying to meet statistical "norms." Kinsey found the average frequency of marital intercourse to be 3.9 times a week for husbands under 20, ranging down to 1.3 times a week for husbands between 51 and 55. But the couples Kinsey interviewed had intercourse varying from "25 times a week" to "hardly ever."

Ebbs and flows are inevitable. A couple's sexual frequency may fall off drastically or virtually cease for weeks or months at a time. A study of husbands and wives, most below the age of 40 and married for an average of 11 years, showed that fully one-third experienced long periods with no sex. For half, sexual activity had ceased for periods of eight weeks or more.

By contrast, couples can find themselves having intercourse more frequently than either really would like. When people engage in intercourse more often than desired, the problem may be unrealistic goals, myths, or one partner's need to prove sexual attractiveness.

Some couples may be pushing their frequency in an effort to achieve the unrealistic goal of simultaneous orgasm. So may a woman who feels that having multiple orgasms is the greatest sign of female sexual achievement.

The same may be true of a man who strains at having intercourse several times a night to demonstrate his masculinity. Multiple ejaculations for a man are relatively rare.

Such pressure to achieve can produce greater frequency—but less enjoyment. In any event, it is wise to be dubious about reports of very high sexual track records. Claims of extreme sexual potency are often wishful thinking.

The best documented high-scorers? Dr. Wardell B. Pomeroy who worked with Kinsey at the Institute for Sex Research at the University of Indiana, reports that the highest rate of ejaculation among 10,000 males was about 6 times per day every day over a period of several years. "For short periods of time," he reports, "the rate would be higher." It is not unusual for adolescent males to report masturbating to orgasm 10 to 15 times a day.

But such sexual marathoners are not necessarily to be envied. Some males who had very frequent orgasms were "compulsive and actually derived very little pleasure from their sexual activity," reports Dr. Pomeroy. "We feel that some high-rating males were so constituted physiologically that a failure to ejaculate at least once a day would leave them tense, nervous, and very uneasy."

Dr. Martin L. Kurland of the Palm Springs Mental Health Clinic in California came across a 41-year-old married man who kept a "sexual track record."

He normally had intercourse four or five times daily, sometimes more. During one 24-hour period he had 17 orgasms, all during intercourse with the same woman. He had had sexual experiences with 377 women.

He came to Dr. Kurland because he was afraid he was "going queer." Lately he was down to having intercourse only once or twice a day.

See also SEX THERAPY; SEXUAL DYSFUNCTION.

"FRIGIDITY" commonly refers to a chronic problem in which the female is unable to respond to any form of sexual stimulation. This is usually accompanied by her inability to reach orgasm. Applied to an individual woman, the preferred term is "nonorgasmic"—or, more optimistically, "*pre*orgasmic." The word "frigid" is avoided as much as possible because of its many negative connotations.

Difficulty in achieving orgasm may be due to physical causes. Among the many medical conditions that may account for the problem are diabetes, spinal cord injuries, alcoholism, multiple sclerosis, and endocrine disorders.

Physiological problems should be ruled out before a woman seeks psychotherapy or sex therapy for orgasmic dysfunction.

Often a woman's inability to respond sexually is due to ignorance about sex or to feelings of guilt and shame inflicted on her in early life. Lack of communication between sex partners is often a major factor in this sexual dysfunction.

General anxiety or hostility toward the sex partner can keep a woman from achieving an orgasm. Sex researchers Dr. William H. Masters and Virginia E. Johnson include distractions, fatigue, and preoccupation with other matters as basic barriers to satisfying sexual experience. Failure to have an orgasm is sometimes due to a woman's fear of letting go or losing control.

Difficulty in reaching orgasm can often be cured through sex reeducation. Some women are able to reach an orgasm for the first time after receiving a simple explanation of female sexual physiology and basic sex instruction.

Many women never achieve an orgasm during penetration but can be brought to climax by stimulation of the clitoris.

Experimenting with different types of touch in a creative, curious manner will enable a woman to develop confidence in herself. Oral sex may bring a woman to orgasm where vaginal intercourse does not.

Women who have found it difficult or impossible to have an orgasm may discover how their bodies work through self-exploration. Dr. Mary S. Calderone, executive director of the Sex Information and Education Council of the United States, advised: "You, yourself, must reawaken your body, rediscover it, reeducate it . . . find out for yourself how it feels to touch yourself in certain places. Find out which places arouse the most pleasure in you when touched. Communicate these discoveries to your husband."

Here are recommendations derived from Masters and Johnson's sexual therapy program. They require the cooperation of a warm, supportive partner:

1. *"Pleasuring"* (or "sensate focus") promotes a loving relationship while freeing a couple from the pressure of performance.

Pleasuring is designed to help a couple communicate and express affection through touching—but at the same time relieve them of the pressure to proceed to sexual intercourse. The goal is to overcome problems and help establish an enduring, mutually satisfying sexual relationship through improved communication.

To engage in pleasuring, the woman and her partner agree to refrain from intercourse deliberately. Instead, for at least 4 days, they set aside an hour or more for love *play*, indulging themselves in the sensation of touching and being touched.

Touching is an important source of sexual stimulation. To express sexual feeling fully, couples must be able to communicate through touching. Touch can convey many emotions: tenderness, affection, comfort, desire, etc.

The couple should communicate in words or gestures what they find pleasurable. They can kiss, stroke, massage, pat each other—but should avoid the breasts and genitals.

Many couples experience a new warmth and closeness through pleasuring.

Even if the man develops an erection they should *not* attempt intercourse. Some couples may feel that it's a shame to let a good erection go to waste, but, among couples who are sexually dysfunctional, attempting intercourse prematurely can result in failure and worsen the problem. A good erection can in itself be pleasurable, both for the man and his partner. Not every erection has to lead to intercourse. By the same token, every time a woman experiences vaginal lubrication, she need not necessarily proceed to sexual intercourse.

2. *Genital play.* On the fourth and fifth days of pleasuring, the woman puts her hand over the man's while he is pleasuring her, and shows him just what she likes by indicating pressure or change of direction. He'll do the same when he is being touched. On or about this session too, they may extend their touching to each other's genitals and other sexually arousing areas. But they do not demand a sexual response from each other, and they make no effort to achieve orgasm.

One good position for a woman to learn what genital play stimulates her is as follows: The man sits at the head of the bed, propped up against pillows. The woman sits leaning against his chest, her head resting against his shoulder:

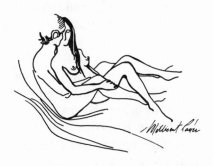

The man should *not* try to second-guess the woman's desires or stimulate her using his choice of approach. In short, he should *not* try

103

to be an "expert at technique" (a common myth of supposed masculinity). The goal for them both is to discover what the woman's actual preferences are, and put them into effect.

Masters and Johnson say the biggest mistake most men make is to manipulate the head of the clitoris as soon as sex play is begun. This can break a woman's individual pattern of sexual responsiveness. The head of the clitoris is extremely sensitive to touch, and direct manipulation can be irritating or painful. Many women may prefer the gentle stroking of the clitora shaft (sides).

Unlike the vagina, the clitoris secretes no lubricant and may be irritated by dry touching. It may help to lubricate it with vaginal fluid, saliva, or a water-soluble jelly or cream like K-Y.

Few women find deep penetration of the vagina with fingers to be sexually stimulating, since the innermost part of the vagina has relatively few nerve endings.

A woman cannot force an orgasm. Orgasm happens spontaneously when a particular woman at a particular time accumulates her maximum amount of sexual stimuli.

In no way should the woman feel pressured to reach orgasm. Nor should she feel disappointed if she fails to reach a climax at this or other sessions. On the contrary she should recognize that nothing is demanded of her, that she has complete freedom to express herself, and that she will soon have another chance.

3. *Insertion.* After the woman has reached satisfaction with genital play, she can go on to the next step: the man lies on his back. She sits astride his thighs facing him. *She inserts his penis.* She holds herself still—and appreciates how the feelings in her vaginal tissue are pleasurable in themselves, without any demand to reach orgasm.

As she wants more stimulation she can move slowly back and forth on the penis. It is helpful for her to think of the penis as hers to play with, to feel and enjoy. It may take a few sessions to develop vaginal feeling.

4. *Thrusting.* Only after the woman develops vaginal feeling should the man thrust his hips in intercourse. At first the thrusting should be slow, with no extra effort to bring about climax.

She should let him know the pace she prefers, by speaking or moving. Helping to regulate his thrusting helps the woman to experience what is happening—a needed change from a habit of merely trying to accommodate to his preferences.

5. *Lateral Coital Position.* The couple can convert from a sitting-astride position to a lateral coital position:

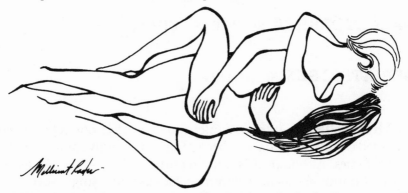

To get into it, the man rests one leg against the bed. The women lies on the inner side of that thigh, straddling his other leg. For traction both of their knees can touch the bed.

Many couples who learn this position prefer it to all others. It allows freedom of movement, ejaculatory control, and excellent opportunity to communicate the desired speed of thrusting.

An electric vibrator can often induce orgasm. The continuous, rhythmic stimulation may be particularly helpful for women who have never experienced orgasm.

However, a nonorgasmic woman had best use a vibrator only as a last resort. Some sex therapists feel that a vibrator can condition a woman to expect the same degree of stimulation with a partner that she receives from her untiring, obliging vibrator.

Once the woman has learned that she is capable of experiencing orgasm, a vibrator can be an enjoyable, useful toy. Vaginal exercises may also aid some women in becoming orgasmic.

Erotic literature or fantasy may also be helpful. Psychologist Albert Ellis advises women who have difficulty in becoming sexually aroused or reaching a climax to "focus, and keep focusing, on something sexually exciting whatever that may be . . . anything, as long as it gets you more interested in your current relations."

Psychotherapy is successful in curing many cases of sexual dysfunction, especially when the woman's inability to have an orgasm results from deep-seated personal problems or hostility toward her sex partner or all males.

See also SEX THERAPY; VAGINAL EXERCISE.

FUNGUS. See YEAST INFECTION.

GALACTORRHEA. See BREAST DISCHARGE.

GERIATRIC SEX. See AGING.

GIARDIASIS is an intestinal infection caused by a one-celled protozoa called *Giardia lamblia*. It is becoming increasingly common in the United States. Although it is not a reportable disease, the Center for Disease Control has identified over 12,000 cases in a single year.

Giardiasis is transmitted through exposure to contaminated feces. This may be by hand-to-mouth contact; by drinking contaminated water; or by eating raw fruits and vegetables exposed to infected feces.

The infection can also be transmitted sexually through anolingual contact or when oral-penile contact follows anal intercourse.

The most common symptom of giardiasis is a watery foul-smelling diarrhea. Others include abdominal pain, loss of appetite, weight loss, nausea, and weakness.

Treatment is usually with the drug quinacrine HCl (Atabrine) for 5 days. Side effects may include dizziness, headache, vomiting, and a yellow tinge to the skin. The extreme bitterness of this drug can be ameliorated by crushing the tablet and mixing it with applesauce. Alternative treatment is with the drug Flagyl.

See also ANAL SEX.

GONADOTROPHIN. See HORMONE DISORDERS.

GONORRHEA ("clap," "dose," "gleet," "strain") is spread almost exclusively through intimate sexual contact. Gonococcus bacteria thrive in the moist, warm mucous membranes that line body openings such as the penis, vagina, and rectum. The gonococci cannot survive long after exposure to air. There is little chance of contracting the disease from public toilets, towels, doorknobs, or other contaminated objects.

If there is any chance that a sex partner has gonorrhea, using a condom can reduce the risk of contracting it. Washing genitals with soap and water both before and after sexual intercourse is also prudent. For a man, urinating directly after intercourse may help ward off infection.

Gonorrhea is epidemic—an estimated 2½ million Americans are infected for the first time each year, making it the most common reportable disease. Among teenagers and young adults, the rate of infection is estimated to range as high as 7 percent.

Contrary to widespread belief, birth control pills do not protect against gonorrhea. Nor does circumcision. Neither does a previous infection confer immunity—a person can get the disease over and over again with every exposure.

Anyone with a suspicion of gonorrhea should go to a doctor or a clinic immediately. Most local health departments have VD clinics that provide free or inexpensive diagnosis and treatment. Many clinics will treat minors without their parents' consent.

Those who have sexual contact with more than one person should have gonorrhea cultures taken routinely. Unmarried women and male homosexuals have the greatest risk of carrying the infection without realizing it.

Grave complications. There is a widespread myth that gonorrhea is a mild disease. Actually, if untreated, gonorrhea can cause severe permanent damage and may be life-threatening. Gonococci usually remain in the genital and urinary tracts, later attacking the internal reproductive organs.

In a woman, gonococci may cause pelvic inflammatory disease (PID), often with fever, abdominal pain, and tenderness. The linings of the Fallopian tubes may become mutilated, blocking the passages through which an egg must pass to be fertilized. About 25 percent of women with gonorrhea eventually need a hysterectomy to arrest the disease.

In a man, gonorrhea can cause sterility by blocking the tubes through which sperm must pass. Further, gonococci may migrate to the prostate and testicles.

When gonorrhea affects the prostate gland, a man's ejaculation may be premature, bloody, or painful. Gonorrheal infection has been implicated as a contributor to the development of cancer of the prostate gland.

GONORRHEA

If gonococci attack a man's urethra (the urinary passage from the bladder through the penis) a permanent narrowing known as urethral stricture may result. The urethra is sealed off by scar tissue, making urination at first difficult and then impossible. Pressure resulting from the buildup of urine in the bladder causes extreme pain. In ongoing, untreated cases, this could lead to kidney failure and death.

Relief is obtained by having the urethra periodically stretched, allowing the passage of urine. For this procedure, anesthetic jelly is applied to a smooth metal instrument called a sound, which is then inserted into the urethra. The physician inserts progressively wider sounds, until the urethra is sufficiently dilated.

Gonorrheal conjunctivitis, a common eye problem of infected infants, can also affect adults. There is a pus-laden dischage from the eye, with red and puffy eyelids. Have such a condition treated immediately—it can cause permanent eye damage within a single day.

Gonococci may invade the bloodstream, causing a systemic infection known as disseminated gonorrhea. Its symptoms are usually fever, malaise, and aches and pains in the joints. There may be skin lesions, mostly on arms and legs. Victims may develop gonococcal arthritis. Knees, wrists, and ankles are most often involved. After a few days, the pain may localize in one joint, with some swelling. Prompt diagnosis and treatment are necessary, since joints can be rapidly damaged by the gonococci.

Symptoms of disseminated gonorrhea usually occur 5 to 7 days after sexual contact, but sometimes not until 2 or 3 weeks later. The condition may mimic other diseases, such as allergy, infectious hepatitis, and systemic lupus erythematosus.

Gonorrhea can develop into endocarditis, an inflammation of the inner lining of the heart. Valves may be affected and may require surgical replacement. If untreated, endocarditis may result in congestive heart failure and stroke.

Gonococci can invade the lining of the brain, leading to meningitis. In the liver, the bacteria can cause hepatitis.

Attacking children. All pregnant women need to be checked for the infection. An infant born to a woman with gonorrhea may contract the infection in the birth canal. The greatest hazard to babies is gonococcal conjunctivitis. Silver nitrate solution is therefore routinely introduced into the eyes of newborns. In babies, gonococci may also cause meningitis and arthritis. The infection has been linked to premature births.

Symptoms may not be noticeable. Men may see the first signs 2 to 10 days after sexual contact with an infected person. There is usually a burning sensation when urinating and a pus-laden discharge from the penis. The man may remain able to spread the disease *for as long as two years* unless he seeks treatment. He remains infectious even though these early symptoms disappear without treatment.

Infected men are usually uncomfortable enough to go to a doctor. But perhaps 1 in 5 men show no symptoms, thus fail to seek treatment. Indeed, asymptomatic gonorrhea in males may be even more common than that.

Most women, on the other hand, have no early symptoms. Those having symptoms usually notice them 7 to 21 days after exposure.

Women with gonorrhea sometimes experience abnormal menstrual bleeding, frequent urination, low fever, rectal discomfort, and light discharge. If ignored, these mild symptoms usually disappear. Thus, estimates the Public Health Service, 9 out of 10 women with gonorrhea do not realize they are infected. Like asymptomatic men, they can nevertheless transmit the disease.

A woman is usually suspected of having the disease only when someone with a diagnosed case names her as a sex partner. It is often weeks or months after first contracting the disease that women experience their first discomfort: pain in the reproductive organs.

The throat may be infected. People who engage in oral sex with an infected partner may acquire pharyngeal gonorrhea: an infection of the pharynx, the region between the mouth and the esophagus.

The disease can be spread from penis to pharynx and from pharynx to penis. The disease can also spread from infected female genitals to the pharynx. There is no case on record of pharyngeal gonorrhea being spread through kissing.

Pharyngeal gonorrhea is seldom seen alone. The victim usually suffers from infected genitals as well. Although some people experience sore throat, pharyngeal gonorrhea is often asymptomatic.

Gonorrhea may infect the rectum. In male homosexuals, rectal infections are common, as they are in women who have multiple partners and who engage in anal intercourse. Some women acquire rectal gonorrhea when their infectious vaginal discharge soils the mucous membrane around the anus, usually during defecation.

Most often, symptoms are mild enough to be ignored, since minor disturbances around the anus are common. Some people suffering from rectal gonorrhea may experience itching, pain, and burning in and around the anus. Sometimes there is bleeding, a creamy pus-laden discharge, and an ineffective urge to produce a bowel movement.

Diagnosis and treatment. The infection is detected by taking a smear of the discharge. The gonococci are identified through cultures and microscopic examination.

It is often very difficult to detect gonorrhea in women, since there may be no discharge or a discharge may not show the presence of gonococci. Making a culture of smears from several different sites (cervix, vagina, urethra, rectum, pharynx) can result in a more accurate diagnosis for women.

The disease can almost always be cured, but organs already damaged cannot be repaired. The usual first treatment is penicillin—taken together with probenecid, a drug that slows body excretion of penicillin. If a person is allergic to penicillin, the drug of choice is tetracycline. Rare strains of gonorrhea, some evidently originating in Southeast Asia, are resistant to the usual treatment. Effective against these infections are such other antibiotics as spectinomycin (Trobicin), cefoxitin (Mefoxin), or trimethoprim-sulfamethoxazole (Bactrim, Septra).

After treatment for gonorrhea, it is wise to get a follow-up check 1 to 2 weeks after completion of treatment. Abatement of symptoms is not sufficient assurance that a gonococcal infection has been eradicated. Even if symptoms were severe, the infection may become silent after treatment. For women, the test should include a rectal as well as a cervical culture.

See also ANAL SEX; PELVIC INFLAMMATORY DISEASE; VENEREAL DISEASE.

GRAFENBERG SPOT. Preliminary research suggests the presence of a female genitourinary structure called the "Grafenberg spot" or "G spot." This focal point for sexual stimulation has been located in several hundred women. Researchers speculate that it may be an erogenous area normally present in virtually all women.

According to findings reported in the *Journal of Sex Research*, the Grafenbery spot is located deep within the upper front wall of the vagina, adjacent to the urethra, about halfway between the pubic bone and the cervix. An oval bean-sized lump, it swells when stimulated. Usually it is stimulated with the partner's fingers, for the spot requires considerable pressure and is difficult for a woman to reach by herself _ when lying down. However, some women report being able to find the spot while seated on the toilet. During intercourse, it is most likely to be stimulated by the penis if the woman is on top.

Evidently, many women can reach orgasm through stimulation of the Grafenberg spot. After an initial feeling of urinary urgency, such women experience an erotic sensation with an orgasm many describe as "deeper" than one attained through clitoral stimulation. This may be the source of the "vaginal orgasm" that was postulated by Freud and others.

About 1 in 10 women apparently ejaculate a milky fluid from the urethra after experiencing orgasm through the Grafenberg spot. Chemical analysis shows this fluid to be different from urine—and to be high in prostatic acid phosphatase, much like the fluid ejaculated by the male. Indeed, the spot is thought to be an analogue in females of the male prostate.

The expelled fluid can vary from a few drops to a few ounces. Many of the women who were found to ejaculate had long suffered embarrassment over "urinating" during orgasm. Some had been diagnosed by physicians as suffering from "stress incontinence." A few had even withdrawn from having orgasms out of fear of releasing this "urine."

See also FEMALE SEXUAL ANATOMY; ORGASM.

HAEMOPHILUS VAGINALIS is a vaginal infection. Caused by a form of rod-shaped bacteria, it is spread primarily by intercourse. It is on the increase mainly because of the rise in adolescent sexual activity.

The organism causes gray, malodorous discharge, occasionally with slight frothiness. A woman may experience mild itching. Treatment usually includes oral ampicillin or tetracycline tablets or suppositories. To avoid an overgrowth of Candida yeast organisms (see YEAST INFECTION) the doctor may prescribe other medications. Nystatin suppositories are advised. Vaginal sulfonamide creams (Sultrin, Vagilia) and suppositories may be less effective but do not cause candidiasis. Furacin cream may also be used.

See also VAGINAL INFECTION.

HAIRINESS. See HIRSUTISM.

HAIR LOSS. See SKIN DISORDERS.

HALLUCINOGENS such as LSD (lysergic acid diethylamide) and mescaline are sometimes lauded as enhancers of sexual activity. Some users report an intensified experience and heightened sensory awareness. Both men and women sometimes report "explosive" orgasm.

On the other hand, in interviews at the Masters and Johnson Institute with 85 men and 55 women who had used LSD on three or more occasions, fewer than 15 percent of each sex claimed that LSD enhanced sexuality. One researcher feels that taking LSD as an aphrodisiac is useless, "because the user can't remain focused on what he started to do."

This variability in sexual response may be attributed to the quality of hallucinogens sold on the street. Often, LSD and mescaline have numerous other drugs and impurities combined with them. Then, too, drug effects are highly variable, differing from person to person and for the same person at different times.

Little scientific research has been done. In male rats, small doses of hallucinogens accelerate sexual behavior, while larger doses completely disrupt sexual behavior.

See also APHRODISIACS.

HEADACHE as an excuse to avoid sex has become a standard joke. In folklore, it is the wife who has the "headache"; in real life it may just as easily be the husband.

Headaches may arise from anxiety, guilt, or tension about sex or from chronic resentment of the partner. Negative emotions about anticipated intercourse can induce physiological reactions, such as contraction of scalp muscles, that may result in a headache as the usual time of intercourse approaches.

Such muscle-contraction headaches may not only result from but also contribute to marital difficulties. When one partner consciously or unconsciously uses a physical symptom to avoid the intimacy of lovemaking, it is almost inevitable that the couple will feel further estranged.

Aggravation of the headache may occur if the sufferer engages in sex despite the headache. Feelings of being used and unloved may add to the level of frustration, anger, and anxiety. If these emotions are not expressed, the muscle tightness may increase, with a heightening of head and neck pains.

Characteristically, muscle-contraction headaches begin with an aching at the nape of the neck or the front part of the head. The pain is usually dull and continuous, sometimes throbbing. It may be accompanied by other psychosomatic problems, such as low-back pain.

The application of heat (compresses or electric pads) and massage will help relieve muscle tightness. Tranquilizers should be used judiciously because of the hazard of drug dependency in patients with chronic tension headaches. Marital counseling or psychotherapy may be useful.

In some people, mounting sexual excitement before orgasm may result in a headache. In straining toward orgasm, they may unconsciously contract the muscles of the head and neck. This type of headache can be prevented or relieved by consciously relaxing those muscles.

People with frequent headaches may avoid sex because of the pain. When the headache is continuous or chronic (very frequent) the sufferer may be feeling ill much of the time. Such chronic or continuous headache is often associated with emotional tension.

People who suffer from frequent disabling migraine (sick headache) may likewise avoid sex because they are often in great pain. Migraine is a severe, throbbing, usually one-sided headache that begins slowly and may last for hours or days. Some sufferers experience flashes of light, numbness, and partial, temporary blindness before an attack. Migraines usually appear at regular intervals, more frequently during periods of emotional stress. They are thought to result from a disorder of blood vessels in the head.

In some people, headaches are a symptom of underlying depression (see entry). Such people often experience loss of sexual desire, which is commonly associated with depressive states.

Headache with orgasm occurs in a small number of people. If such headaches occur frequently, or if they become increasingly frequent or severe, a complete neurological examination is in order. The headache could be caused by a blood clot in one of the cerebral blood vessels or by a brain tumor or abscess.

Hypertension may produce a headache at orgasm resulting from physical or emotional excitement, particularly among people with

113

poorly controlled or undetected high blood pressure. The pain may be severe, diffuse, and throbbing and may persist for many hours. Other possible causes of headache at orgasm include diabetes and thyroid disease. A small number of people who suffer such headaches are found to have low spinal fluid pressure. For them quick relief may be obtained by lying on the back.

Migraine is sometimes aggravated by intercourse. At the moment of orgasm, some migraine sufferers experience the classic throbbing associated with localized migraine. Such headaches result from the vasodilation of small arteries in the pain-sensitive portions of the head. If the pain persists, it may be relieved by vasoconstricting drugs. Biofeedback techniques have been useful in controlling migraine in some patients.

Occasionally, angina pectoris may account for headache at orgasm. Sexual intercourse may precipitate angina, which is sometimes manifested by jaw or neck pain. The pain is usually severe and subsides very gradually.

Most orgasmic headaches are benign. No physiological condition can be found to account for the pain. The cause may be excessive excitement or effort during intercourse that may cause blood pressure to rise beyond normal levels. It has also been speculated that hormone-like chemicals called prostaglandins, which are produced in both males and females, may be responsible.

Characteristically, headache at orgasm is extremely severe, persistent, and on both sides of the head. Usually, the headaches last an hour or two, but some sufferers have a dull ache of the scalp or neck for several days. For most people, the pain does not occur after every orgasm.

To help prevent orgasm-induced headache, patients are often advised to avoid alcohol before sexual relations. Alcohol has a tendency to exaggerate enlargement of blood vessels, which may contribute to headache. Drugs such as propranolol and indomethacin have sometimes been used successfully as preventives.

See also BACKACHE; HYPERTENSION.

HEART DISEASE need not be a reason for abstaining from sexual activity. Because sexual intercourse increases heart rate, blood pressure, and breathing, many heart patients withdraw from sex out of fear of bringing on a heart attack. The patient's wife (or husband, or other sex partner) is often the one with this anxiety. Resulting frustration and marital conflicts may worsen the cardiac condition.

Resuming sexual activity depends on how well a heart patient has recovered. Only a physician familiar with a particular patient's condition can give him specific advice. But, to get it, the patient may need to ask. Masters and Johnson found that two-thirds of patients who had suffered a heart attack received no sexual advice at all during their medical treatment. The advice given the remaining third was so vague as to be useless.

In general, following heart attack or heart surgery, a patient should resume less-taxing forms of sexual activity on returning home from the hospital (touching, cuddling, stroking). This gentle activity, without expectation of intercourse, helps relieve anxieties that can result in impotence. It can boost confidence and ease the resumption of intercourse.

A patient can safely go on to masturbation or oral sex as soon as he can tolerate an accelerated heart rate of 130 beats per minute. In an uncomplicated recovery, this usually occurs after four to eight weeks.

Intercourse takes much less effort than is popularly believed. Often heart rate rises more from driving a car than from intercourse. A heart patient can usually resume intercourse when he is able to climb one or two flights of stairs or walk several blocks at a brisk pace. The average patient achieves this at about 16 weeks after a heart attack.

A patient can closely assess how much sexual activity he can tolerate by undergoing a standard series of stress tests followed by electrocardiograms. From the ECGs, a doctor can tell what a patient's maximum heart rate can safely be. He can then estimate if his heart rate during intercourse falls within safe limits.

For an even more precise determination of how sex affects his heart, a patient can get a Hellerstein Sexercise Tolerance Test, using a miniature ECG recorder at home while making love. Such objective measurements can help give a worried patient the confidence to return quickly to his former level of sexual activity. Most doctors will recommend an exercise program to improve general cardiovascular condition. Any increase in such tolerance for exercise can also speed a patient's resumption of sex.

The doctor should be informed of any chest pain that occurs during or after intercourse. Nitroglycerin immediately before making love may be prescribed. Other danger signs should also be reported: palpita-

115

tion that continues for 15 minutes or more after intercourse; sleeplessness caused by sexual exertion; or marked fatigue on the day after intercourse.

For safer sex. At least at first, a heart patient is advised to take it easy during intercourse—to be pleasurable, sex does not have to be athletic. By using restraint, a patient can ordinarily remain within his exercise tolerance.

The best time for intercourse is in the morning after a restful night's sleep. The room should be reasonably cool. Hot humid weather can make intercourse risky. So can unaccustomed high altitudes (above 5,000 feet).

Three positions which lessen cardiac workload are recommended for the heart patient. These are (1) lying on the side, in face-to-face position; (2) lying on the back, with the partner on top; and (3) sitting on a wide chair, low enough for the feet to touch the ground.

A heart patient should refrain from having intercourse for three hours after eating a heavy meal, or drinking alcohol. Food, especially an elaborate dinner, increases the workload on the heart. Alcohol also raises demands on the heart; moreover, even a small amount can dull sexual responsiveness—and so bring about frantic activity.

Sex with a new partner—or with an extramarital partner—can be extremely taxing. A heart patient is likely to be under emotional stress from guilt, unfamiliar surroundings, and anxiety over performing. In addition, such an encounter frequently follows an evening of heavy eating and drinking.

Death during intercourse? Many heart patients fear they will have an attack and die during intercourse. That is very rare, reports cardiologist Herman K. Hellerstein of Case Western Reserve University. Sexual activity was associated with sudden death in only 3 of 500 heart patients he studied.

A heart patient may suffer sexual impediments from loss of self-esteem since such a condition can make him weak and dependent, unable to do productive work. Insomnia, anxiety, and depression often follow. These states may result in sexual dysfunction.

Impotence may follow a heart attack or heart surgery. In most cases, the impotence is of psychological origin—not surprising in view of the enormous physical and psychological stress the victim's been subjected to. A woman's fears about sexual activity may make her inhibited and unresponsive, with difficulties in achieving orgasm.

Sexual problems can be caused by medication. Some drugs used to treat heart disease or hypertension interfere with sexual activity. Impotence is an especially common side effect and often can be remedied by a change of drugs.

Some heart patients unconsciously use their medical condition as an excuse to retire from an active sex life. Professional counseling may be desirable.

See also IMPOTENCE.

HEMATOSPERMIA. See EJACULATION, BLOODY.

HEMODIALYSIS. See KIDNEY DISEASE.

HEMORRHOIDS (piles) are swollen veins in the rectum. They
affect perhaps 1 in 3 Americans.

Common symptoms of hemorrhoids are rectal bleeding, pain, and itching. Sometimes the enlarged veins protrude out of the rectum.

Untreated hemorrhoids can result in severe complications. Anemia may develop from recurrent bleeding. An extremely painful blood clot can form on the hemorrhoids. Infection can develop. The hemorrhoids can rupture and hemorrhage.

For a mild case of hemorrhoids, a physician may recommend soothing creams, suppositories, or ointments. Bathing in warm water 3 or 4 times a day may provide relief.

Medication to shrink blood vessels may be prescribed, as may drugs that soften stools. Surgery is usually recommended for a severe case with pain, bleeding, and infection. In most cases, it is a permanent cure. But even after surgery some people develop more hemorrhoids since not all rectal veins can be removed.

Women may develop hemorrhoids during pregnancy, when the enlarged uterus may press on veins, interfering with the blood supply and causing irritation.

Chronic coughing and jobs involving heavy lifting or long standing can predispose a person to hemorrhoids. People with chronic constipation who frequently strain to pass hard, dry stools are also prone to the condition.

117

Hemorrhoids can occur when a tumor presses on veins in the rectum or when circulation is slowed because of heart disease. People who are overweight are more likely to develop hemorrhoids than people of normal weight.

Some people who self-diagnose hemorrhoids are actually suffering from venereal warts—and spreading the infection. Anyone with persistent rectal symptoms should consult a physician.

People with hemorrhoids should avoid anal penetration.

See also ANAL SEX; WARTS, VENEREAL.

HEPATITIS. Sexual activities may lead to hepatitis B (genital), a virus inflammation of the liver. It is caused by the same organism as serum hepatitis, the most injurious and lethal form of the disease.

Sexual intercourse appears to be a method of transmission. But oral and anal sex evidently spread far more cases.

The first symptom may be yellowing of the whites of the eyes. This results from bile pigments entering the blood from the diseased liver. The skin may acquire a yellowish "jaundice" color, but many hepatitis victims never develop this sign.

Other signs include tiredness, loss of appetite, and upset stomach with or without vomiting. There also may be itching, headache, and pain in the right side of the abdomen. A fever may occur at first but generally stops in a few days. The liver may enlarge and become tender. Urine becomes darker until it resembles diluted coffee. One curious symptom is that smokers may find tobacco so nauseating that they give up smoking.

Hepatitis requires a physician's care. The diagnosis is confirmed by a laboratory test of blood serum. Treatment in most cases is bed rest. Getting up too soon or being too active may cause permanent, possibly severe liver damage, especially if there is jaundice. A neglected case can lead to death.

A vaccine against hepatitis B is now available. Given in 3 injections over 6 months, it is thought to give protection for at least 5 years. The vaccine is recommended for those considered at high risk of infection: medical workers, kidney dialysis patients and others who need frequent blood transfusions, those in close contact with infected people, narcotics addicts, and people with numerous sexual contacts.

See also ANAL SEX; ORAL SEX; VENEREAL DISEASE.

HERNIA (rupture) is due to a weakness or opening in the muscle of the abdominal wall, allowing intestines or other organs to bulge out.

Abdominal wall weakness is thought to be a birth defect, although a hernia may not develop for many years, if at all.

When a great deal of the intestine pushes through, there is the danger that the hernia may become strangulated: its blood supply is cut off and gangrene may result. Emergency surgery is necessary to save life.

Inguinal hernia—the most common type—occurs low in the abdomen, at the groin. In boys, it can extend into the scrotum. A child with an inguinal hernia may experience vomiting and fever. Men will often complain of pain in the groin, but a hernia can be present with no pain. Frequently there is a swelling or lump in the groin. The condition is very rare in females.

Inguinal hernia may develop from the pressure of chronic constipation, or from prostate enlargement, in which the man must strain to urinate. Any condition that causes frequent coughing may lead to a hernia. It may also result from intestinal obstruction or from straining to lift heavy objects.

Surgery is the recommended treatment. Local anesthesia is widely used because it allows the doctor to check the hernia repair under stress: still on the operating table, the man is asked to cough. Hernia patients who have had local anesthesia often walk from the operating table and resume normal activity within 3 days.

In cases where the patient is a poor surgical risk, a sick older man, for example, the physician may recommend a truss—a corsetlike garment with pressure pads—until the surgery can be performed. A truss should be specially fitted to the individual—never bought by mail-order.

There may be danger in engaging in sexual intercourse while having an inguinal hernia. The exertion of intercourse could force the large intestine into the scrotum, causing pain and possible strangulation of the intestine.

If a patient refuses surgery, he should at least wear a truss while having intercourse. He can also reduce hazardous exertion if he avoids the male-superior position in favor of lying on his side or having his partner on top.

HEROIN addiction commonly interferes with sexual functioning in both men and women. Men often experience decreased sexual desire

119

and impotence or other potency problems, such as retarded ejaculation or failure to ejaculate.

Female heroin addicts frequently suffer from infertility. Many stop menstruating. Depressed sexual desire is often reported, as is a reduction in breast size. Heroin seems to predispose an addict to sexual difficulties by interfering with sex hormone production. Methadone is thought to exert a similar influence, although usually not as severe.

When the heroin addict stops using the drug, sexual functioning and fertility are not immediately restored. Endocrine problems may persist for several months. Psychological problems may similarly persist and may interfere with sexual functioning.

See also APHRODISIACS.

HERPES GENITALIS. Herpes simplex virus (HSV) can attack the coverings and linings of the sex organs, and can be transmitted through sexual intercourse. Genital herpes is a common—and dangerous— venereal disease. It is also painful and returns over and over again.

HSV type 1 is generally responsible for "cold sores" and "fever blisters," type 2 for genital infections. Both types of herpes simplex can be spread through oral sex. Type 1 can cause painful genital sores. Conversely, type 2 can infect lips, mouth, and tongue. So it is unwise to engage in oral sex when either partner has a cold sore. In general, however, type 1 is considerably less serious than type 2.

A genital herpes infection can be serious for a woman since it seems to be associated with a greater incidence of cancer of the cervix. The virus has been isolated from cervical cancer cells. In large part because of the link with HSV, cancer of the cervix is considered to be a venereal disease. It is most prevalent in women who engage in intercourse at an early age and with numerous sexual partners. It is practically unheard of in nuns or celibate women.

The virus may also attack the eyes, nose, mouth, throat, lungs, intestines, and the central nervous system, including the brain. If a woman is pregnant, her baby's life is especially threatened by the disease, principally by spontaneous abortion or by herpes encephalitis—a crippling, often fatal brain infection. She can usually have a baby by vaginal delivery if she has no active sores in her vagina or on her labia. But if such sores are present, she may require a caesarean birth—delivery through an abdominal incision—so that the baby will not be exposed to the herpes virus as it passes through the birth canal.

Herpes sores first appear in the genital area three to six days after sexual contact. They sometimes itch, but they are more likely to go unnoticed until they ulcerate and become painful, especially while one is walking or urinating.

The first attack may last a month or so. Then, at unpredictable intervals, attacks are likely to recur—each lasting from a few days to two weeks. An attack may start with tightness, stinging, tingling, or burning of infected areas. Clusters of small blisters usually follow. These break down in a couple of days, becoming crusty-looking sores. During an attack of herpes, there may be a fever, swollen glands, and a feeling as though one were coming down with flu. Attacks may be triggered by fever, sunburn, or premenstrual changes.

Sexual intercourse or other skin contact should be avoided until sores have healed entirely. The disease can spread easily between sex partners. A woman may be a silent carrier of the disease. She may have no symptoms, yet the virus is in her sex organs and can spread to others. The infection can be detected through a Pap smear.

Large doses of the amino acid lysine (about 1,000 milligrams per day) appear to promote healing and retard recurrence, according to research reports. Recovery also seems to be speeded by contraceptive creams and foams containing nonoxynol 9 and by exposing the sores to fluorescent light and keeping them dry and aerated. Acyclovir (Zovirax) may make outbreaks shorter and less painful.

See also CERVICAL CANCER; VENEREAL DISEASE.

HIGH BLOOD PRESSURE. See HYPERTENSION.

HIRSUTISM (hairiness, hypertrichosis) in women may be biologically normal though contrary to fashion. Some ethnic groups have more noticeable hair growth than others, which may in comparison appear excessive. Mediterranean and Semitic peoples, for example, are generally hairier than Anglo-Saxons.

Many women normally develop some hair on the upper lip or chin following menopause. A glandular disorder may be present, however, if a young woman has a sudden increase of hair on the face, chest, abdomen, or extremities. She should see an endocrinologist, a specialist in glandular problems. An endocrinologist should be consulted if a child, regardless of sex, develops hirsutism.

In some women, hirsutism is accompanied by other male secondary sex characteristics: male-pattern balding, deepening of the voice, and increased musculature with male body contours. At the same time, the women's breasts may shrink and their clitoris enlarge.

Tumors on the adrenal glands or the ovaries may account for such changes. With proper medical care, the process can usually be reversed.

Hirsutism may also be a symptom of a glandular disorder called Cushing's syndrome. Excess hair can be a side effect of taking steroids and streptomycin. An excess growth of hair is occasionally induced by X-ray therapy or by plaster casts or heavy straps that rub against the skin.

It is a myth that facial creams can cause excess hair. Often women start using such creams around their menopause when skin dryness is likely to become a problem, and hair resulting from menopause may be attributed to the creams. (Hormone therapy for menopause does not reduce or reverse unwanted hair growth.)

What to do about excess hair? When, as in the great majority of cases, it is a cosmetic rather than a medical problem, a woman has the following choices:

● *Bleaching* is the simplest cosmetic aid and is harmless to the average skin. At best it conceals hair, particularly on the upper lip and arm. At worst it may cause the hair to break off, or it may color the skin slightly. Excessive hair bleaching may make hair harsh and strawlike.

Before bleaching it is a good idea to degrease hair with acetone (nail polish remover), then rub it off. A woman can use a commercially prepared bleach or home preparation: one ounce of 6 percent hydrogen peroxide (20 volume peroxide), 20 drops of household ammonia, and a few soap chips to form a paste. The solution should be tested on a patch of skin for possible irritation.

● *Shaving* is the best and fastest method for removing leg and arm hair. Despite a near taboo against a woman's shaving her face, there is nothing medically harmful in it.

Shaving's only disadvantage is that it must be done frequently and carefully. Cuts can be minimized by wetting the skin, applying shaving cream, and shaving in broad strokes in the direction of hair growth.

It is a fallacy that shaving coarsens or darkens hair. Every hair, whether it be dark or light, long or short, is darker and thicker in the portion closest to the skin. The root, which determines hair structure, is unaffected by anything done to the hair above the skin's surface.

• *Tweezing* may be best for facial hair since it retards regrowth. It is recommended for long solitary hairs such as on breasts.

It is wise to apply a hot cloth to the area to be tweezed. A magnifying mirror aids in plucking hair on the brows or face. Hair should be tweezed in the direction the hair grows or the follicle will become enlarged. Tweezing is the best method for shaping eyebrows.

Tweezed hairs do not grow back thicker than before, although it may appear that way. Shorter hair is always rougher. Tweezing removes the hair just above the papilla or root of the hair follicle. Nor is it true that tweezing promotes cancer of the skin. Since an irritation may develop from tweezing hairs in moles, clipping mole hairs is preferred.

• *Waxing* (zipping) is a method of plucking hair en masse, if a bit painfully. A thin layer of melted wax is applied to the skin and allowed to cool with a cloth laid over it. As the cloth is stripped off, the hair embedded in the wax is plucked out. It should be stripped off quickly against the direction of hair growth or the hair will stretch, become distorted, or break off above the skin. Wax should not be too hot.

Female hormones (estrogens) do not make waxing creams any more effective, despite advertisers' claims. The American Medical Association can find no scientific evidence to support claims that the use of estrogen creams in conjunction with zipping would result in permanent hair removal.

• *Chemical depilatories* can be dangerous on the face besides being messy and time consuming. Thioglycolate, the basic ingredient, reduces protein bonds and dissolves the hair.

Instructions on the package should be followed carefully to avoid such reactions as eczema or contact dermatitis. Milk and cold compresses relieve irritation, as do steroid ointments.

• *Abrasion* with pumice is rarely a good idea. It is impractical for large areas. If used too vigorously, it may cause irritation. After hair removal with a pumice, cream or lotion should be applied.

Electrolysis is the only permanent method to remove hair. One method, electrocoagulation, is done by inserting a thin needle down the hair shaft to the follicle base and sending a short-wave heat-producing current to burst the cell of the root. It is a long, expensive, and sometimes uncomfortable process.

Properly performed by a licensed operator, it is safe. But the destruction rate is only 30 to 50 percent of the hairs treated. If it is 100 percent, too high a current was used. Electrolysis does not work very well on fine hair.

The operator should be licensed, should use sterilized needles, and should have adequate lighting. A shallowly implanted needle does not destroy the root. One planted too deeply destroys healthy tissue. Improper electrolysis can cause infection, distorted hair growth, or pitting and scarring.

Home electrolysis devices should be avoided. "Even if the machines could work successfully," warns Consumers Union, "it would be impossible for a woman to treat herself by electrical methods without risking damage to the skin."

The likelihood of regrowth and scarring is great since it is difficult for an untrained person to gauge the direction of the hair follicle, locate the base of the hair, and judge the amount of current needed. At best, such devices are suited for removal of hair on readily accessible parts of the arms and legs.

Consumers Union further warns against using X rays to destroy hair follicles. No matter how carefully they are administered there is serious risk of permanent skin damage and possibly skin cancer.

See also BREAST HAIR.

HOMOSEXUALITY is the attraction to members of the same sex. It may also include the practice of sexual relations. In common usage, the term is usually applied only to males. Lesbianism is the term used for same-sex contacts among females.

Homosexuals are thought to constitute about 4 percent of the adult male population; lesbians, about 1 or 2 percent of the female population.

Why do some people become homosexual? No one really knows. Homosexuality is thought to be determined by a multiplicity of factors, including a person's milieu, his psychological makeup, and his relationships with his family and others.

The American Psychiatric Association no longer considers homosexuality as an illness in itself; the American Medical Association similarly no longer considers it a disease syndrome.

Homosexuals exist in every social class and occupation. They hold responsible jobs. Many are married or have been married. They are no more emotionally unstable than the rest of the population.

Indeed, most homosexuals cannot be distinguished from heterosexuals. The cliché of a limp-wristed, effeminate homosexual is more the exception than the rule. This stereotype constitutes only a small minority (perhaps 15 percent) of the homosexual population. The great majority are as masculine-looking as the typical heterosexual male. Nor do most lesbians fit the stereotype of the mannish woman.

Homosexuals and disease. As a group, sexually active homosexual males suffer a relatively high rate of venereal disease.

Homosexuals in a monogamous relationship will naturally have little risk of contracting sexually transmitted diseases. But those who have many different partners are at particularly high risk for gonorrhea, nongonococcal urethritis, syphilis, hepatitis, and genital herpes.

These venereal diseases often go unnoticed, or are misdiagnosed. They tend to be in unusual sites—such as the throat and rectum—and are frequently asymptomatic. To aid a physician in making a proper diagnosis, it is wise for a patient to let the doctor know he is a homosexual. Without this knowledge, the physician can easily mistake oral gonorrhea for a simple sore throat.

Men who have oral-genital or anal sex with many partners are advised to have cultures of the pharynx, urethra, and rectum taken every 3 to 6 months in order to detect gonorrhea. Homosexuals with many contacts should consider being vaccinated against hepatitis B.

Other infections common among homosexuals include amebiasis and giardiasis, both caused by intestinal protozoa. Anal intercourse followed by oral-genital or oral-anal contact is thought to be the mode of transmission. Also transmitted among homosexuals are such intestinal infections as salmonellosis and shigellosis, which cause diarrhea.

Anal intercourse may result in rectal injury (see ANAL SEX). Venereal warts and pubic lice are also frequently seen among homosexuals.

Lesbians have a much lower incidence of sexually transmitted diseases than heterosexual women or homosexual males. But lesbians who have multiple partners and those who occasionally have sexual contact with men are at risk of contracting venereal diseases.

See also AMEBIASIS; ANAL SEX; GIARDIASIS; GONORRHEA; HEPATITIS; HERPES GENITALIS; VENEREAL DISEASE; WARTS, VENEREAL.

HORMONE DISORDERS. The endocrine system helps coordinate the life processes of the body, maintain a stable balance in the internal environment, and enable the body to respond to the external environment.

It consists of about ten ductless glands that produce hormones—chemical substances that are carried by the blood to other parts of the body where they either stimulate or inhibit activity.

Many endocrine glands affect one another so as to form an interrelated system. Thus a disorder of one gland often stimulates or inhibits the mechanisms of other glands, with varied effects on the body. Some of these are sexual.

PITUITARY DISORDERS. The pituitary gland, a pea-sized organ at the base of the brain, produces hormones that affect many other endocrine glands. Among the pituitary's hormones are the growth hormone, thyrotrophic hormone, lactogenic hormone, gonadotrophic hormones, and ACTH.

The growth hormone regulates the body's growth by stimulating the growth of the long bones. Thyrotrophic hormone (or Thyroid Stimulating Hormone) stimulates the thyroid to produce its own hormone. Lactogenic hormone (prolactin) stimulates the mammary glands in the breasts to secrete milk.

The gonadotrophic hormones affect the gonads (the testes in the male, the ovaries in the female) in a complicated cycle of interrelationships that is essential to reproduction as well as other sexual processes. ACTH (Adrenocorticotrophic hormone) stimulates the adrenal glands.

The pituitary may underfunction because of tumors on or near the gland, radiation therapy, blood clots, surgery, or other problems.

Pituitary tumors produce significant hormonal deficiencies in about 60 percent of cases. The first sign is typically hypogonadism, a deficiency of hormones produced by the testes and ovaries. This causes disruptions in reproduction and sexual functioning. Other common symptoms include loss of vision, headaches, and sleep or appetite disturbances.

126

In Sheehan's syndrome, which usually occurs after postpartum hemorrhage, the pituitary deficiency results from destruction of tissue. The first sign of this problem is usually failure to produce breast milk. Recovery from the bleeding is extremely slow. Lack of menstruation or very sparce menstruation is common, and fertility problems are frequent. There is also commonly evidence of thyroid and adrenal insufficiency.

When there is no pituitary gonadotrophin production, both sexes may suffer severe atrophy of the gonads. In men, sperm production stops, and sexual desire and potency decrease. Often, the ability to ejaculate is lost. Facial hair growth ceases, and body hair decreases. Men typically also suffer from weakness, weight loss, and decreased muscle mass.

Many of these problems are easily reversible with testosterone therapy. Gonadotrophin stimulation is necessary for reversing atrophy of the testes and restoring sperm production. Fertility can in many instances be restored by the administration of a combination of hormones.

In women, pituitary deficiency typically leads to infertility resulting from failure to ovulate and estrogen deficiency. Estrogen deficiency may also result in atrophy of the vaginal mucosa and breast tissue. Most women experience decreased sexual desire, and orgasmic response is ofter impaired.

Sometimes, the pituitary overfunctions. Acromegaly is the result of a pituitary tumor that leads to excess amounts of growth hormone. Typically, the first symptoms of this disorder are headache, visual disturbances, coarsening of facial features, a thickening of the skull, prominence of the jaw, and enlargement of the hands and feet.

If the disorder occurs before puberty, the result is gigantism, excessive growth of the long bones in the body resulting in pathologically tall stature.

In women with this disorder, there are commonly menstrual irregularities or the cessation of menstruation. Many experience low sex drive. Prolactin levels may be elevated, with breast milk discharge.

In men, most suffer from diminished sex drive—although early in the course of the disease there is sometimes increased sexual desire. Impotence is common, affecting 30 to 40 percent of men with acromegaly.

About 15 to 20 percent of people with this disorder suffer from diabetes, which may contribute to their sexual problems.

Successful treatment of acromegaly is difficult. Treatment approaches include surgery, radiation therapy, and medication. The associated sexual problems may not always be reversed with treatment. Hormone therapy may improve sexual functioning.

ISLANDS OF LANGERHANS DISORDER. Part of the pancreas is a ductless gland named the Islands of Langerhans. This gland secretes the hormones insulin and glucagon. Insulin helps regulate carbohydrate metabolism, causing glucose to be converted to glycogen, and controlling the oxidation of glucose in the cells. Insufficient insulin causes a concentration of glucose in the blood. The disease that results is called diabetes and is associated with a number of sexual effects (see DIABETES).

THYROID DISORDER. The thyroid gland is an H-shaped structure located in the neck on both sides of the trachea. Its hormone, thyroxin, regulates the general rate of the body's metabolism.

In hypothyroidism, an undersecretion of thyroxin, the rate of metabolism is lowered. Thyroid deficiency may result either from a defect in the gland itself or from a disorder of the pituitary or hypothalamus.

A thyroid deficiency from birth results in cretinism—characterized by mental retardation, dwarfism, and a disproportionate body. Puberty is either delayed or incomplete. Thyroid hormone replacement will bring on sexual maturation.

Myxedema is a thyroid-deficiency disease of adults typified by a slowing of mental processes, lowered metabolic rates, and swelling of the face and body.

With hypothyroidism, there may also be weakness, easy fatigability, dry or coarse skin, intolerance to cold, slow speech, impaired memory, constipation, and muscular aching.

Deficiency of thyroid hormone is commonly associated with disruptions in sexual functioning. In men, about 80 percent experience decreased sexual desire and 40 to 50 percent have erectile difficulties. Depressed sperm production is common.

Difficulty in becoming sexually aroused is experienced by some women with hypothyroidism. There may also be difficulty in attaining orgasm. About 35 percent experience extremely heavy menstruation; some fail to menstruate. When the hypothyroidism is moderate to severe, fertility is often impaired.

The decreased sexual functioning associated with hypothyroidism is largely due to the disorder's cumulative effect on body systems and symptoms such as weakness and muscular aches.

Hypothyroidism can be successfully treated with thyroid hormone. There is almost always a dramatic improvement in sexual functioning after therapy.

When too much thyroxin is secreted—a condition called hyper-thyroidism—the individual's rate of metabolism is increased, resulting in tremendous energy and restlessness. The condition may result in exophthalmic goiter, in which the thyroid gland swells and the eyeballs protrude.

Hyperthyroidism may also be accompanied by weakness, fatigue, tremor, weight loss with increased appetite, heartbeat irregularities, great mood swings, warm and moist skin.

Sexual desire is usually unaltered or diminished—although increased libido is sometimes seen in patients with milder disease, but this is sometimes accompanied by impotence. Indeed, impotence occurs in about 40 percent of men with hyperthyroidism.

In women, menstrual flow is usually disrupted, often absent. Cycles typically become erratic. Orgasmic response is usually unimpaired.

Hyperthyroidism may be treated by surgical removal of part of the thyroid or by various drugs or the use of radioactive iodides. Sexual functioning is usually corrected with treatment.

ADRENAL DISORDER. The adrenal glands, one on top of each kidney, consist of the medulla, or inner part, and the cortex, or outer layer. The adrenal medulla secretes adrenalin and noradrenalin, which have metabolic effects that prepare the body for emergencies. Under stress there is an adrenalin surge that causes the fight-or-flight reaction: the heart beats more rapidly and vigorously, the rate of breathing increases, the blood clots more rapidly, and digestion slows.

The adrenal cortex secretes cortin, which is composed of at least six active hormones. (The one most commonly known is cortisone.) They increase the amount of glucose in the blood by assisting in the change of glycogen, proteins, and fat to glucose. Some adrenal cortex hormones have effects similar to those of male sex hormones.

An insufficiency of adrenal cortex hormones may be due to destruction of the adrenal glands themselves or to disorders of the pituitary or hypothalamus.

Addison's disease is chronic adrenocortical insufficiency. It commonly causes fatigue, weight loss, low blood pressure, increased skin pigmentation, poor appetite, nausea, abdominal pain, and personality changes.

In women, there may be a decrease in body hair. Often, there is a significant decrease in sexual desire. About 30 to 40 percent of women with Addison's disease report diminished capacity for orgasm or the inability to attain orgasm. With treatment, sexual functioning often improves.

Men usually experience diminished interest in sex and about 35 percent become impotent. Treatment for Addison's disease usually brings dramatic improvement in strength and a sense of well-being, with an associated improvement in sexual functioning.

Overproduction of cortisol, one of the adrenal cortex hormones, results in a condition called Cushing's syndrome—often caused by an adrenal tumor.

The syndrome causes many changes in physical appearance, including obesity, purple streaks on the abdomen, excessive bruising, increased skin pigmentation, and excessive hairiness. In both men and women, diminished physical attractiveness resulting from the disorder may have a negative effect on sexual functioning.

There may also be muscular weakness, high blood pressure, diabetes, and alterations of personality.

Women with Cushing's syndrome often stop menstruating, and they have a predisposition to vaginal infection.

Men with Cushing's syndrome usually report diminished sexual desire. They may also experience difficulty in erectile functioning.

Sexual changes are usually correctable when the disease is brought under control. But impotence may persist if the diabetes brought on by the syndrome does not significantly improve. Medication used to treat the high blood pressure may also contribute to impotence.

The adrenogenital syndrome results when the adrenal cortex produces excessive androgens (male sex hormones) because of a genetic enzyme defect. When this occurs in a genetic female during fetal development and early childhood, the girl usually has ambiguous genitals.

Effects range from mild clitoral enlargement to what looks like a normal-sized penis. Internal reproductive structures are normal, but the vagina is sometimes closed.

Without treatment, the child will most likely develop a male appear-

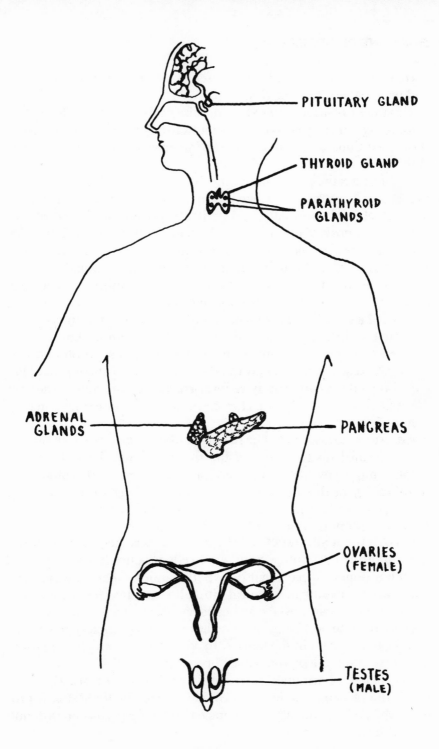

PITUITARY GLAND

THYROID GLAND

PARATHYROID GLANDS

ADRENAL GLANDS

PANCREAS

OVARIES (FEMALE)

TESTES (MALE)

ance, with a broad chest, heavy muscular development, narrow hips, and male pattern hair development.

Treatment is surgery to reduce the size of the clitoris at the earliest possible age. If surgery to construct a vaginal opening is necessary, it should be done after puberty—scarring may result if it is done in childhood.

Steroid therapy, preferably begun before the age of six, suppresses the excessive output of androgen. Female secondary sex characteristics develop relatively normally, and fertility is possible for the majority.

If the diagnosis is not made until later in childhood, and the child has been raised as a boy, it will be traumatic to reassign sex. After 2½ years of age, the child should continue to be raised as a male.

When the adrenogenital syndrome occurs in adulthood, a woman may develop acne, increased body and facial hair, and an enlarged clitoris. She typically stops menstruating and ovulating, thus becoming infertile. Increased sexual drive is another common sign.

These changes almost invariably cause the woman profound psychological distress, which may interfere with sexual functioning. Masculinizing effects can usually be reversed with corticosteroid therapy. Treatment is commonly given for one or two years; sometimes, lifelong therapy is necessary.

PARATHYROID DISORDER. The parathyroids are a group of four minute glands located on the lobes of the thyroid gland. Their hormone, parathormone, regulates the amount of calcium in the blood. An insufficiency of this hormone causes increased nervousness and the tendency to violent muscular contractions and spasms, which may interfere with normal sexual function.

HYPOTHALAMUS DISORDER. The hypothalamus is a region in the lower portion of the cerebrum whose nerve cells produce hormones called neurohormones. Impairment of hypothalamic functioning can produce extreme obesity; mechanical difficulties can interfere with sexual functioning. So can lowered self-esteem associated with obesity.

GONAD DISORDER. The gonads are the two testes (testicles) in the male and the two ovaries in the female. In addition to producing sperm or ova, these glands also produce sex hormones.

The male sex hormones collectively are called androgens. Testosterone is the principal male sex hormone secreted by the testes. It produces the male secondary sex characteristics—deep voice, beard, and masculine body form.

The ovaries produce estrogen and progesterone. Estrogen is responsible for the development of secondary sex characteristics such as the growth of breasts and the widening of the hips. Progesterone, along with estrogen, controls the production of ova by the ovaries and the associated changes in the uterus that result in the menstrual cycle.

When the testes fail to function properly, a male experiences decreased production of testosterone or impaired sperm production or both—a condition called **MALE HYPOGONADISM.**

Various disorders may result in hypogonadism. These include congenital absence of the testes, inflammation resulting from mumps or gonorrhea, disorders of the pituitary or hypothalamus, spinal-cord injury, and a number of special syndromes.

When the testosterone deficiency occurs in a young boy, he typically fails to experience the usual changes of puberty. The child will retain an infantile penis, small soft testes, underdeveloped muscles, and a high-pitched voice.

When the deficiency occurs in adulthood, there is usually decreased sexual desire and potency. With prolonged deficiency, the male secondary sex characteristics begin to regress. In most cases of testosterone deficiency, the problem can be corrected with testosterone replacement therapy.

One common condition associated with male hypogonadism is *Klinefelter's syndrome*—occurring once in every 500 live male births. Infants with this syndrome are born with abnormal chromosome patterns.

Testosterone levels are usually subnormal. The testes are commonly very small, and produce no sperm.

In adulthood, a man with Klinefelter's syndrome has a characteristic body type: he is tall with very long limbs; his muscle development is poor; he has some breast development; his face and body hair are sparce.

Generally, men with this syndrome have low sex drive and varying degrees of impotence. There is a greater proportion of mental retardation and behavioral disturbances associated with Klinefelter's syndrome.

Low sex drive and impotence will usually improve with testosterone replacement therapy when there is a testosterone deficiency.

In a much less common condition of male hypogonadism—*testicular feminization syndrome*—a genetic male fetus produces a normal amount of testosterone. But it fails to have the usual effect, for the tissues of the fetus are insensitive to it.

The child is born with external genitals that appear female, with labia, a vagina, and a clitoris. But there are no true uterus, cervix, or Fallopian tubes, and the vagina is typically shortened.

While these genetic males look like normal females, they have functioning testicles—most often in the abdomen or incompletely descended. Fertility is not possible.

Children with testicular feminization syndrome are almost always raised as girls, and generally have normal childhoods. It is considered a mistake to raise them as boys, for they will always have a female appearance.

At puberty, the usual male changes do not occur. On the contrary, children with this syndrome develop normal female breast growth, and are usually strongly feminine in attitudes and behavior. Such children can be told that they have a disorder involving hormones in the gonads, and that they will not menstruate or be able to bear children because the uterus has not developed properly.

When the ovaries fail to function, a girl will not experience normal sexual maturation; her uterus will not enlarge, her breasts will not develop, she will have no growth of pubic or axillary hair, and menstruation will not occur.

Ovarian insufficiency may result from many disorders, including congenital absence of the ovaries, surgery, irradiation, and tumors of the hypothalamus or pituitary. Other endocrine or metabolic disturbances may also result in failure of sexual maturation, as may chronic diseases such as diabetes or kidney diseases or obesity or malnutrition.

One fairly common cause of female hypogonadism—occurring once in 2,500 female births—is *Turner's syndrome.* This disorder is characterized by the absence or minimal development of the gonads because one sex chromosome is missing.

Infants with Turner's syndrome have normal looking external genitals. But their vaginas are often shallow and their uteruses small. They have no functioning ovarian tissue.

Girls with this syndrome have an abnormally short stature (average adult height is 55 inches)—and generally at least two of the following: webbed neck, prominent low-set ears, childlike chest with widely spaced nipples, senile face, high-arched palate, low hairline, high blood pressure, and heart abnormalities. Intelligence may be normal or slightly below normal.

Often, the syndrome is not diagnosed until the teenage years, when the girl fails to menstruate. Replacement therapy will bring on secondary sex characteristics, but fertility is impossible. Sex drive is often moderately to severely depressed, and orgasmic dysfunction is common.

Ovarian failure in adulthood may be due to disorders of the ovaries, hypothalamus, or other endocrine glands. Chronic debilitating disease may also interfere with functioning. Most commonly, ovarian failure is due to a disruption of the normal relationship between the hypothalamus, the pituitary, and the ovaries, without any demonstrable organic disease. Sometimes, the problem follows acute psychological stress. In some cases, an ovarian tumor is responsible for failure of the ovaries to function.

See also DIABETES.

HORMONES. See HORMONE DISORDERS.

HYMEN PROBLEMS. The hymen is a thin membrane partially blocking the vaginal opening. It serves no physiological function. Normal hymens have a great variation in thickness, size, and the shape of the opening.

An intact hymen is no proof of virginity—nor is a torn or stretched hymen a proof of sexual experience. A few women are born without hymens.

Girls often worry that the hymen will cause them pain and bleeding during their first intercourse. This is likely if the hymen breaks or tears on penetration.

Ideally, the hymen should be slowly stretched over a period of time. This often happens when teenage girls use tampons during menstruation. Over the months, the tampons stretch the hymenal opening, making the initial penetration easier.

Girls can also self-dilate their hymens. Every day for two weeks while in the bathtub the young woman can exert pressure along her posterior vaginal wall for about 20 seconds.

If the hymen opening is unusually small, the physician may recommend dilation, an office procedure. On two or three office visits, the hymen is stretched with the doctor's fingers or with instruments until the opening can accommodate the full width of two fingers. Local and/or topical anesthesia is used.

In rare cases, a female has a hymen with no opening (imperforate). Menstrual blood has no outlet, and accumulates in the vagina. The usual complaint is periodic abdominal pain. Intercourse is not possible, and surgical correction is necessary.

Some women have very thick hymens, which are incapable of stretching. This condition makes sexual intercourse difficult or impossible and requires surgery. Surgery may also be needed for other hymen abnormalities—such as one or more bands of hymenal tissue obstructing the vagina.

The hymen may become irritated because of allergic reaction or inflammation from douching solutions, feminine hygiene sprays, or detergents. Vaginal infections may also affect the hymen. Herpes genitalis can cause extreme pain when it affects the hymen and labia.

Intercourse may be painful for women who have irritated hymenal remnants or other hymen problems. Their fear of pain may cause contractions of the vagina to guard against abrupt penile entry. When women experience such vaginal spasm (vaginismus), hymen abnormalities are explored as a possible source of the problem.

See also INTERCOURSE, PAINFUL; VAGINAL SPASM.

HYPERSEXUALITY is pathologically excessive sexual interest or activity. In men, this condition is called satyriasis; in women, nymphomania.

Satyriasis is characterized by an uncontrollable sexual appetite, an overpowering drive for sexual satisfaction. Sex is the dominant drive in the man's life. His seeking after sexual gratification is compulsive and indiscriminate.

The Don Juan syndrome refers to a particular type of male hypersexuality. For the Don Juan, sexual activity is unconsciously aimed toward overcoming inferiority feelings with proof of sexual success. The Don Juan is not interested in his partner of the moment. Once having proved he can excite and conquer her, he is compelled to move on to the next woman. His compulsion is fueled by intense narcissistic needs. In some, this frenzied heterosexual drive is thought to be a defense against unconscious homosexual impulses.

Nymphomania is characterized by a woman's inability to be sexually satisfied. She is thus constantly striving toward sexual gratification. Some women with this condition are unable to reach orgasm; they seek the possibility of orgasmic release with one partner after another. Others may have multiple orgasms, but never become satisfied.

Most commonly, hypersexuality is psychogenic in origin. The compulsive need for sex is often a compensation for feelings of inferiority. This sort of hypersexuality is considered a type of compulsive neurosis.

Psychosis accounts for hypersexuality in some patients. Both men and women who are suffering from mania are likely to show hypersexual symptoms since ordinary social and sexual inhibitions typically weaken during a manic episode. The patient may take multiple, impulsively chosen sexual partners, and may undress or masturbate in public. Such hypersexual behavior in mania often abates with phenothiazine therapy.

In men, hypersexuality is sometimes thought to be associated with genetic factors, such as chromosomal abnormalities. In women, the condition occasionally arises because of a tumor on the adrenal glands or ovaries.

Brain dysfunction may account for hypersexuality. Disorders of the temporal lobe of the brain occasionally cause compulsive sexual activity in both men and women. The patient may exhibit unusual sexual behavior, such as the sudden need for indiscriminate sex, or exhibitionism, or fetishism. Disorders of the frontal lobe of the brain, by reducing normal inhibitions, may similarly result in excessive, inappropriate sexual behavior. If these brain disorders can be successfully treated, the sexual symptoms usually disappear.

Hypersexuality of psychogenic origin is often treated by psychotherapy. For some men, oral contraceptives taken daily or every other day may reduce sex drive. For women, treatment may include progesterone and tranquilizers.

HYPERTENSION (high blood pressure) patients may fear that sexual intercourse is a danger for them since intercourse raises blood pressure.

Actually, while blood pressure is normally elevated during the sexual response cycle, the effect is only transient and has nothing to do with cardiovascular hypertensive disease.

Hypertension is a major health problem in this country. About 23 million Americans suffer from the condition, many without being aware of it. In a small percentage of cases, the condition can be traced to a specific disease—such as kidney disease, tumors of the adrenal gland, or abnormalities of the large arteries.

By far the most common kind of hypertension is "essential" or "primary" hypertension, which does not seem to be related to any other disease and for which the cause is not known.

Blood pressure is a measure of the force of the blood through the arteries. Normally, the pressure in the arteries ranges between 100 and 140 systolic (contraction pressure) and between 70 and 90 diastolic (relaxation pressure)—although these limits vary at different times and in different people. Blood pressures up to 140/90 or 150/90 are usually considered normal.

Heredity predisposes a person to develop hypertension, but such factors as obesity, emotional stress, and excessive sodium consumption may aggravate or precipitate the condition.

Hypertension is called a "silent disease." It generally has no symptoms until complications develop—and these complications are likely to be serious. Hypertension may lead to heart disease, arteriosclerosis, kidney failure, and cerebral hemorrhage (stroke).

Indeed, a person with severe, untreated hypertension is at great risk of suffering a stroke, especially with acute exertion. Very active sexual intercourse may constitute just such an exertion.

The possibility of stroke as a result of intercourse is considerably reduced if the hypertension is controlled by medication. It may also be possible for the medication to be timed to assure maximum effectiveness during the time of usual sexual activity. Further, a supervised program of conditioning exercises will allow for greater tolerance for exertion and will also help reduce blood pressure.

Hypertension medication may interfere with sexual functioning. Although there is no cure for primary hypertension, appropriate therapy can considerably reduce its risks. Drugs are a major part of hypertension treatment. (Other measures may include weight reduction, exercise, rest, psychotherapy, and giving up smoking.)

Unfortunately, the medications used in the treatment of hypertension sometimes have a negative effect on sexual response. Among men, delayed sexual response, reduced sexual desire, and impotence may result.

Switching medications may relieve the problem. Drug reactions are unpredictable and highly individual. A patient who has problems with one of them may well be quite unaffected by another.

Often a man used to a rapid response panics. He either becomes psychogenically impotent or stops taking the medication. It may help him to know that the drugs may merely delay his response and that, with prolonged stimulation, he may achieve erection and orgasm despite his slowed reaction time.

For women, antihypertensives have been implicated in decreased vaginal lubrication and inability to reach orgasm. Some women on antihypertensives also experience a decrease in libido; others retain their strong desire for intercourse but are frustrated by their physiological incapacity to be aroused.

Methyldopa (Aldoclor, Aldomet, Aldoril) is one antihypertensive whose adverse effects on female sexual response have been well documented. Guanethidine (Ismelin) causes failure to ejaculate in men and is thought to have a comparable effect on women. The problem often can be relieved by modifying the dosage or switching from one type of antihypertensive to another.

Among both men and women, the difficulty may not arise from the drug alone—but from the drug in combination with such other factors as fatigue, emotional stress, marital discord, alcohol consumption, and concurrent illnesses and medications. If these contributing causes are reduced, the patient's sexual functioning may be restored even while taking antihypertensives.

See also ARTERIOSCLEROSIS; IMPOTENCE; STROKE.

HYPERTHYROIDISM. See HORMONE DISORDERS.

HYPERTRICHOSIS. See HIRSUTISM.

HYPOSPADIAS. See PENIS MALFORMATION.

HYPOTHYROIDISM. See HORMONE DISORDERS.

HYSTERECTOMY is the surgical removal of the uterus. If a woman is told she needs one, she should feel she has the option to get another doctor's opinion.

Some hysterectomies are unnecessary—a situation ethical gynecologists call the "rape of the pelvis." A study of 246 hysterectomies at 10 hospitals found that fully 31 percent of the uteri removed were normal. In more than 9 percent of the cases, the hysterectomies were performed for such nonspecific complaints as irritability, fatigue, and headache. An additional 17 percent of the patients had no complaints at all.

Dr. Norman F. Miller of the University of Michigan School of Medicine called such operations "hip-pocket hysterectomies," beneficial only to where a knife-happy surgeon keeps his money. Some women in what Dr. Miller called this "surgical racket" are rushed into such operations even though their complaints are entirely unrelated to gynecology.

Such abuses, of course, are the exceptions rather than the rule. Still, a second opinion should be considered. A woman is best off consulting a board certified obstetrician-gynecologist who is a fellow of the American College of Obstetricians and Gynecologists.

Fibroid tumors may not be large enough to justify the hazards of surgery. Fibroids, the commonest reason for hysterectomies, are hard, noncancerous growths ranging from grape- to grapefruit-size. Their cause is unknown. They usually appear between ages 35 and 40.

It is estimated that 1 out of every 4 or 5 women have fibroid tumors. If they cause no pain or discomfort, most physicians prefer to do nothing about them, since after menopause the fibroids may disappear.

In some cases, the fibroid may push against the lining of the uterus, causing heavy bleeding during menstruation or between periods. If the tumor presses against the bladder it may cause frequent urination; if against the rectum, it may cause constipation. Rapidly enlarging tumors are an indication for surgery.

Sometimes fibroids can be removed without removing the uterus. This procedure—called a myomectomy—is a good alternative for a woman who may wish to bear children in the future. If a woman becomes pregnant after a myomectomy, her uterine walls may be weakened, and her baby will most likely need to be delivered by caesarean section.

Other common reasons for hysterectomy include severe menstrual disorders, pelvic inflammatory disease, and cancer of the cervix.

Removal of the uterus terminates menstruation and brings an end to childbearing. But unlike tubal sterilization, hysterectomy is not a preferred surgical method of birth control.

Hysterectomy need not affect the ability to enjoy sex. The vagina and the clitoris, which respond to sexual stimuli, are not affected by removal of the uterus. In fact, many couples find increased pleasure in sex once the possibility of pregnancy is eliminated.

A woman's ovaries are not removed in a simple hysterectomy. If the ovaries are diseased and must be removed at the same time as the uterus, the operation is known as an oophorectomy and hysterectomy. Removal of the ovaries will bring about premature menopause.

Removal of the uterus alone does not bring on premature menopausal problems. Contrary to widespread misapprehension, a hysterectomy will not cause wrinkles or hairiness. It is also untrue that either type of hysterectomy makes a woman grow fat, shrinks her breasts, or necessarily causes emotional problems.

A woman may prefer a vaginal rather than an abdominal incision. The vaginal hysterectomy requires more skill than the abdominal but is generally considered quicker and safer. It often requires a briefer hospital stay and a briefer convalescence than the abdominal hysterectomy. A hysterectomy usually requires about a week in the hospital and about 3 to 4 weeks for recovery.

See-also AGING; CERVICAL CANCER; MENOPAUSE.

IMPOTENCE (erectile dysfunction). A man almost inevitably experiences times when he is impotent—unable to achieve or sustain an erection. Contrary to the myth of the ever-ready male, such episodes of "transient" or "acute" impotence are part of normal male sexuality.

In addition, penises normally wax and wane during lovemaking, often becoming firm and limp several times. But if a man becomes anxious about his supposed failure, emotional stress is likely to build up. With persistent "performance anxiety," impotence may become chronic.

Erections develop when arteries increase blood flow to the penis, filling spongy tissue and balloonlike chambers. This engorgement causes the penis to enlarge and stiffen. If a man is suffering from impotence, a multitude of factors can be interfering with his erection.

Is he ill? Any debilitating acute illness—a bad cold, for example—can render a man incapable of intercourse until his recovery is complete. Diabetes-related impotence is thought to afflict more than 2 million men—but an estimated half of them don't realize that their impotence springs from their diagnosed medical condition. A wide range of other illnesses can cause impotence (see pp. 151-53).

Is medication blocking him? Drugs for lowering high blood pressure commonly have impotence as a side effect. So do amphetamines and many tranquilizers and antidepressants (see p. 151).

Ending use of the drug may produce rapid cure. Merely switching to another medication for the same condition may restore potency.

Is he tired? Fatigue—from overwork and everyday stress—is one of the commonest causes of impotence. Often the condition can be relieved simply by catching up on sleep—and having intercourse rested and relaxed.

Has he drunk too much? As few as two drinks can block an erection. That explains why, after returning from a party, a man may be disappointed if he tries to make love.

Many men try to overcome inhibition or sexual difficulty by drinking to loosen up. But they continue to have trouble, so they drink more and the pattern then becomes reinforcing. Alcohol is self-defeating. Indeed, chronic impotence is an early sign of alcoholism.

Has he overeaten? After a heavy meal, the blood rushes to the stomach, liver, and intestines. The increased volume of blood elsewhere in the body may make it difficult to sustain an erection.

Overweight and a poor physical condition can also impair sexual performance. Active sexual intercourse requires a vigorous body.

Is he trying too hard? Cultural upbringing makes sexual prowess essential to the self-esteem of most men. This attitude is reflected in everyday language: "impotent" also means "helpless."

The villain in many cases of impotence is a mythic great lover whom sex therapists often refer to as "Super Stud." This fantasy bedroom athlete—with his push-button erection, monumental staying power, and *Kama Sutra* know-how—is what many men and women expect the male to be. Alas, though he has as little relation to real-life lovemaking

142

as Batman has to crime-fighting, Super Stud may set the standard for a man's sex life.

Such unrealistic expectations can place tremendous pressure on men. Impotence is commonly caused by fear of failure. If a man regards sex as a performance rather than a pleasure, he can easily fall into anxiety over not meeting an imaginary standard.

Pressures to achieve an erection tend to have the opposite effect. No man can will an erection. The very attempt breeds failure. He then may feel pressured to try again—and his emotional stress renders him impotent. Each failure to perform weakens his confidence and makes his next attempt all the more difficult. Two or three such episodes within 72 hours can be so traumatic that the man's potency thereafter is defeated by his anxiety.

Similarly, a man may not be attracted to his partner, yet feel under pressure to perform anyway—an invitation to impotence.

Or a man may be impotent because he is trying to have intercourse more often than he really wants to. Sex drive varies enormously among normal men and can rise and fall in response to other aspects of life. If physically and emotionally a man would be satisfied with making love once or twice a week (or less often), he is likely to have trouble maintaining an erection on a three-times-a-week schedule.

Is he too goal-oriented? A man may see sex as a series of tasks to be performed toward a particular end. He is likely to be observing himself—sex therapists call it spectatoring—as he strives toward his goal of obtaining an erection and ejaculating. Such an emphasis on sex as a goal rather than a process can render a man impotent.

Is he feeling inadequate? Job tensions can leave a man feeling worthless and unable to perform. Often impotence follows a symbolic loss of potency in work: not getting a raise, losing a job, being passed over for promotion.

"Making it" has both vocational and sexual connotations. Some men who are extremely ambitious become severely depressed when they don't have the successes they strive for. Such losses often result in reduced self-confidence and impaired sexual functioning.

Some authorities speculate about a "new impotence" caused by men's reactions to women's sexual expectations. More women are aware of their sexuality—and their desires for sexual gratification have intensified the pressure on some men. Under such pressure, some men may experience impotence.

143

Does he worry about aging? Once impotent under any circumstances, many older men conclude, "It's all over for me." They withdraw from sexual intercourse altogether rather than face the ego-shattering experience of repeated impotence.

In fact, a man can remain sexually active through his 80s, at least. Starting around 40 or so, he may notice it takes him longer to achieve an erection and it may be somewhat softer. He may not ejaculate every time he has intercourse, or ejaculation may take longer. A man can think of this as a delightful prolongation of an always-pleasurable act. The changes need not interfere with his pleasure in intercourse.

Is he depressed? A man may not be aware of an underlying mental depression. But it may result in his losing his desire or ability for sex. The condition often occurs in the 40s or 50s as part of a midlife crisis when a man may feel he has peaked out at work and everything—job, home life, health—is downhill from now on.

Other signs pointing to mental depression: Impaired energy; difficulty getting to sleep or getting up; forgetfulness; bouts of agitated behavior. The proper antidepressant can usually clear up impotence from this cause.

Other types of emotional stress may similarly make a man impotent. Among such stressful situations are the illness or death of a loved one, moving to a new home, trouble with the law, or any severe financial reversal. Several lesser emotional problems can render a man impotent from the combined stress.

Does he harbor resentment? A man and his partner may have disagreements over money, family problems, or whatever. It is wise to resolve these conflicts before attempting intercourse. Any unresolved hostility can contribute to impotence.

Finding the cause. If a man suffers from recurrent impotence, he needs to consult a physician. This may be difficult for him to do since most men regard impotence as an aspersion on their masculinity and are reluctant to reveal the problem even to a doctor.

To broach the subject painlessly, a man might ask the doctor "Do you treat sexual difficulties?" Many men are vague out of embarrassment and merely throw out hints like "I have no energy," or "I'm not the man I used to be." The doctor may not pick up the clue.

Before a doctor can treat impotence, he needs to determine if its origins are emotional or physical, or both. One tip-off to psychogenic impotence: it is selective, affecting a man under some circumstances but not others. He may be able to masturbate but not penetrate a vagina. He may be impotent with one woman but not another. He may be able to get an erection in a hotel but not at home, or vice versa.

Indeed, any erection a man has at any time shows that his genitals can respond and that his impotence is most likely psychogenic. Typically, if impotence is of emotional origin, a man has erections in his sleep, when his inhibitions are dozing—or on awakening, before urinating. An erection may also occur at such times if impotence is induced by fatigue, alcohol, or drugs.

By contrast, damage from disease or injury is likely to block erections even during sleep. To determine if that is the case, the doctor may ask the patient to use a portable device called a nocturnal penile tumescence (NPT) monitor. The device attaches to his penis and, while he is sleeping, measures the extent to which he gets erections.

Organic causes were long thought to account for only about 10 percent of cases of impotence. Now impotence is being increasingly recognized as a common effect of disease and drugs. Researchers at the University of Pittsburgh School of Medicine examined men who complained of impotence. More than half had significant, previously undetected physical abnormalities that may have contributed to it.

Even when an organic condition is not the sole cause of impotence, it can make a man more vulnerable to emotional stress. The combination of psychological and physical factors can add up to an impeded erection.

To help pin down the cause of impotence, a thorough physical examination is necessary. It should include a double check for diabetes: a fasting blood sugar test plus a glucose tolerance test. Other musts for accurate diagnosis are a complete blood count and urinalysis, tests of thyroid and sex hormone production, and a survey of neurological functions (including senses, reflexes, balance, and coordination). The physician may also check the penis with a stethoscope, listening for the two dorsal arteries of the penis. If no pulse is heard, there is likely an obstruction of the arteries feeding the penis.

An X-ray procedure in which a contrast medium is injected into one of the penis's hollow chambers can show defects of Peyronie's disease (see entry) or reveal a leakage resulting from a pelvic fracture. Bladder studies may help assess the nerve supply of the penis.

For organic impotence. Prospects for relief depend on the cause of a man's impotence. Treatment with testosterone and gonadotropin is available if he has low levels of these androgens (male sex hormones).

Androgens mostly benefit older men whose hormone production has declined with age. Younger men often need androgens if their hormone production is reduced by liver disease or by undescended testicles or other genital disorders.

If a man takes androgens, he should be checked regularly for cancer of the prostate and of the breast, the growth of which is speeded up by the hormones. He may also develop priapism (a persistent abnormal erection) and edema, the retaining of excessive amounts of body fluid. These should be called to a doctor's attention.

Should all else fail, a man may consider a surgical implant. A penile prosthesis can give the shape and consistency of a normal erection. The penis can be inserted into a vagina, and a man can usually experience orgasm and ejaculation. (See PENILE PROSTHESES.)

The Small-Carrion prosthesis is made up of a pair of silicone sponges implanted in the corpora cavernosa, the twin chambers in the penis that normally engorge with blood. A man gets a permanent erection, which is flexible enough to be inconspicuous under his clothing. The implant is simple and relatively inexpensive, and results are generally excellent. The major disadvantage springs from the permanent erection. It makes routine cystoscopy (examination of the bladder) and some types of urological surgery difficult if not impossible.

The Scott inflatable prosthesis is a hydraulic system that fills with fluid small balloons implanted in the corpora cavernosa. (The fluid is radiopaque—capable of being seen on X ray.) When a man wants an erection, he compresses a small bulb implanted in his scrotum. Releasing the bulb makes the erection subside. However, the hydraulics make the system relatively expensive and subject to mechanical failure.

Most users of implants have organic causes for their impotence. But an implant may be suitable if a man suffers from psychogenic impotence that resists adequate psychotherapy, including couples therapy. The implant makes it possible for him to attain orgasm and ejaculation.

Implants are also recommended for some men whose impotence is caused purely by medication for high blood pressure. These men may stop taking antihypertensive drugs, preferring the disease to the impotence. For them an implant can be a lifesaver.

Impotence sufferers should beware of do-it-yourself devices. It is dangerous to apply a rubber band or other constriction to the base of the penis in the hope that it will maintain an erection. The penis can be injured—indeed, nearly severed. In any event, blood flow to the corpora is deep within the tissue, so it is not affected by such external constriction.

External penile splints are rarely satisfactory. Those intended to support a limp or semilimp penis are generally uncomfortable for both partners and often slip off. Sheathlike devices are sold to encase the penis. Inserting this artificial device may provide some pleasure for the woman but does little to stimulate the man wearing it.

If impotence is psychogenic, a man may have difficulty accepting that his impotence has emotional causes. Men with impotence often want to believe they have a medical problem rather than a psychological one. To support that delusion, a man may find himself hoping he has an abnormal blood sugar reading. He may search for a doctor who will find a physical cause.

Failing to find an organic problem, some men seek to blame their impotence on being "too busy" or "too tired"—rather than confront a deeper reason. This can prolong the problem by delaying proper treatment.

Accurate sex information may help overcome unrealistic expectations and resulting performance anxiety. It may be beneficial for a man to have a frank talk with a carefully selected physician—one who has experience in dealing with sexual problems. (See SEX THERAPY for tips on finding such a physician.) Ideally, the sex partner should be present, for an informed and supportive partner is a valuable asset in overcoming impotence. The physician may also help the man recognize stresses in his life that impede his erection and counsel him on resolving them.

If the man is amenable to sex therapy, he may benefit from a program aimed at reducing anxieties and improving sexual communication. A couple typically start with pleasuring, in which they refrain from intercourse but engage in love play. In steps, they proceed to insertion and orgasm. Many couples are successful applying this technique to themselves. (See "FRIGIDITY" for detailed instructions.)

147

Another technique that works for many couples is "stuffing." The man lies on his back, and his partner sits straddling his hips. She stuffs his penis into her vagina—proving that an erection is not necessary for entry. The increased sensation brought on by the vaginal containment is often enough to produce erection.

Chances for overcoming impotence through sex therapy are greatest if the man is free of other profound psychological disturbances and if he has a cooperative partner. He also stands the best chance of success if his impotence is "secondary"—he has had intercourse before problems developed with his erections—rather than "primary" (he has never had intercourse).

If impotence persists because of hidden emotional factors, psychotherapy may be beneficial. To treat impotence, a man generally must first deal with his underlying emotional conflicts.

Go to a prostitute? Some men attempt do-it-yourself sex therapy by going to a prostitute. In theory this can work because a woman can often help a man solve his problem of impotence—if she is sensitive, caring, and sexually mature.

Some prostitutes may well fill the bill. But usually, far from helping impotent men, encounters with prostitutes can be extremely stressful and themselves the cause of impotence. Prostitutes often hate men, are motivated only by money, and demand quick performance. These conditions can cause difficulty for any man, and worsen the impotent man's feelings of inadequacy.

Potency frauds. Quackery runs amok in this field. An impotent man would be wise to steer clear of unlicensed "practitioners" and "sex counselors." Impotent men often suffer further psychological damage at the hands of unscrupulous promoters.

To relieve impotence, a quack may offer a man a "shot" of a promised cure—often merely vitamins or just plain distilled water.

It may seem to work because of a placebo effect—if a person believes something increases potency, it well may do so, at least temporarily. But the placebo (from the Latin for "I shall please") can reinforce a man's belief that there is an organic basis to psychological impotence. He may thus become dependent on the shots.

Impotent men should also steer clear of gadgets that are advertised to bring on erection. Sold in sex shops or through catalogs, these devices are ineffective—and may be dangerous. The "erection ring," for example, is a plastic device that encircles the base of a man's penis. Presumably, it helps him gain and maintain an erection. In fact, if the gadget is put on tight enough to impede the blood supply to the penis, it may cause permanent injury (see PENIS INJURY).

All advertised drugs are junk, despite their suggestive brand names. Most such products do not explicitly promise to cure impotence, but their very names imply a cure. In a fraud order against a product called Stagg Bullets, for example, postal authorities commented, "The word sex is not used, but one does not need a magnifying glass to see it." Other supposed medications that have come under attack for mail fraud bear names like Viri-tabs, Instant Erection, and Hard-on Powder.

Recently multivitamin and mineral preparations have been promoted as aids to sexual vigor. While supplementary vitamins and minerals may improve a man's general state of health, they are no direct cure for impotence. One supposed impotence pill widely sold at health food stores contained such useless ingredients as papaya leaves, prickly ash bark, ground cockleburrs, and radish powder.

Royal jelly, from bees, is worthless for restoring potency. Products that contain male hormones can be dangerous if used without medical supervision. Their value in the treatment of impotence is limited to specific medical conditions.

No food has any value as a sexual stimulator. Olives, ginseng, plover's eggs, oysters, radishes, mangoes, pumpkin seeds, and countless other edibles and not-so-edibles have been used as aphrodisiacs. There is no evidence that any have more than a placebo effect.

Magic impotence cures are offered by some practitioners of the occult: hiding a dead bat under the bed; sprinkling the walls of the house with the blood and bile of a male dog; anointing the genitals with sesame oil. These are neither more nor less effective than any other quack remedy.

Advice for women: If a woman's sex partner fails to achieve or sustain an erection, her positive attitude can do much to keep his transient impotence from becoming chronic. She should refrain from such comments as, "Don't worry, everything will be okay, dear." This only reinforces the fear that something is wrong. Many statements made at this moment are likely to be interpreted injuriously.

Her best bet may be to express without words comfort, tenderness, and emotional warmth. She will be of great help doing whatever she can to make the man understand that the physical act of intercourse is secondary to the emotional act of loving.

If the man wants to discuss the episode, she can encourage him to verbalize his fears and embarrassment. She may say matter-of-factly that this is something that happens and the problem is minor and temporary, conveying the message: "Let's wait till another time." This takes the pressure off the moment and implies her continued confidence in him.

A woman may be able to relieve her partner's performance anxiety by encouraging him to focus on her. There is a sexual give-to-get response: by pleasing the woman, the man is likely to become aroused himself. Being guided by feeling—rather than achieving—also can free him from the spectator role, in which he worries if he is reaching a sexual "goal."

Further, a woman can explore ways of gaining pleasure that don't require his erect penis: oral or manual stimulation or mutual masturbation. These help take the pressure off the male partner, and his potency may return.

She should not try to seduce him. To kindle his ardor, she may be tempted to put on suggestive clothing or extra makeup. He may find these clichés unattractive to begin with. Worse yet, he is likely to feel under greater pressure than ever. His impotence will be intensified. So will be the woman's frustration.

It is wise for a woman to beware of reacting with hostility. Nagging is one form hostility often takes. Needling him is another—not only about his sexual prowess but about his abilities as a husband, father, breadwinner, and householder. All this tends to further lower his self-respect and inhibits his erection even more.

A woman's own self-image is likely to be threatened by her sex partner's impotence. Mistakenly, she may blame herself for not arousing him, for failing in her "feminine role." Some women pursue extramarital affairs—to reassure themselves, to obtain sexual satisfaction, or to vent their anger at their husbands.

A woman's physical and psychological discomfort may be so great that, intentionally or not, she avoids contact with her sex partner. She may protest illness or pick a fight whenever a sexual encounter seems imminent. She may engage in a flurry of activities that keep her out of the house. His response may be, "She doesn't love me anymore," worsening his impotence and possibly ending the marriage.

Both partners may benefit from professional counseling, ideally taken jointly. Both may need reassurance that their respective reactions, however extreme, are understandable in light of a painful and seemingly uncontrollable situation. They thereby may break patterns of denigrating themselves and each other—and proceed constructively toward establishing an improved emotional and sexual relationship.

See also AGING; APHRODISIACS; DIABETES; MEDICATIONS; PENILE PROSTHESES; PEYRONIE'S DISEASE.

These Drugs Can Cause Impotence

addictive drugs
alcohol
amphetamines
anticholinergics
antidepressants
antihypertensives
atropine
barbiturates
chlordiazepoxide
chlorprothixene
digitalis
diuretics
estrogen
guanethidine
hypnotics
imipramine
methadone
methantheline bromide
monoamine oxidase inhibitors
nicotine
phenothiazines
reserpine
sedatives
spironolactone
thioridazine
tranquilizers

Impotence May Be Due to These Medical Conditions
Here is a list of the most common medical and surgical causes of impotence.

IMPOTENCE

Anatomic
congenital deformities
hydrocele
testicular fibrosis

Cardiorespiratory
angina pectoris
coronary insufficiency
emphysema
myocardial infarction
pulmonary insufficiency
rheumatic fever

Endocrine
acromegaly
Addison's disease
adrenal neoplasms
castration
chromophobe adenoma
craniopharyngioma
diabetes mellitus
eunuchoidism (including Klinefelter's syndrome)
feminizing interstitial-cell testicular tumors
infantilism
ingestion of female hormones (estrogen)
myxedema
obesity
thyrotoxicosis

Genitourinary
perineal prostatectomy
prostatitis
phimosis
priapism
suprapubic and transurethral prostatectomy
urethritis

Hematologic
Hodgkin's disease

leukemia, acute and chronic
pernicious anemia
sickle cell anemia

Infectious
genital tuberculosis
gonorrhea
mumps

Miscellaneous Causes
chronic renal failure
cirrhosis
toxicologic agents (lead, herbicides)

Neurologic
amyotrophic lateral sclerosis
cord tumors or transection
electric shock therapy
multiple sclerosis
nutritional deficiencies
parkinsonism
peripheral neuropathies
spina bifida
sympathectomy
tabes dorsalis
temporal lobe lesions

Vascular
aneurysm
arteritis
sclerosis
thrombotic obstruction of aortic bifurcation

INCEST is sex between family members.

Ranging from sexual fondling to vaginal intercourse and anal and oral sex, it is a phenomenon that cuts across class, race, and ethnic lines.

It occurs in rich as well as in poor families, in well-educated as well as in illiterate families, in white as well as in black families.

Further, incest is much more common than most people suspect. It may occur in as many as 1 in 10 families nationwide. Estimates are that 25 million American women have been sexually abused by their fathers, stepfathers, or older brothers.

It is not uncommon for brothers and sisters to have a sexual relationship. This type of sibling incest is estimated at five times more common that father-daughter incest, the most frequently reported type. Father-son incest is an increasingly reported act.

A girl sexually abused by her father usually suffers a great psychological burden. She frequently feels betrayed by her mother, subtly pushed into a sexual relationship with the father to take the mother's place. She may thus feel abandoned and isolated. She knows she is engaging in a secretive act that is wrong, and she may become controlling and manipulative toward her father. If sexual attention is the only sign of affection she receives from her father, she may be ambivalent about the experience and hence feel guilty.

Alcoholism and incest are often related. In many incestuous families, the father is an alcoholic. He may approach his daughter sexually only when he is drunk.

It is not unusual for a girl to feel that it is her obligation to submit in order to hold the family together. If she finally divulges her guilty secret, perhaps after 4 or 5 years of sexual victimization, she may indeed find that the family comes apart and that she herself is blamed.

A girl who has been sexually abused by her father is likely to suffer severe emotional repercussions. She may experience lifelong feelings of shame, self-loathing, alienation, and contamination. It is common for the victim of incest to sexualize all relationships and thus have trouble developing intimate friendships with both men and women. Her premature heightened awareness of sex tends to push her into extremes of sexual adaptation, such as promiscuity or prostitution. Sexual dysfunction in adulthood is common.

Incest is increasingly recognized as a problem that has its roots in the family and for which the whole family needs treatment. Counseling—available through county or state mental health departments or private agencies—can help the victim of incest avert lifelong repercussions. The family can be helped to understand the family dynamics that led to incest and how to be alert to them in the future. They require help in deciding whether the family might be able to remain intact and how the adult offender may be rehabilitated.

See also PEDOPHILIA; RAPE.

INFERTILITY (sterility) affects about 1 in 8 United States couples of childbearing age. A couple are considered infertile when pregnancy has not occurred after a year of normal sexual relations without the use of birth control.

If a couple have been trying unsuccessfully to conceive for a year, they should see a doctor. If the woman is over 35, she should see a doctor after 6 months. With treatment, perhaps half of infertile couples may be able to conceive.

For a pregnancy to occur, a man must produce and discharge an adequate number of normal, moving sperm cells. The woman must ovulate, expelling a normal egg from the ovary. This egg must pass through the Fallopian tubes, be fertilized by the sperm, carried to the uterus, and embedded there. Any disruption in this series of events can result in infertility.

The causes of infertility may lie in the man or woman or both. Both husband and wife need to undergo physical examination plus examination of their reproductive organs. For a doctor who specializes in fertility problems, a man should seek a board-certified urologist; for the woman, a board-certified gynecologist. Many hospitals have outpatient fertility clinics. Some physicians specialize in fertility problems.

Chronic medical problems may contribute to infertility. Endocrine disturbances, such as hypothyroidism, can affect fertility. Deficiencies in the hormones from the pituitary, adrenal, and reproductive glands may prevent conception. Often the trouble may be traced to chronic infections, malnutrition, overweight, anemia, and various metabolic problems.

Excessive smoking and use of alcohol may also affect fertility. Many of these problems can be fairly easily corrected, and pregnancy may result within a few months.

Severe emotional stress can slow or stop the flow of hormones, inhibiting ovulation or sperm production. Often the stress has to do with the prospect of pregnancy. Men and women may suffer from an unconscious fear of pregnancy and doubts about becoming parents.

Overwork and career tensions often contribute to the stressful situation. While emotional problems alone rarely cause infertility, they comprise an important element that needs to be considered in diagnosis and treatment.

Women may have more trouble conceiving in their thirties. A recent study reported in the *New England Journal of Medicine* suggests that there is a decrease in fertility in women after age 30.

Couples may be helped by altering habits surrounding intercourse. The couple should have intercourse at times of the month the woman is most likely to conceive. This is when she is ovulating (when her ovary has discharged an egg), about 2 weeks before her next menstrual period. In a woman with a 28-day menstrual cycle, ovulation would most likely occur at about 14 days. Couples are advised to abstain for 3 days before ovulation. A man who travels a lot may need to schedule his trips so that he will be home when his wife is ovulating.

A woman who wishes to become pregnant does well to lie in bed for a while after intercourse. If she immediately gets up and washes, she loses a lot of semen, thereby reducing her chances of conceiving.

A man might try having intercourse no more than every second or third day. More frequent intercourse can cause his sperm to be ejaculated before they have matured. Conversely, of course, excessively infrequent intercourse reduces chances of conception.

Sperm are damaged by excessive heat. A man should avoid taking long hot baths, which can interfere with sperm production. Men who work in extremely high temperatures sometimes need to change jobs to resolve an infertility problem.

A woman who would like to establish the probable time of her ovulation can keep a temperature graph. Just before ovulation, body temperature dips, then shows a rise that remains fairly stable until the next menstruation. Charted over several months, the graph can help a woman become familiar with her ovulatory pattern.

A woman can also find out when she is ovulating by checking the consistency of her vaginal mucus. Pre- and post-ovulatory mucus is described as sticky or tacky. Just before and at the time of ovulation, the mucus is thin, clear, and stretchy (see NATURAL FAMILY PLANNING).

The male-superior position of sexual intercourse, with the man on top and the woman below, is thought to be best for conception. This position allows the sperm to be delivered high in the cervical canal and makes it less likely that semen will leak out.

If a woman is told by her physician that her uterus is severely tilted, her best position for conception may be the knee-chest position: She rests on her knees and her chest, while her partner enters her from behind.

Blockage of the Fallopian tubes is a common cause of infertility. An obstruction may result from infection or the effects of gonorrhea. Emotional stress can cause the tubes to go into spasm.

Mildly blocked Fallopian tubes frequently open during the examination procedure. Several types of surgery are used—with varying degrees of success—to treat severely blocked tubes.

For women with severely blocked Fallopian tubes that cannot be surgically opened, physicians are experimenting with a new and promising procedure: the egg can sometimes be fertilized with the husband's sperm in the laboratory, then injected into the woman's uterus.

About 1 in 5 infertile women cannot become pregnant because they fail to ovulate. Or a woman may ovulate but produce an abnormal egg. In some cases, the uterus may not be properly prepared for accepting the fertilized egg because of an inadequate secretion of the female hormone progesterone. Tumors, polyps, or infections in the uterus may also prevent pregnancy. A small or tilted uterus alone will rarely keep a woman from conceiving.

For the woman who fails to ovulate, drugs that stimulate the ovaries to produce mature eggs are available. These drugs sometimes induce multiple ovulation and may lead to twins, triplets, or other multiple births.

Sometimes a woman has thick mucus obstructing the cervix, instead of the thin, clear mucus needed for conception. Or sperm may be repelled or destroyed by the chemical nature of the mucus or by bacteria or other organisms. Some women develop antibodies to their husband's sperm; in effect, they become immune to conception.

Cervical mucus hostile to sperm is usually treated with the female hormone estrogen. Or the husband's semen may be injected directly into the wife's uterus. Antibiotics are used to treat any bacterial infections that may be interfering with conception.

Men are responsible for or contribute to more than 40 percent of the cases of infertility. A common cause of male infertility is the inadequate development or quantity of sperm cells. A small number of men produce no sperm at all.

Mumps may have injured the testicles, destroying their ability to produce adequate sperm. Scars from venereal disease may be obstructing the tubes through which sperm pass.

Many infertile men have congenital defects in their reproductive system. Chronic infection of the prostate may be a cause of infertility. So may undescended testicles.

Men commonly confuse infertility and virility, considering a diagnosis of sterility a blow to their manhood. Actually, a sexually active male may have poor semen, while a man with little interest in sex can be perfectly fertile.

When a man has a low sperm count, it may be possible to achieve a pregnancy by obtaining a split ejaculate: the first part of the ejaculated semen—which has the highest number of active healthy sperm—is caught in a container and transferred directly into the cervical canal.

If the wife is fertile but the husband is not, the couple may consider artificial insemination in which a donor's sperm is injected into the woman's uterus. About 10,000 such infants are born in the United States yearly.

Trying to conceive may cause sexual problems. Having to make love by the calendar is likely to add tension to an already tense situation. Couples who are striving to conceive often lose sight of the pleasurable spects of lovemaking in focusing on achieving pregnancy. Decreased sexual desire, temporary impotence, and an inability to achieve orgasm are common problems among such couples. Both partners may bring guilt, blame, depression, inadequacy, or anger to the sexual relationship.

It is best for couples trying to conceive to be as spontaneous in their sex lives as they can manage. As far as possible, they should try to concentrate on the pleasurable process of lovemaking—rather than on its intended goal. Diagnostic tests—such as temperature charts—should be discontinued as soon as they have served their purpose.

Many couples find self-help discussion groups an excellent tool for venting their feelings about fertility problems. Group therapeutic counseling can also be beneficial. For information about support groups for infertile couples, contact Resolve, Inc., P. O. Box 2038, Washington, D. C. 20013-20838.

INHIBITED EJACULATION. See EJACULATION, RE-TARDED.

INTERCOURSE, PAINFUL (dyspareunia). Both men and women may find intercourse painful for a wide variety of reasons.

Among men, poor hygiene may be a cause of painful intercourse. For the uncircumcised, if the foreskin is not frequently retracted to remove smegma, inflammation and infection may occur. An unretractable foreskin is also likely to cause painful intercourse.

Allergic reactions to contraceptive creams, foams, or jellies, or to douching preparations may cause inflammation and blistering of the penis. Intercourse can be extremely painful, especially if the blisters break.

Vaginal infections can infect the man's penis and urethra, causing burning and itching after intercourse. Many venereal diseases can cause painful intercourse. Gonorrhea typically causes severe pain during and right after ejaculation.

Men who have sustained an injury to the penis may find intercourse painful. So may men who suffer from testicle inflammation or prostatitis.

Some men experience painful intercourse because of congenital malformations of the penis that make it curve. Acquired conditions such as Peyronie's disease (see entry) may also result in penile curvature and may make intercourse painful.

Men who suffer from tumors of the testicles or penis may find sex painful. Priapism, a persistent abnormal erection, frequently causes uncomfortable intercourse.

Conditions inside the woman's vagina may cause the man distress. The tail of a woman's IUD occasionally disturbs the tip of her partner's penis. Sometimes, a man finds intercourse uncomfortable because of the woman's improperly fitted or poorly positioned diaphragm.

If a woman's vaginal hysterectomy has been improperly repaired, the man can feel discomfort. Inadequate vaginal lubrication causes discomfort for both partners. Congenital malformations of the vagina may also do so.

A woman who suffers from the venereal disease lymphogranuloma venereum may have scarring, ulceration, and swelling of the vagina. Her male partner commonly feels a scratching sensation. Tumors of the vagina can cause a similar sensation. A few men are unable to tolerate normal vaginal secretions. The head of the penis may blister and peel after intercourse. In a small number of cases, psychological factors may account for painful intercourse.

INTERCOURSE, PAINFUL

Among women, vaginal infection is a common cause of painful intercourse. A burning sensation may persist after intercourse. Some venereal diseases cause sores that may make intercourse painful.

Women may find intercourse painful because of allergic reactions to chemical contraceptives, douche preparations, rubber in diaphragms or condoms, feminine hygiene sprays, or bubble bath. Some women have an allergic sensitivity to semen.

Intercourse may be painful when a woman's vagina does not adequately lubricate. Sometimes this is due to medication (such as the use of antihistamines) or the effects of aging. In most cases, however, the cause is insufficient sexual arousal before penetration.

Intercourse may also be painful because of congenital abnormalities or tumors of the genitals. Hymen problems, such as a rigid or thick hymenal ring, sometimes account for uncomfortable intercourse.

A woman who suffers from rectal or intestinal problems may find sex painful. So may a woman with urinary tract infection. Pelvic inflammatory disease or cysts on the ovaries may cause a woman to feel lower abdominal pain induced by the man's thrusting.

After childbirth, a poorly healed episiotomy may cause a sharp pain at the vaginal opening.

Endometriosis—in which tissue from the uterine lining occurs in abnormal places—commonly causes pain with deep thrusting. It is usually most severe just before menstruation.

Any irritation, scrape, or cut on the vulva or vagina is likely to result in painful intercourse. Abscesses often cause sharp, localized pain, with burning or searing.

In the case of women who suffer from vaginal spasm, penetration may be difficult or impossible, and there may be pain at the vaginal opening. This condition is usually thought to be psychogenic, but may be related to previous vaginal trauma. Psychological factors may also contribute to other causes of painful intercourse.

In view of the diverse causes of painful intercourse—some minor, others very serious—early and accurate diagnosis is most important. It is recommended that a man consult a urologist; a woman, a gynecologist.

See also ENDOMETRIOSIS; PENIS INFLAMMATION; PENIS INJURY; PENIS MALFORMATION; PRIAPISM; SEMEN ALLERGY; VAGINAL DRYNESS; VAGINAL INFECTION; VAGINAL SPASM; VENEREAL DISEASE.

ITCHING. See LICE; PINWORMS; SCABIES; VAGINAL IN-FECTION.

IUDs are small, flexible plastic or metal devices that are inserted into the uterus.

IUDs are 95-99 percent effective. With an intrauterine device (also called a loop, or coil), a woman is provided with automatic protection. Other than sterilization and the Pill, the IUD is the only means of contraception that does not require some preparation by the user. Hence, it will not interfere with sexual spontaneity.

The exact mechanism of the IUD is not fully understood. The IUD is thought to prevent pregnancy by causing changes in the endometrium (the lining of the uterus), possibly altering the time of month when it is ready to accept implantation. The IUD may also affect the Fallopian tubes by increasing the speed at which the egg is transported, hence preventing fertilization. It is also possible that the IUD is an abortive agent: if the egg does become fertilized, it may not be able to implant because of increased contractions of the tubes and uterus.

An IUD is a poor choice for a woman if she dislikes the thought of a foreign object inside her.

A woman who opts for an IUD has a choice of a plastic device (such as the Lippes Loop or Saf-T-Coil) or a copper-containing device (such as the Copper T and the Cu 7). Unlike plastic IUDs, which can stay in place indefinitely, a copper device must be replaced every two or three years.

IUDs come in several sizes. Smaller IUDs are suitable for women who have never been pregnant.

The insertion of an IUD requires a complete gynecological examination. The doctor opens the woman's vagina with a speculum, a duck-billed instrument, and prepares to insert the IUD with a tube-shaped introducer. Doctors prefer to insert IUDs during menstruation, when there is no chance of a woman's being pregnant and when insertion is most comfortable because her cervix is soft.

The IUD has a string tail that stays outside the cervix. If the string is reasonably long and silky, neither the woman nor her partner should feel it. At least once a week during the first month and after each period, she needs to check the string with her finger to see if it is still in place.

If the string disappears, or if she feels the device in her cervix, she needs to see her doctor. An expulsion is more likely to occur during menstruation, so she should check her sanitary napkins or tampons to make sure the IUD has not been passed out. If she expels one type of IUD, she may be able to retain a different type.

She should make an appointment to be reexamined within three months, preferably shortly after the first menstrual period following insertion. Annual examinations are usually sufficient after this unless trouble develops.

As a common reaction, she may experience increased discharge—watery, clear, mucuslike, and odorless—with the IUD. If she experiences an unpleasant odor from the discharge, it may be a sign of infection that she should report to her doctor.

A woman can expect some spotting of blood for a week or two after the IUD is inserted. Menstrual-type cramps and backache are also common. The first few menstrual periods after insertion are likely to be earlier, heavier, and longer. There may be spotting between periods. These discomforts tend to disappear after a few months.

To make her IUD nearly foolproof, a woman can use a vaginal spermicide for seven to ten days during the high-fertility midpoint between her periods. This is especially important during the first year, when most failures of IUDs occur.

Despite the IUD's advantages, it may cause side effects. A small percentage of users suffer severe cramps and bleeding from the IUD and must have it removed. After a while, some users complain of an unpleasant vaginal odor, possibly resulting from bacteria encrusting the IUD tail. This usually clears up quickly with a vaginal antibiotic.

It is estimated that IUD users are four times more susceptible to pelvic inflammatory disease (PID) than nonusers. Some physicians feel that a woman who has never been pregnant should not use an IUD if she has more than one partner, thereby increasing the possibility of PID that might lead to infertility or even the necessity for hysterectomy. Some doctors prefer not to recommend IUDs at all until after the woman has had at least one successful pregnancy.

Infections tend to occur during menstruation. If a woman experiences unusual pain during her period, she needs a prompt examination for pelvic inflammation. Often this is a relapse of a previous infection. Most such infections can be treated with antibiotics. Removal of the IUD is generally advisable.

An extremely rare complication of the IUD, occurring about once in every 2500 insertions, is perforation of the uterus—the device penetrates the uterine wall. In most instances there is no pain or any other symptom. Perforation of the uterus may be the result of faulty insertion. An IUD that has entered the abdominal cavity should be surgically removed.

If a woman has an abnormally small or irregularly shaped uterus, she may not be able to use the device. IUDs are generally not recommended for women who have had recent pelvic inflammatory disease, venereal disease, or other gynecological infections. The IUD is also ruled out for women who have severe anemia, heavy menstrual bleeding or abnormal uterine bleeding, cancer of the uterus, or fibroid tumors in the uterus. There are no known cases of uterine or cervical cancer resulting from the device. The IUD has no effect on fertility after it is removed, providing there were no complications while the IUD was in place.

See also CONTRACEPTION; PELVIC INFLAMMATORY DISEASE.

KIDNEY DISEASE (chronic renal failure) is twice as likely to affect men as women.

Sexual problems are common among kidney patients. In men, uremia from renal failure commonly causes decreased libido and difficulty in obtaining or sustaining an erection. As a result of lowered sperm production, men may be infertile.

Women frequently report difficulty in becoming sexually aroused and reduced frequency or intensity of orgasm. Some women are no longer able to achieve orgasm. Changes in the menstrual cycle are common. Ovulation may be irregular, and pregnancy is rare.

Underlying diseases leading to the chronic renal failure—such as diabetes mellitus, systemic lupus erythematosus, and tuberculosis—may adversely affect sexual functioning independent of kidney damage.

Hemodialysis often worsens sexual problems. When people are maintained on kidney machines, sexual functioning already impaired from chronic renal failure may further decline.

An estimated 7 out of 10 men on hemodialysis suffer from impotence and loss of sexual desire. These sexual problems result from a combination of physiological and psychological factors. Hemodialysis is often associated with chronic anemia, decreased levels of blood zinc, and increased levels of parathyroid hormone—any of which can contribute to impotence.

Patients on hemodialysis are often hypertensive. Medications to control their elevated blood pressure may contribute to potency problems. Hemodialysis itself is an exhausting procedure and may leave the patient too weak for intercourse several days a week.

Hemodialysis puts a great strain on marital relationships. The spouse of a hemodialysis patient is often burdened with extra responsibilities—which can result in exhaustion, resentment, and guilt. Family life is in turmoil. There is bound to be great anxiety about the illness. These stresses cannot help but affect sexual functioning.

Further, the patient on hemodialysis may be depressed—half of dialysis patients are. Depression typically diminishes libido and disturbs sexual functioning.

Men and women who undergo dialysis may become infertile. Women may stop menstruating. Men often experience a reduction in the quantity and quality of sperm.

Some men masturbate while undergoing the dialysis procedure. They report that masturbating helps relieve anxieties about hemodialysis. If they can do so discreetly, hospital personnel should have no objection.

Intercourse among couples in which one spouse is on maintenance hemodialysis is frequently either nonexistent or rare. Of 17 such couples in one study, 7 did not engage in intercourse at all, and 6 had intercourse less than once a month. Only 2 couples reported having intercourse at least once a week.

Counseling often improves family functioning and sexual communication. Group therapy with other dialysis couples may be the best approach. Medication can relieve depression.

After a kidney transplant some patients report improvement in sexual activity. Women are more likely than men to return to their preillness levels of sexual function.

Sexual desire frequently returns. Men may regain their fertility. Some women with kidney transplants have achieved pregnancy.

Transplant patients may suffer from sexual problems that are largely psychogenic. It is not uncommon for patients to fear that vigorous sex will dislodge the transplanted kidney. Most transplant patients have considerable anxiety that the kidney will be rejected. Economic insecurities and family difficulties may remain, adding to sexual problems. Body image disturbances plague some patients after surgery. So, too, steroid medication to suppress rejection may have negative sexual consequences.

For many couples, stress on the relationship persists after successful surgery. New expectations place demands on both partners. Both the patient and the spouse who has been the caretaker must make the transition to once again being lovers.

Support groups, couple counseling, and in some cases individual as well as conjoint marital therapy may be required.

See also STEROIDS.

KIDNEY TRANSPLANT. See KIDNEY DISEASE.

KLINEFELTER'S SYNDROME. See HORMONE DISORDERS.

LABIA. See FEMALE SEXUAL ANATOMY.

LESBIANISM. See HOMOSEXUALITY.

LICE (pediculosis pubis, pubic lice, crab lice, crabs) are transmitted during sexual intercourse or other close physical contact. The lice can also spread through contaminated clothing, bedding, toilet seats, and the like.

Sufferers usually experience intense itching. The crab louse is most likely to inhabit genital and anal hair. But it is also at home in the short hairs of underarms, eyebrows, eyelashes, chest, beard, and moustache. Scratching may result in infection or open sores.

The crab louse can be observed with a strong light and a magnifying lens. It looks like a graying flake of dandruff attached to the thick hairs close to the skin. Louse eggs (nits) are usually firmly attached to the base of the hairs. Unlike dandruff flakes, nits adhere when brushed.

Another clue to infestation: brown dustlike louse excreta on underpants. There may also be gray-blue marks, ¼ to 1¼ inches in diameter, on the trunk, thighs, and underarms—a systemic reaction to the lice's saliva.

Standard treatment is a hot soapy bath or shower, followed by an application of 1 percent gamma benzene hexachloride (Kwell) cream or lotion, which must be prescribed by a physician. An over-the-counter product—*Rid*—is also effective. Medication should be washed off after 12 to 24 hours, then reapplied if needed at weekly intervals. Bug spray, turpentine, or other home remedies should be avoided. These may cause reactions worse than the original problem. To prevent reinfection, clothes, bedding, and towels should be dry-cleaned or machine-washed. Possible infection in other family members and sex partners should be considered. Those who engage in sexual activity with many partners would be wise to be checked for gonorrhea, which often accompanies pubic lice under such circumstances.

LIVER DISEASE. See ALCOHOLISM; HEPATITIS.

LSD. See HALLUCINOGENS.

LUPUS. See SYSTEMIC LUPUS ERYTHEMATOSUS.

LYMPHOGRANULOMA VENEREUM (LGV) is a venereal disease marked by swelling and ulceration of the lymph nodes in the groin. Large masses form, pouring out pus.

The infection, caused by a member of the chlamydia group, may spread to the rectal area, with bleeding, discharge, and scarring. The first swellings appear seven to twenty-eight days after intercourse. Early treatment with tetracycline can prevent permanent damage, which includes scarring, rectal tightening, and abnormal enlargement of the genitals.

See also VENEREAL DISEASE.

MALE CLIMACTERIC. While men do experience some changes in sexual responsiveness and sperm production with aging, they go through nothing as dramatic and conclusive as the female's menopause. There is no such thing as a "male hormonal menopause."

A small number of men over 60 suffer what some clinicians have termed the "male climacteric syndrome." It is characterized by four or more of the following: listlessness; weight loss and/or poor appetite; decreased interest in sex, often with loss of potency; impaired ability to concentrate; tiredness; weakness; and irritability.

Such nonspecific symptoms may result from a variety of medical problems, which should be ruled out. These may include depression, severe chronic anemia, or cancer of the gastrointestinal tract.

Men suffering from this syndrome have a markedly subnormal testosterone level in the blood. Within two months after receiving testosterone replacement therapy, their symptoms significantly abate. Educating and reassuring the patient and his sex partner may also lead to a significant decrease in symptoms.

The terms male climacteric or male menopause have also been applied to a crisis that many men undergo sometime between ages 40 and 60—the so-called mid-life crisis. This is a time when a man may begin to feel that his sexual attractiveness is on the wane. He may re-examine his career, his relationships with family and friends, his worth as a human being. In an attempt to reassure himself about his sexual attractiveness, a man may seek out much younger women as sexual partners. Some men require counseling to help them through a mid-life crisis.

See also AGING; MENOPAUSE.

MALE MENOPAUSE. See AGING; MALE CLIMACTERIC.

MALE SEXUAL ANATOMY. The male external genitals include the penis, testicles, scrotum, and epididymis.

The *penis* consists of the glans, or head; the shaft, or trunk; and the bulb, or base. At the tip of the glans is the urethral opening (meatus), the external opening of the urethra, the tube through which urine and semen pass.

Within the penis are the *corpora cavernosa* and the *corpus spongiosum,* sometimes called the spongy bodies. These are composed of erectile tissue and fill with blood to bring about an erection.

The *two testicles* (or testes) are oval glands about 1½ inches long.

167

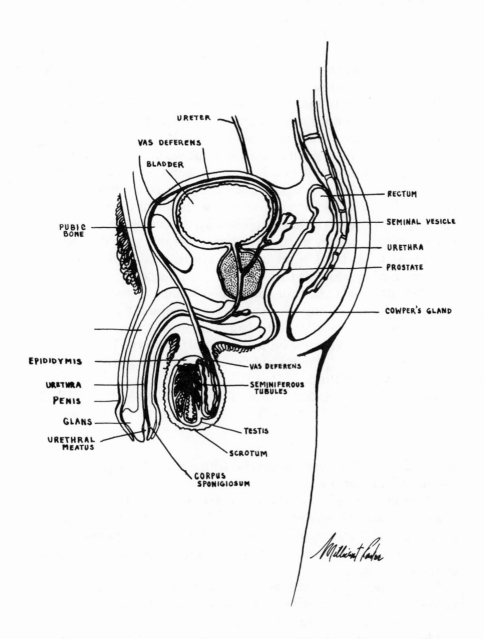

URETER

VAS DEFERENS

BLADDER

PUBIC
BONE

RECTUM

SEMINAL VESICLE

URETHRA

PROSTATE

COWPER'S GLAND

EPIDIDYMIS

URETHRA

PENIS

GLANS

URETHRAL
MEATUS

CORPUS
SPONIGIOSUM

VAS DEFERENS

SEMINIFEROUS
TUBULES

TESTIS

SCROTUM

Within the testicles are the *seminiferous tubules,* which produce the *sperm* cells, the male reproductive cells. At ejaculation, as many as 300 million sperm cells are contained in the *semen.* Besides sperm, semen contains fluid secreted by several reproductive organs.

The testicles are also involved in the production of the male hormone testosterone. Each testicle (or testis) lies in a thin sac of skin called the *scrotum.* In addition to the testicle, each scrotum contains an *epididymis.* This is a small tube which is part of the channel through which sperm pass during ejaculation. The epididymis stores sperm prior to ejaculation, and contributes some fluid for semen.

The male's internal genitals consist of the vas deferens, the seminal vesicles, the ejaculatory ducts, the prostate, and the Cowper's glands.

The *vas deferens* are a pair of tubes that form a continuation of the epididymis. Each vas deferens connects with one of the two *seminal vesicles,* convoluted pouches that join with the end of the vas deferens to form the *ejaculatory ducts,* two short tubes that pass through the prostate gland and end in the urethra. The seminal vesicles secrete a fluid containing nutrients that support sperm metabolism.

The *prostate* is a chestnut-sized gland located directly below the bladder and surrounding the urethra. Just behind the prostate is the rectum, the lowest portion of the large intestine.

The prostate provides the bulk of the fluid for semen. The *Cowper's glands,* two pea-sized glands just below the prostate, contribute a small amount of seminal fluid.

See also FEMALE SEXUAL ANATOMY; ORGASM; PROSTATE ENLARGEMENT; PROSTATITIS.

MARIJUANA is closely associated with sex in the minds of many of its millions of users in America.

The drug, derived from the *Cannabis* plant, is often reported to enhance sexual feelings and experiences. Some researchers feel that this effect is due to heightened suggestibility caused by marijuana. People may experience alterations in time perception and in the perception of tactile sensations.

But such perceptions may be misleading. The marijuana user may perceive an enhancing effect on sex, but in reality sexual performance may be unchanged or even impaired.

The Masters and Johnson Institute interviewed 800 men and 500 women aged 18 to 30 about the effects of marijuana on sex. Four out of five users of both sexes reported that the drug enhanced the enjoyment of sex for them.

But further questioning revealed that their impression of improved sexual functioning was more imagined than real. For most men reported that marijuana did *not* increase their sexual desire. Nor did it increase the firmness of their erections or make it easier to get or maintain erections. The drug did not give them a greater degree of control over ejaculation or intensify their orgasms.

Women reported similar experiences. The drug did *not* increase sexual desire or the amount of vaginal lubrication. Nor did it heighten orgasm or induce multiple orgasm.

Rather, the men and women reported, the drug's sex-enhancing qualities can be attributed to a greater degree of relaxation and an increased sense of touch. In some people who are normally very anxious or guilty about sex, the drug may enhance the experience by relaxing inhibitions and loosening their ordinary restraint.

Rigorous scientific studies of the effect of marijuana on sex have been scanty. Animal studies show that the drug affects the endocrine system and can interfere with the production of sex hormones. Marijuana—or its active ingredients—decreases copulation in male rats and inhibits sperm production. It decreases circulating levels of the male sex hormone testosterone and reduces the weight of some sex organs. In female rats, the drug interferes with sex hormone levels and egg production.

Similar effects have been observed in some human marijuana users. Some studies have shown decreased circulating testosterone levels in healthy young men who are chronic users. Very high single doses produce similar results.

While lower levels of testosterone may not have any sexual effects, some men who are chronic users show decreased sperm production. Some suffer impotence; their potency returns within a few weeks after discontinuing the use of marijuana.

Among women, the studies suggest, marijuana may also affect sex hormones and reproduction. One study of women in the 18-30 age group who were heavy smokers (four times a week) showed shorter menstrual cycles and a higher incidence of cycles without ovulation. In rhesus monkeys, whose reproductive process closely resembles that of humans, those with moderate-to-heavy doses showed a high incidence of miscarriage or stillbirth—40 percent of all conceptions as compared with 8 percent in the control group.

Taken as a whole, the accumulating data from animal and human studies suggest that chronic heavy use may have adverse effects on the glands and hormones involved in growth and reproduction.

MASOCHISM. See SADOMASOCHISM.

MASTECTOMY (breast amputation for breast cancer) is usually experienced as a devastating loss. It is almost inevitably equated with a loss of femininity and sexual attractiveness.

Several different types of mastectomy are now being performed. The treatment of choice has been the *radical mastectomy*—removal of the involved breast, the underlying pectoral muscles, and the lymph nodes under the arms.

Modified radical mastectomy is increasingly accepted as an alternative to radical mastectomy. In this operation, the breast and underarm lymph nodes are removed, but pectoral muscles are left intact. The cosmetic result of this surgery is far superior, and the cure rate for the two operations is nearly identical.

In the simple mastectomy, the breast is removed and a sampling of the underarm lymph nodes is taken. This and other less radical procedures (such as the lumpectomy) are still considered controversial.

In many relationships, breast stimulation plays an important role in erotic play. Some women respond intensely to breast stroking and sucking. Breasts also serve as a source of sexual arousal for the man.

Moreover, our culture puts a great emphasis on the breast as an erotic symbol. Thus, it's no wonder that loss of a breast is so often followed by fear, anxiety, and depression—and great concern about possible sexual rejection.

Yet the impact of mastectomy on a woman's sexual life is rarely addressed. In a Masters and Johnson Institute pilot study, only 4 of 60 women reported having had discussions prior to the surgery about how it might affect their sexuality. Many of the women wanted such counseling but assumed it was inappropriate since no health professionals brought up the topic.

Many mastectomy patients report that the surgery has a negative effect on their sex lives. In the Masters and Johnson study, frequency of intercourse generally decreased. Women who frequently initiated intercourse before surgery rarely did so afterward. The frequency of

172

breast stimulation as a part of sexual activity declined. (Stimulation of one breast has the same sexual effect as stimulation of both.)

Mastectomy patients need an opportunity to ventilate their anxieties. Typically, a woman's greatest concern is fear of rejection by her husband or other sex partner. She may also fear his pity, which implies a belief that she has indeed been diminished.

It is usually wise for the husband to view the surgical scar as soon as possible after the surgery. Once over this hurdle, many couples find sexual adjustment easier.

A single woman may feel that her ability to attract men has now been destroyed. She may wonder how and when to inform a potential sex partner about her mastectomy.

After mastectomy, women may hesitate to resume intercourse. Some women prefer to have intercourse in the dark because they are uneasy about their sex partner's viewing the amputation. Others may keep brassieres on or wear clothing on the upper part of the body.

In general, some studies show, those older women who had little psychological investment in their breasts and understanding husbands or close friends to confide in adjusted fairly easily to mastectomy. Younger women for whom an active sexual relationship was important, who considered breast size essential for attractiveness, and who perceived husbands or friends as unsupportive, had a difficult time adjusting.

One invaluable resource for both emotional and practical support is the Reach to Recovery program of the American Cancer Society. Volunteers—mastectomy patients themselves—visit the patient shortly after her operation. During two visits, the volunteer discusses such things as exercises, cosmetic devices, and clothing adjustment, and lets the patient ventilate her concerns. More information about this program can be obtained by contacting the local division of the American Cancer Society.

Sexual intercourse can resume as soon as the incision is well-healed and painless. There is little chance of damaging the surgical site during lovemaking. The couple may use any comfortable position. The male-superior position, with the man supporting himself on his hands and knees, may initially be the safest and most comfortable for the woman. Another preferred position is for both partners to lie on their sides facing each other, with the woman's surgical site away from the bed. Other acceptable positions are the female-superior or the reverse female-superior—with the woman astride the male facing his feet.

173

It is wise for a mastectomy patient's husband or other sex partner to be involved in discussions about sexual problems—with a nurse, social worker, psychotherapist, or other health professional.

To a great extent, of course, a couple's sexual adjustment after mastectomy depends on the relationship they shared before the operation. But sexual problems can beset even the most loving couple.

A loving, supportive husband may have unexpected reactions to the surgery. He may feel revulsed and repulsed. Trying to hide these feelings may make him feel guilty and resentful. Or the wound may provoke anxiety about mutilation, causing him to withdraw unconsciously from sexual relations.

One common scenario: a mastectomy patient sees herself as mutilated and repulsive. She thus withdraws from sexual contact with her husband. He, feeling rejected, eventually stops approaching her, helping to perpetuate a cycle of misunderstanding. Couples should make a great effort to speak freely to each other about sex-related concerns. Discussions with a counselor or physician may also prove helpful.

Reconstructive surgery of the breast is an option for many women with modified radical mastectomy and for some with radical mastectomy. A silicone gel prosthesis can be implanted, and an areola constructed of tissue from the vulva. Some surgeons save the nipple with this in mind. In some cases, the reconstructive surgery can be done at the same time as the mastectomy. Many women report increased feelings of self-esteem and sexual desirability after reconstructive breast surgery.

See also BREAST CANCER; CANCER.

MASTURBATION (self-stimulation) is giving oneself sexual pleasure.

Among children. Infants begin to explore their bodies at a few months of age, discovering fingers, toes, hair. A male infant who by chance grasps his penis may find it pleasurable to fondle. Frequently, he will fondle it to erection.

Girl infants are less likely to find their genitals during body exploration. Yet it has been observed that baby girls as young as a few months exhibit orgasmlike reactions by pressing and/or rubbing their legs together.

Preschoolers often discover the pleasure of rubbing a soft doll or other soft toy against their genitals. Young children may masturbate when they are tired, bored, or irritable.

The activity will not harm the child either physically or mentally. The only injury that could result is the child's feeling guilty and anxious if a parent reacts by scolding or punishing.

Most infants who masturbate soon stop the practice. A bored child can be distracted with a game or toy. If an older child masturbates in public, the parent can explain: "To touch your body and know how good it feels is okay. But, like other bodily functions, it's the sort of thing people do in private." If the child is discreet, there is rarely reason to discuss the matter further.

Infrequently, a child's masturbation can be a sign of psychological problems requiring professional assistance. One clue is where the child masturbates. An emotional disturbance is suggested by persistent masturbation in public places or in plain view of other members of the family or of authorities at school. The more flaunting or provocative a child's masturbation, the more likely it is that the child is using it as a weapon against parents.

Pinworms or genital infections can cause itching or burning, leading to a great deal of genital touching that appears as compulsive masturbation. Such organic problems should be ruled out before psychological remedies are considered.

Masturbation is a form of sexual experience shared by 95 percent of men and 80 percent of women. Kinsey reported those—and the following—statistics by way of demonstrating the universality of masturbation as a sexual outlet.

Males generally begin masturbating in early adolescence—80 percent start before age 15. Usually a boy is told how to do it by friends. His first ejaculation typically comes from masturbating.

Most females learn how to masturbate not from friends but accidentally while exploring their genitals. Women tend to begin masturbating at a later age than men.

Mythical damage. The supposed injuries caused by masturbation in large part are imagined punishments.

Masturbation is a religious offense, and Judeo-Christian teachings are imbued with prohibitions against it. The condemnation is rooted in the crime of Onan (Gen. 38:9). Under the Biblical law of levirate marriage, Onan was required to wed his late brother's wife and give her a child. However, Onan performed coitus interruptus and spilled his semen on the ground. Angry, God slew him.

The ancient Jews evolved a blanket prohibition against the "vain effusion" of semen. The severity of Onan's punishment caused the offense to be considered of paramount gravity. Violators were cast out of the community with the anathema, "Your hands are filled with blood."

To discourage masturbating, it was forbidden for a man to sleep on his back. He was not to sleep alone in a room. Unless his wife was available for intercourse, he was not to hold his penis while urinating. He was not to eat fat meats, cheese, eggs, or garlic—foods that were thought to heat the body, and thereby cause commission of the crime.

There is no escaping a taboo so strong, not even by the irreligious. In the last century, physicians believed they were offering a scientific view of masturbation. "It's not a sin," they declared. "It's a disease."

Doctors developed drugs, devices, even surgery for its "cure." Medical journals and texts advised corrosives and cauterizing to blister the penis or clitoris. Diagrams showed how to pin or wire the foreskin or labia. Difficult cases called for clitoridectomy or castration. Even today medical journals still carry letters from doctors who use words like "slavery" to describe masturbation.

Since we live in a society where many view masturbation as a sin—and where many believe it has severe physical and emotional consequences as well—it is no surprise if many people experience emotional conflicts over masturbating. In many instances, the major harm coming from masturbation is the guilt it generates.

Is masturbation a symptom? Since masturbation is so charged with emotion, it has a complex relationship with mental health, sometimes as a symptom of an underlying disorder.

Some suffer from the rare syndrome of compulsive masturbation. In such cases, the masturbation is but one sign of a state of chronic anxiety. Compulsive masturbation is accompanied by a pervasive feeling of nameless dread. The masturbating is mechanical, driven, and essentially joyless.

The problem is not the masturbation but the pressures that lead to the compulsion. A physician should be consulted. Tranquilizers can usually help relieve anxiety while counseling gets at its cause.

Some people feel depressed after masturbating. They may actually be experiencing the state of relaxation that generally occurs after orgasm. If they are apprehensive, they may misread this enjoyable psychophysical response as a defect.

Depression may follow masturbation if it is associated with failure. To the extent that masturbation is a solitary act, it brings into sharp focus any unfulfilled yearnings. It may be a painful reminder of what a person is missing or is afraid to see.

In the pleasurable excitation of masturbating, some people feel temporary release from their strivings for love, friendship, health, beauty, and money. But an orgasm must inevitably be followed by disappointment when these questions return as painful as ever.

Yet another function masturbation can serve is the relief of nonsexual tensions. Masturbation can have a sedative effect; it may help bring on sleep.

In marriage, masturbation is another sexual option. It can provide a change in sensation from the orgasm of intercourse. Among married couples, masturbation is probably more frequent during periods when one spouse is absent, ill, or otherwise sexually unavailable.

In some marriages, masturbation—mutual or solitary—may substitute for intercourse during the wife's menstruation or after the birth of a baby. A man who is prone to quick ejaculation may find that masturbating before intercourse may help to delay climax. Masturbation may provide an option in a marriage where one partner prefers greater sexual frequency than the other. A wife may masturbate if her husband suffers from impotence or premature ejaculation. A frequently impotent man may find that masturbation is his most reliable sexual outlet.

In marriage, masturbation may be evidence of underlying problems if it is frequent, habitual, or preferred to sexual intercourse. A disorder exists only if the attempted solution is unsatisfactory to one or both partners.

In some marriages, masturbation is accompanied by many negative feelings. The person who masturbates may feel guilty and frequently resentful toward the partner who has "driven" him (or her) to it. The nonmasturbating partner may feel rejected and unloved or feel that the masturbating partner is "abnormal."

Married couples may retreat from each other sexually and practice masturbation when there are grave problems in the marriage. It is a common expression of hostility for one partner to withhold sex and flaunt this by masturbating in view of the other.

Professional counseling, possibly including sex therapy, may be required to help resolve such problems.

Masturbation sometimes causes medical problems. Rubbing can irritate the genitals. A water-soluble lubricant often avoids soreness. A man with a tight, chronically irritated foreskin may need circumcision.

Someone who uses a vibrator or artificial penis may get an allergic reaction from its plastic, rubber, or metal parts. Those who have suffered contact dermatitis elsewhere on the body, as from nickel jewelry or rubber gloves, should be especially wary.

Some people may masturbate by using a vibrator in the anus, then applying it to the genitals. Unless it is washed after being in the anus, they are in danger of infection from rectal bacteria and parasites.

It may likewise be dangerous to insert foreign objects into body orifices. Ice cubes or various types of vegetables—cucumbers, celery sticks, carrots—can scratch and irritate the vaginal walls.

A sharp or breakable object is especially hazardous. If it perforates to the abdomen, peritonitis may develop. It is often fatal. A sharp object that cannot be easily retrieved is a medical emergency.

Medical realities. Masturbation has never been proven to impair health or fertility in any way—no matter how often it is practiced. Physiologically, there is no such thing as "excessive" masturbation. A person generally stops when it is no longer pleasurable and resumes when it is enjoyable again—all safely and without further consequences.

Masturbation will not cause acne, warts, hairy palms, gonorrhea, epilepsy, bedwetting, consumption, insanity, or blindness. In healthy people, it will not decrease initiative; it will not sidetrack the desire to meet members of the opposite sex.

The exploration of the body and its sexual sensations can be a healthy growth process, leading to enhanced sexual responsiveness. Conversely, a resistance to masturbation may result from excessive control and inhibition that can cause sexual difficulties.

Heightened sensation. If masturbation has been among an individual's sexual outlets, Kinsey found, he or she is more likely than non-masturbators to enjoy heightened sexual sensation in marriage.

Masturbation is likely to provide a more intense physiological response than intercourse, for an individual can concentrate entirely on personal sensations, without having to think about a partner. Thus, masturbators can experience self-centered activity, supported by fantasies and unencumbered by any consideration of another person's feelings, desires, or pleasure.

With masturbation, a person often has less self-consciousness about letting go. Masturbation-techniques are limited only by human imagination. Males commonly masturbate by lubricating the shaft of the penis and making rhythmic motions up and down. Many men and boys also manipulate their testicles, anus, nipples, and any other parts of the body they find a source of erotic sensation.

Most women and girls masturbate by stimulating the clitoris and labia with a hand or some other object. The index and middle finger of the dominant hand are most often used. Some women can reach orgasm merely by pressing their thighs together or by rhythmically contracting and releasing the vagina.

Many women achieve orgasm by breast stimulation alone. The hands or other objects (such as vibrators) may be used to stimulate the whole breast or just the areola-nipple portion. The breasts may be pressed against a surface such as a bed.

Masters and Johnson have found that the intensity of the first three phases of sexual response is greater during masturbation than during intercourse. During orgasm, masturbation produces stronger spasmodic contractions of the pubococcygeus muscle in the pelvis of the female. In the male, masturbation causes greater contractions of the urethra and prostate. These contractions heighten orgasmic sensations.

By concentrating only on their own sexual demands, without the distraction of a partner, women are often able to remain at a high level of sexual tension—going from one climax to another, without allowing the sexual tension to diminish below the plateau level. Note Masters and Johnson: "Usually physical exhaustion alone terminates such an active masturbatory session."

A woman may be able to reach orgasm more quickly during masturbation than during intercourse. She controls the pressure and rhythm. She knows exactly what she enjoys—and she can avoid what she finds distracting or painful.

The knowledge about her body that a woman gains through masturbation also makes her better able to communicate her preferences to her partner. Doing so is a sign that she takes responsibility for her own sexual pleasure—rather than assuming that her partner will intuitively know what she likes and dislikes.

This lifts a burden that many males have carried throughout their married lives. If the man did not receive sexual satisfaction, it was his own fault. If his partner was not satisfied, that was his fault as well.

179

When each partner accepts his or her own ultimate responsibility for sexual satisfaction, the relationship benefits.

MEDICATIONS sometimes have a negative effect on sexual functioning.

The sexual side effects of drugs vary greatly from person to person—depending on such factors as absorption rate, body weight, metabolism rate, length of use, excretion rate, dosage, and interactions with other drugs.

It is thus impossible to predict with any reliability precisely what sexual consequences a particular drug will have. All sexual side effects of medications are *potential*, rather than expected or invariable. Further, little systematic research has been done on most drugs and their effect on sexuality; while interest has increased in recent years, this is still a largely unexplored area.

Some physicians regularly prescribe medications without being aware of their possible sexual sequelae. Others may withhold information about potential sexual side effects because they fear that suggestible patients will have sexual reactions they might not otherwise have had. Physicians also may worry that patients will not take the medication if they are concerned that it will impair their sexual functioning.

On the other hand, many patients suffer from sexual difficulties without realizing that they may be due to medication. The best course is for a doctor to be forthright and say, "Certain sexual problems sometimes occur with people taking this drug. Please let me know if this happens with you, so I can make an adjustment in your medication."

Patients should realize that drug-related sexual effects are often reversible. In many instances they can be minimized or eliminated by changing the drug or reducing the dosage. Sometimes, sexual problems can be relieved by substituting a combination of drugs for a single drug.

Patients should not assume that a sexual difficulty is necessarily caused by a drug they are taking. The difficulty may be due to such other factors as illness, marital difficulties, the effects of aging, alcohol, or social drug use. The problem should be discussed with the physician.

Following is a chart of common medications and their potential sexual side effects:

DRUG

Class of drug	Generic name	Major brand names	Major uses	Possible effects on sexuality
Amphetamines	methamphetamine	Ambar	Appetite suppressants, central nervous system depression, hyperactivity in children, narcolepsy	Impotence; decreased sexual desire, particularly in women
		Desbutal		
	chlorphentermine	Pre-Sate		
	fenfluramine	Pondimin		
	diethylpropion	Tenuate		
		Tepanil		
	dextroamphetamine	Amodex		
		Benzedrine		
Antidepressants	*Tricyclic antidepressants:*			
	imipramine	Tofranil	Endogenous depression	Delayed ejaculation; failure to ejaculate; erectile difficulties; delayed orgasm in women
	desipramine	Norpramin		
	amitriptyline	Elavil		
	protriptyline	Vivactil		

DRUG

Class of drug	Generic name	Major brand names	Major uses	Possible effects on sexuality
	MAO inhibitors:		Depressive states	Delayed ejaculation; impotence; failure to ejaculate; delayed orgasm in women; increased sexual desire possibly due to improvement of depression
	tranylcypromine	Parnate		
	phenelzine	Nardil		
	pargyline	Eutonyl		
	isocarboxazid	Marplan		
	lithium	Lithonate	Manic depression	Impotence
		Lithane		
Antilipemics	clofibrate	Atromid-S	Hyperlipoprotein-emia (or excess of lipoproteins in the blood)	Impotence
Antihypertensive	phenoxybenzamine	Debenzyline	Preoperative man-agement of pheochromo-cytoma, a tumor of the sympathetic nervous system; treatment of	Impotence; inhibited ejaculation; "dry" ejaculation

Generic	Brand	Use	Side effects
			excessive tachycardia (rapid heartbeat)
methyldopa	Aldomet	Hypertension (high blood pressure)	Inability to maintain erection; failure to ejaculate; decreased sexual desire in both men and women; in rare cases, milky breast discharge
guanethidine	Ismelin	Hypertension	Failure to ejaculate; in rare cases, erectile dysfunction; decreased sexual desire; decreased emission of semen; "dry" ejaculation
reserpine	Demi-Regroton, Diupres, Rau-Sed, Sandril, Ser-Ap-Es, Serposil	Hypertension, Huntington's chorea	erectile dysfunction; bizarre erotic dreams; depressive psychosis

183

DRUG

Class of drug	Generic name	Major brand names	Major uses	Possible effects on sexuality
	propranolol	Inderal	Hypertension, angina, migraine, abnormal heart beat, familial (hereditary) tremor	Erectile dysfunction
		Inderide		
	clonidine	Catapres	Hypertension	Erectile dysfunction
Antiparkinsonians	levodopa	L-dopa	Parkinsonism	Increased sexual desire
		Dopar		
		Larodopa		
Antipsychotics	thioridazine	Mellaril	Schizophrenia, depression, itching, nausea, various neurological disorders	Inhibition of ejaculation; failure to ejaculate; erectile dysfunction; changes in sexual desire; decreased sperm count; failure to menstruate; milky breast discharge; breast development
	chlorpromazine	Thorazine		
	chlorprothixene	Taractan		
	promazine	Sparine		
	prochlorperazine	Compazine		
	trifluoperazine	Stelazine		

Class	Generic	Brand	Indications	Effects
	triflupromazine	Vesprin		in male; decreased serum testosterone
	perphenazine	Trilafon		
	fluphenazine	Prolixin		
	haloperidol	Haldol		
	piperacetazine	Quide		
Antispasmodics	methantheline	Banthine	Peptic ulcer, functional gastrointestinal disturbances	Impotence
	propantheline	Pro-Banthine		
	isopropamide	Darbid		
Anxiolytics, sedatives, hypnotics	chlordiazepoxide	Librium	Anxiety, sexual dysfunction, muscle spasm, insomnia, medication before surgery or medical procedures	Increased and decreased sexual desire; failure to ejaculate; failure to menstruate; milky breast discharge; decreased testosterone levels
	diazepam	Valium		
	oxazepam	Serax		
	meprobamate	Equanil		
		Miltown		

DRUG

Class of drug	Generic name	Major brand names	Major uses	Possible effects on sexuality
Cytotoxics, cancer drugs	*Alkylating Agents:* busulfan	Myleran	Cancer, psoriasis	Failure to menstruate; decreased sperm production; sterility; decreased sexual desire; impotence
	carmustine (BCNU)	BiCNU		
	chlorambucil	Leukeran		
	cisplatin	Platinol		
	cyclophosphamide	Cytoxan		
		Procytox		
	dacarbazine	DTIC-Dome		
	lomustine (CCNU)	CeeNU		
	mechlorethamine hydrochloride	Mustargen		
	melphalan	Alkeran		

pipobroman	Vercyte
thiotepa	Thiotepa

Antimetabolites:

azathioprine	Imuran
cytarabine	Cytosar
floxuridine	FUDR
fluorouracil	Adrucil
hydroxyurea	Hydrea
mercaptopurine	Purinethol
methotrexate	Mexate
thioguanine	Lanvis

Antitumor Antibiotics:

bleomycin sulfate	Blenoxane
dactinomycin	Cosmegen

187

DRUG

Class of drug	Generic name	Major brand names	Major uses	Possible effects on sexuality
	doxorubicin hydrochloride	Adriamycin		
	mithramycin	Mithracin		
	mitomycin	Mutamycin		
	procarbazine hydrochloride	Matulane Natulan		
Diuretic	spironolactone	Aldactone	Hypertension, congestive heart failure, fluid retention, potassium sparing effects with other diuretics	Impotence; failure to menstruate; male breast development
	Thiazides:			
	hydrochloro-thiazide	HydroDiuril	Hypertension, congestive heart failure, fluid retention, kidney failure	Impotence
	chlorthalidone	Hygroton		

Ganglionic blockers	mecamylamine	Inversine	Hypertensive crisis	Erectile dysfunction; failure to ejaculate; decreased emission of semen
	trimethaphan	Arfonad		
Steroids	*Estrogens:*			
	chlorotrianisene	Tace	Oral contraceptives, replacement therapy in deficiency or menopause, osteoporosis, painful menstruation, prostate cancer, suppression of breast milk	Depression; increased sexual desire in women; decreased in men
	dienestrol	Dienestrol Cream		
	diethylstilbestrol	DES		
		Synestrin		
	esterified estrogens	Amnestrogen		
		Climestrone		
		Estratab		
		Estrofol		
		Evex		
		Menest		

189

Class of drug	DRUG		Major uses	Possible effects on sexuality
	Generic name	Major brand names		
	estradiol	Aquagen		Decreased sexual desire in both men and women
		Estrace		
		Progynon		
	estrone	Estrovarin		
Progestins:				
	dydrogesterone	Duphaston	Oral contraceptives, painful menstruation, endometriosis, infertility	
		Gynorest		
	ethisterone	Lutocylol		
		Progestolets		
	norethindrone	Norlutin		
	norgestrel	Ovrette		
	progesterone	Lipo-Lutin		
		Progelan		

190

Progestasert

Progestilin

Progestin

Androgens and Anabolic Steroids:		Replacement for deficiency, postpartum breast milk suppression, anemia, osteoporosis, contraceptive in men, breast cancer	Increased sexual desire in men and women; in women, masculinization, with hair growth, failure to menstruate, enlargement of clitoris
danazol	Cyclomen		
	Danocrine		
ethylestrenol	Maxibolin		
stanozolol	Winstrol		
testosterone	Android-T		
	Androlan		
	Andronaq		
	Dura-Testrone		
	Histerone		

DRUG

Class of drug	Generic name	Major brand names	Major uses	Possible effects on sexuality
		Testo-Med		
		Testrone		
Miscellaneous	trimeprazine	Temaril	Itching	Inhibition of ejaculation; male breast development; milky breast discharge; menstrual irregularities
	disulfiram	Antabuse	Alcoholism	Impotence in rare cases
	aminocaproic acid	Amicar	Hemophilia, coagulation problems	Ejaculation may be inhibited

See also AMPHETAMINES; AMYL NITRITE; APHRODISIACS; COCAINE; DEPRESSION; HALLUCINOGENS; HEROIN; IMPOTENCE; MARIJUANA; STEROIDS; TRANQUILIZERS.

MENOPAUSE is the permanent cessation of menstruation. Thereafter, a woman can no longer bear children.

There is a 2 to 5 year span—called the perimenopause—during which a woman's body undergoes the physiological changes leading to menopause. A woman is considered to have reached menopause when she has not menstruated for 6 months to a year. The period thereafter is known as the postmenopause.

Most women experience menopause between 44 and 53 although it may begin as early as 36 or as late as the 60s. The age when a woman began menstruating—be it early or late—gives no clue as to when she will reach menopause. There is some evidence that smoking precipitates earlier menopause.

Normal sex urges remain after menopause. In one respect, menopause may even enhance the enjoyment of sex in later years: many couples welcome release from the possibility of pregnancy.

Since the ovarian cycle is unpredictable during menopause, it is wise to use contraception for a year after the last menstrual period. A woman taking birth control pills will continue to menstruate.

A woman often recognizes the onset of menopause by changes in her menstrual pattern. She may have a heavier or lighter flow than normal. She may completely miss periods. These indicate that changes are taking place in her endocrine system.

As a woman approaches menopause, her ovaries produce less and less estrogen, the principal female sex hormone. Ovulation stops, and the production of the hormone progesterone abruptly declines. The pituitary reacts by attempting to stimulate production of these hormones. The intricate glandular balance of the body goes into turmoil, attempting to achieve a new balance.

The most common symptom of the menopause is the hot flash or flush. Flashes consist of a feeling of heat that spreads over the body. A woman may have visible blushing which starts at her chest and rises up to her neck, face, and head. From there it may spread all over her body. She may alternately sweat and shiver. If she takes her temperature during an episode, she will find that she does not have any real fever.

193

These hot flashes may start from 2 to 5 years before the actual menopause and may continue for several years thereafter. They may occur by day or night. Some women experience as many as 20 or more a day and may be awakened by this sensation several times a night.

The hot flashes are caused by the sudden excessive dilation of small blood vessels close to the skin's surface. This results in more blood being brought to the area, which produces increased local heat and activates sweat glands. The instability of the blood vessels is believed to be due to changes in the production of various hormones in the female sexual cycle, spurred by the decrease in estrogen production.

Other symptoms associated with menopause: dizziness, weakness, insomnia, nervousness, headache, backache, and vaginal dryness. A woman may experience sharp changes in blood pressure, heart palpitations, and stomach upsets. There may be weight gain or redistribution of weight, and breast pains. Brown patches may develop, especially in areas exposed to light, such as in the face, hands, arms, or legs. A woman may also experience a recurrence of skin allergy.

After several months or a year or more, a woman's body adjusts to the hormonal changes, and the menopause-related symptoms disappear. Many women report a new vigor and excellent health after menopause.

It is dangerous for a woman to assume that all physical symptoms are related to menopause. This is the time of life when diabetes, cancer, high blood pressure, and other diseases are most likely to occur.

All symptoms should be reported to a doctor, especially heavy bleeding between periods, and any vaginal bleeding after periods have stopped. After menopause, women should continue to have periodic pelvic examinations.

Anxiety and depression often afflict menopausal women. Emotional stress may result from a multitude of changes, in addition to menopause, facing a woman at this time of her life.

A woman who devoted her life to raising a family suddenly finds herself with grown children who do not need her. A career woman may find herself pressured by younger women. A woman may find herself depressed by wrinkles and overweight in a culture that puts a premium on youth. She may be depressed by the realization that she will never again be able to bear children. Depression characteristic of the menopause usually comes on gradually and with no history of previous depression.

For a woman who was anxious before menopause, the psychological implications and annoying physical symptoms of menopause may lead to severe psychological symptoms. A small number of menopausal women develop a depressive psychosis called involutional melancholia.

A hormonal deficiency may sometimes contribute to a woman's depression and can be relieved by estrogen therapy. Psychotherapy may be needed for a woman suffering severe emotional disturbances.

Some women, on the other hand, go through the menopause without any negative psychological symptoms. These are usually women who have managed other stressful situations effectively.

Estrogen replacement therapy can help relieve menopause symptoms but can be hazardous. It is helpful in the treatment of hot flashes and atrophic vaginitis and may possibly help osteoporosis, a bone problem often accelerating at menopause.

But *The Medical Letter* advises against routine prescribing of estrogens for menopausal women. There is strong evidence that women on long-term estrogen therapy have a five to eight times greater chance of developing endometrial (lining of the uterus) cancer. A woman who is considering estrogen replacement therapy is advised to first undergo examination of the endometrium to detect cancerous or precancerous changes. Some doctors recommend an annual examination.

Estrogen may also accelerate existing cancers, increase the size of uterine fibroid tumors, and aggravate cysts in the breasts.

Estrogen therapy may cause irregular vaginal bleeding. Some doctors control this by purposely producing bleeding by prescribing progesterone in addition to estrogen. (This combination is thought to be safer than estrogen alone.) This results in artificial menstrual periods. Other side effects of estrogen therapy may include nausea, fluid retention, breast tenderness, gall bladder disease, abnormal blood clotting, and elevated blood pressure.

A younger woman who has had both ovaries surgically removed will go through a so-called artificial menopause. Hormone therapy is usually called for.

The Food and Drug Administration recommends that women should not be on estrogen therapy if they have cancer of the uterus or breast (except in some special cases where the drug is used to treat breast cancer). Estrogen should also be avoided when a woman has undiagnosed vaginal bleeding, clotting in the legs or lungs, or a history of stroke, angina, or heart attack.

In view of the risks of estrogen replacement therapy, women should use it only for the relief of severe menopausal symptoms—in as small a dose as possible for the shortest possible time.

See also AGING; MENSTRUATION.

MENSES. See MENSTRUATION.

MENSTRUATION (period) is the monthly shedding of the uterus from puberty until menopause. Menstrual flow contains blood plus cells and tissue from the degenerating layers of the endometrium, the lining of the uterus. Each month, the uterus prepares for a potential fertilized egg. If pregnancy does not occur, some endometrial layers are expelled in the menstrual flow.

Without being aware of it, most people have been affected by centuries of religious teaching about this bodily function.

Leviticus (15:19-32) proclaims that a woman who has an "issue" of blood shall be put apart for seven days. "And everything that she lieth upon in her separation shall be unclean." Whoever touches her or her bed or other objects shall be "unclean" until evening and must wash himself and his clothes. After seven days have elapsed, and a woman's period is over, she is commanded to bring sacrifices to a priest, who "shall make an atonement for her before the Lord for the issue of her uncleanness."

Sages interpreted these passages into a host of intricate rules governing conduct during menstruation. A husband who has intercourse with his wife while she is menstruating is punishable with being "cut off from his people," declares one code of Jewish law; she is subject to the same punishment. To touch her in a caressing manner is punishable with whipping. "He is not permitted to come in contact with her, even with her little finger."

Even contact far short of intercourse was denied a couple during menstruation. They should not hand anything to each other. They should not eat at the same table, unless their dishes are separated by a physical barrier. They may not fill each other's cup. If she is sick, he is not permitted to attend her "even without touching her unless in a case of extreme necessity." It is proper for her to wear special clothes during the days of "her uncleanliness" so that both of them "be ever reminded that she is menstrually unclean."

Among Orthodox Jews, intercourse remains forbidden during menstruation. But such beliefs still linger even among the irreligious. Many women have heard superstitions about menstruation: a permanent wave will not take on a menstruating woman; her plants will die; her meat will spoil; her bread will fail to rise. Further, menstruation is often presented to young girls in a negative way: is it "the curse," a time when a woman is "unwell."

It is thus no wonder that sex during menstruation retains an aura of taboo. Despite widely held fears, menstrual blood is not "unclean" or in any way harmful to either partner. Nor is it likely that coital thrusting will force menstrual fluid into the Fallopian tubes.

Some couples find intercourse especially enjoyable during menstruation. The very moist vagina can enhance sensation, and the woman's pelvic vasocongestion (engorgement with blood) may heighten her orgasm. This, in turn, may relieve her menstrual cramps, which are in part caused by the vasocongestion. Many women experience an increase in sexual desire at the start of a period.

Couples may be put off by the potential messiness of intercourse during menstruation. If a woman uses a diaphragm, she can insert it before intercourse. Towels under the couple can protect the bedding. And, because many a man is put off by the prospect of finding his penis blood-smeared, it is a good idea to keep a damp washcloth near the bed.

It is unusual for a woman to conceive during her menstrual period. But it is not impossible. If a woman's menstrual period is very long, ovulation may begin even while the last traces of blood are showing, and there is a chance that sperm could survive long enough for fertilization to take place. It is thus wise to use contraception after the first few days—or, better still, all during the menstrual period.

Hygienic care. Many women consider tampons more esthetic, and less messy, than sanitary napkins. A young woman who uses tampons is likely to become acquainted with her reproductive anatomy and to become comfortable about touching her genitals. Thus, use of tampons often promotes a girl's positive adjustment to menstruation. Moreover, the use of tampons tends to gradually stretch the hymen, which will ease first intercourse.

To ease insertion of a tampon, a water-soluble lubricant like K-Y is recommended. The tampon is inserted at an angle toward the small of the back, not upward. Deodorant tampons may cause an allergic reaction and should be avoided. For days of heaviest flow, a tampon plus a minipad may afford the best protection.

To avoid the slight possibility of toxic shock syndrome—a new disease frequently associated with tampon use—it is wise for a woman to change tampons frequently and to alternate the use of sanitary pads and tampons in the course of each menstrual cycle. Pads can most easily be used at night. Tampons made with cotton, rather than synthetics, should be used.

Most girls begin menstruating between 11 and 13½. But it is not uncommon for girls to start as early as 9 or as late as 17. Most girls get their first periods 2 to 3 years after their first breast buds appear. A physician should check a girl who is not menstruating 4 years after her breast budding. Women normally continue to menstruate at monthly intervals until menopause—except during pregnancy or sometimes while breastfeeding.

A girl who is 18 or over and has never menstruated requires a physician's attention. Her failure to menstruate, termed primary amenorrhea, may be due to a large number of physiological conditions, many of them genetic. She may have an obstruction of the cervix or the vagina. She may have been born with a deformed or missing uterus, or her ovaries may be malfunctioning. She may be suffering from hormonal deficiencies. Psychological stress may also play a part.

Secondary amenorrhea, in which a menstrual pattern becomes established, then ceases for 6 or more cycles, may also be due to a variety of conditions. Often, it is due to weight loss. Young girls suffering from anorexia nervosa, in which self-starvation causes acute loss of weight, almost always stop menstruating. Otherwise normal young women who are extremely lean—gymnasts, ballet dancers, track-team members—often fail to menstruate. This is so because at least 10 percent of a female's body weight must be fat, or her estrogen will be too low for her to ovulate and menstruate.

In almost all such cases, the amenorrhea is reversible. Soon after gaining the proper amount of weight, a woman will begin menstruating. It may take some months for her periods to become regular. She should use contraception even if she is not menstruating, since ovulation can occur unpredictably.

Emotional stress is responsible in a large number of cases of secondary amenorrhea. The condition may also be due to an ovarian cyst or a pituitary or ovarian tumor. Other possibilities include diabetes, hyperthyroidism, heart disease, and tuberculosis.

Premenstrual tension affects some women. Irritability just before the period begins is believed to be caused by an imbalance of hormones or a retention of sodium and water. There is almost always striking relief once the period begins. Women who suffer more serious psychological problems before menstruation—such as severe anxiety and depression—should consult a doctor.

Severe menstrual pain (dysmenorrhea) requires a physician's attention. Many women experience a dull ache in the lower abdomen and mild cramping. These menstrual cramps usually abate after the start of the flow.

Aspirin can help relieve cramping pain. Its anticoagulant properties may help prevent clots some women are prone to. Such clots are expelled by painful contractions of the uterus.

Some women, however, have menstrual pain so severe that it interferes with their daily activities. Agonizing cramps may keep them in bed for one or two days every month. There may also be nausea, vomiting, diarrhea, headache, lethargy, fainting, and flushing.

In some women with severe menstrual pain, no physiological problems can be found. Emotional factors, such as fear or the feeling of disgust, often contribute to menstrual discomfort. Severe cramps may be caused by excessive production of prostaglandins, which cause the uterine muscles to contract.

Dysmenorrhea is usually treated with analgesics to relieve the pain. Physicians may also prescribe hormones and tranquilizers. The drugs ibuprofen (Motrin) and mefenamic acid (Ponstel) can often relieve the menstrual pain by inhibiting prostaglandin production.

In some cases, dysmenorrhea may be due to organic causes. The condition may be caused by uterine abnormalities.

Dysmenorrhea can also result from infections, tumors, or pelvic inflammatory disease. Polyps, endometriosis, and IUD problems may account for the condition.

Excessive menstruation (menorrhagia) also requires a doctor's care. A woman should be concerned if pads or tampons changed several times a day do not afford protection, or if the menstrual blood forms into large clots. Emotional stress may precipitate excessive menstruation. But menorrhagia can be caused by hormone disorders and abnormalities of the reproductive organs. It may also be due to polyps, inflammations, and diseases such as rheumatic fever.

A woman should also see a doctor if she bleeds between periods.

A good diet aids in the proper functioning of the menstrual cycle. Supplemental intake of vitamin B6 (pyridoxine) and vitamin C has helped some women overcome menstrual bloatedness by serving as a natural diuretic. Some women have responded to increased intake of minerals such as calcium prior to the onset of menstruation to promote rhythmic—as opposed to spastic—contractions of the uterus.

See also ENDOMETRIOSIS; MENOPAUSE; PUBERTY; VAGINAL BLEEDING.

MENTAL RETARDATION afflicts over 6 million people in this country. Between 100,000 and 200,000 babies born each year are mentally retarded.

A child who is mentally retarded has unusual difficulty in learning and in coping with the problems of everyday life. Depending on the degree of retardation, he may seem just mildly slower than other children, or he may be incapable of doing virtually any tasks for himself. He may have problems of speech, vision, and hearing and impairments of motor coordination.

While there is no cure, most retarded children can be helped through special classes and vocational training centers. Most states have clinics for diagnosis and evaluation of mentally retarded children. Counselors can advise whether the child should be placed in an institution or raised at home, now the recommendation in most cases.

No specific cause can be found for most mental retardation. Sometimes the retardation is due to birth defects such as Down's syndrome or hydrocephalus. About half the children born with cerebral palsy are mentally retarded. Metabolic problems such as PKU can lead to mental retardation.

Retardation has also been traced to diseases in the mother during early pregnancy, such as rubella, meningitis, or toxoplasmosis. Syphilis in the mother and Rh disease can also result in retardation.

A mother in poor health and poor nutrition runs a higher than average risk of having a retarded infant. Retardation is often accompanied by premature delivery and low birth weight. Problems during delivery can injure the child's brain, causing retardation. Some kinds of retardation are due to hereditary factors.

Sexuality of the mentally retarded. Two myths are associated with sex and retarded people: One is that they are completely asexual. The other is that they are highly sexual and likely to be impulsive, or even dangerous, in their sexual advances to other people. Since the range of mental retardation is so great, these stereotypes are meaningless.

Little scientific research has been done on sex and the mentally retarded. In general, retarded people, like others, usually have a need for a relationship with another human being. Touching and physical closeness are very important. Sexual contact is often an important factor in their lives.

In institutions, the sexual needs of retarded people have generally been denied. The retarded are usually segregated by sex and almost completely deprived of contact with the opposite sex. In such situations, close physical relationships with same-sex members often develop. These may or may not include genital sexual activity. Masturbation may also be used as a sexual outlet.

It is important for mentally retarded children to be taught about sex in language they can understand. The information may have to be repeated many times before it is comprehended.

For many retarded adolescents, learning social skills is an important part of sex education. They should also be taught under what circumstances certain kinds of sexual behavior are acceptable. Retarded girls should learn how to avoid being sexually exploited. Retarded children can often be taught that masturbation and other sexual behavior should be conducted in privacy. For the mentally retarded in institutions, provision should be made for privacy for sexual purposes.

Contraception often presents a problem. Some conditions that cause mental retardation are also associated with infertility. The majority of the mentally retarded, however, are considered fertile but would be unable to care for a child. The choice of an appropriate contraceptive is thus of primary importance.

For most retarded women, the IUD is considered the best contraceptive. Some mildly retarded women may be able to use oral contraceptives. A small number of mildly retarded men may be able to use condoms effectively—but most cannot do so reliably.

Sterilization procedures—such as tubal ligation and vasectomy—

provide maximum protection against pregnancy and may be a solution for many retarded men and women. But since the retarded are usually not judged competent to give informed consent to such procedures, sterilization remains a difficult legal and ethical problem.

MESCALINE. See HALLUCINOGENS.

METHADONE. See HEROIN.

MICROPENIS. See PENIS SMALLNESS.

MIGRAINE. See HEADACHE.

MISCARRIAGE. See ABORTION.

MOLLUSCUM CONTAGIOSUM is a viral disease of the skin and mucous membranes.

The virus is spread through direct sexual contact, or through close physical contact such as wrestling. Epidemics sometimes occur in institutions.

Most cases of molluscum contagiosum occur among young adults and children. The virus usually appears as multiple flesh-colored or pearly pimples with a depression in the middle of each. The most common sites are the trunk and genitals. Eyelids are often affected. Pimples may also occur on the mucous membranes of the mouth or rectum.

The disease is usually self-healing. Although the virus may persist for many months, in most cases it will spontaneously disappear. When a diagnosis is made, treatment consists usually in removing the pimples with a sharp curette, a scraping device. Bleeding is easily controlled with direct pressure, and anesthesia is not required.

See also VENEREAL DISEASE.

MULTIPLE SCLEROSIS is a neurological disorder that typically strikes young adults between 20 and 40. It is characterized by periods of exacerbation and remission which leave cumulative damage. Over many years, the victim usually becomes progressively more disabled—although mild forms of the disorder are becoming increasingly recognized.

Sexual dysfunction is a prominent symptom. Other signs of multiple sclerosis may include visual impairment (sudden blindness, double vision, eye pain, tremors), sensory alterations, bladder dysfunction, paraplegia, and speech disturbances.

Sexual disturbances may be temporary in the early stages of the disease if there is a remission. As the disease progresses, however, the sexual impairment is likely to become permanent.

In men, impaired potency is common. They may get erections but not be able to sustain them. Some suffer from premature ejaculation or retarded ejaculation. Men with potency problems may benefit from the use of a surgically implanted penile prosthesis.

Women with multiple sclerosis often report a decreased interest in sex and problems in attaining orgasm. If vaginal dryness makes intercourse painful, a woman can use a lubricant such as K-Y jelly.

Both men and women may find sexual activity difficult because of motor disturbances, such as weakness, difficulty in movement, and spasms.

Sensory disturbances may similarly interfere with sexual functioning. Genital numbness is common. A man with multiple sclerosis may be capable of erection, but not be able to feel his penis in his partner's vagina. A woman may have no feeling in her vagina or clitoris. Conversely, there may be a hypersensitivity in the genitals which may make sexual activity unpleasant. If the oversensitive area is in the external genitals, a topical anesthetic cream applied before intercourse may relieve the problem.

Psychological disturbances may contribute to sexual dysfunction. Most people assume that a diagnosis of multiple sclerosis inevitably means eventually being confined to a wheelchair, helpless. Anxiety, depression, and fear are common reactions, and usually interfere with sexual functioning.

Group counseling benefits many multiple sclerosis patients. Therapists can help patients adjust to the uneven course of the disease and cope with progressive disability.

Patients should bear in mind that neurologic symptoms—including sexual responsiveness and functioning—fluctuate in the course of the disease. Sexual capacity may return during a remission.

If the ability to have intercourse is permanently lost, couples can experiment with other ways of gratifying each other sexually, such as manual or oral stimulation.

The cause of multiple sclerosis is not known, nor is there a cure. Some patients respond well to therapy with adrenocorticotropin.

See also IMPOTENCE; ORAL SEX; PRIAPISM.

NATURAL FAMILY PLANNING (rhythm method, fertility awareness). All four methods of natural family planning involve calculating the fertile days within the menstrual cycle and abstaining from sexual intercourse for a certain number of days.

Calendar Rhythm Method. This method is based on three assumptions: 1) that ovulation (release of the egg from the ovary) occurs some 12 to 16 days before the beginning of menstruation; 2) that the egg survives for 24 hours; and 3) that sperm are capable of fertilizing an egg for a period of 48 to 72 hours.

The calendar method is based not on signs and symptoms of ovulation, but rather on mathematical calculations involving the length of at least 6 to 12 previous menstrual cycles.

Once a woman observes the longest and the shortest cycles, she then calculates that her fertile period begins on the 18th day before the end of the shortest likely cycle. The last day of the fertile period is calculated by figuring the longest cycle minus 11 days.

Thus, a woman whose menstruation begins every 28 to 32 days must abstain from intercourse on the 10th through the 21st day after her period starts. (She subtracts 18 from 28 to get 10; then subtracts 11 from 32 to get 21.)

The disadvantage of this method is that there is always the possibility that there will be a change in the length of the menstrual cycle, thus resulting in miscalculation of the fertile time. The calendar method, although practiced by many couples for many years as the only form of natural family planning, is now considered obsolete.

Basal Body Temperature Method. This method involves charting on a temperature graph the changes in body temperature, which may indicate fertile and infertile days.

While this method cannot identify exactly when ovulation occurs, a slight rise in temperature usually means that a woman has started to ovulate. Before ovulation, her temperature is likely to range from 96.6 F to 98.2 F. During and after ovulation, the range is 97.6 F to 99.2 F. A woman should not engage in intercourse until 3 consecutive days after this temperature rise.

The temperature is best taken by a basal body temperature thermometer, which is calibrated in tenths of a degree, and measures temperatures between 96 and 100 degrees Fahrenheit. Temperature can be taken either orally, rectally, vaginally, or under the arm—but it should be taken at the same site and at the same time daily, preferably in the morning on awakening.

Fluctuations in temperature may be influenced by illness, stress, drugs, alcohol, and sleeplessness. These factors should also be noted on the temperature chart.

Ovulation Method. This method is based on the changes that occur in the mucus of the cervix in the course of a woman's menstrual cycle.

Also called the vaginal mucus method, it requires a woman to examine her cervical mucus for changes. Following her menstrual period, the mucus will be scant. After that, she will have a sticky discharge. As she draws closer to ovulation, her mucus increases in amount. A clear, slippery mucus that looks like egg white and can be stretched between the fingers indicates the peak period in which she can conceive. About the fourth day after ovulation, the mucus becomes cloudy and sticky and reduces in volume or dries up entirely. This shows her safe period for intercourse, which lasts until her next menstrual period.

When a woman first begins the method, she must abstain from sexual intercourse for one month. This allows her to become aware of how her cervical mucus changes in the course of her menstrual cycle. During her menstrual flow and the first phase of her cycle, she should abstain every other day, so that she can accurately identify the fertile mucus when it occurs. After she identifies the fertile mucus, she should wait 4 days before engaging in intercourse.

Sympto-Thermal Method. This is a combination of methods to help a woman identify her time of ovulation. She can observe changes in her cervix and cervical mucus; basal body temperature changes; and secondary signs of ovulation which may include increased sexual desire, breast tenderness, abdominal bloating, vulvar swelling, slight pain in the ovary, and some vaginal spotting.

At the time of ovulation, the cervix thickens and increases its slippery mucus discharge. It also elevates and dilates slightly. A couple can observe and record these and other signs of ovulation and should abstain from intercourse until a few days after these changes occur.

As with all forms of birth control, natural family planning has its advantages and disadvantages.

Among its advantages are: freedom from chemicals and foreign bodies; increased fertility awareness and greater knowledge of the anatomy and physiology of the female body; increased communication and cooperation required of both partners to use these methods successfully; increased use of other options for sexual expression and affection when intercourse is prohibited.

Among its disadvantages are: interference with the spontaneity of sexual desire and fulfillment; a sense of programming sexual response on infertile days; the need to record consistently and accurately the changes in bodily signs.

Failure of the methods can occur if a woman misreads or misunderstands the various changes. They may be complicated by such factors as illness, a change in climate, changes in geographic location, and stresses such as family problems, job tensions, and school exams.

A couple considering family planning methods requires instruction in their use. Further information, counseling, and instruction may be obtained by consulting the following:

Human Life and Natural Family Planning Foundation
1511 K Street, NW
Washington, DC 20005

National Family Planning Federation of America, Inc.
1221 Massachusetts Avenue, NW
Washington, DC 20005

Human Life Foundation
1776 K Street, NW
Washington, DC 20006

Couple to Couple League
3621 Glenmore Avenue
Cincinnati, Ohio 42511

See also CONTRACEPTION.

NEPHRITIS. See KIDNEY DISEASE.

NGU. See NONGONOCOCCAL URETHRITIS.

NOCTURNAL EMISSION (wet dream) is the spontaneous discharge of semen during sleep.

A boy's first nocturnal emission usually occurs when he is between 12½ and 14 years old. Before this age, a boy should be told by his parents to expect nocturnal emissions, that most boys experience them during adolescence, and that they are normal and harmless. Without such preparation, emissions may produce guilt and anxiety. Boys also need to be told that some males never experience nocturnal emissions and that this is likewise normal.

Parents should stress that the experience of nocturnal emissions is extremely variable. For some males, emissions occur periodically throughout adulthood. For others, emissions occur only during adolescence. Some adolescent boys have emissions nearly every night; others at intervals of weeks, months, or years.

Emissions are thought to occur as a result of erotic dreams. Without any penile manipulation, erection occurs. Orgasm and ejaculation may cause some males to awaken briefly. Others may have no recollection of the dream or the orgasm. The only evidence of the emission may be stained pajamas or sheets.

NONGONOCOCCAL URETHRITIS (NGU) presents urinary symptoms like those of gonorrhea but without the gonorrhea bacteria.

Victims may suffer burning, frequent urination, and a whitish discharge. NGU now accounts for over half the male urethritis cases seen at VD clinics.

The most frequent culprits are chlamydia trachomatis organisms, bacterialike parasites that multiply within human cells. Symptoms may appear one to three weeks after contact—which can occur either through sex or in contaminated swimming pools. An inflammation of the eye—"swimming pool conjunctivitis"—also may be picked up in unchlorinated pools.

In adults, the genital infection is apparently not serious. In babies, it may cause an eye infection similar to that caused by gonorrhea, but usually less destructive. If untreated, the baby may develop pneumonia. Chlamydia infections are curable with tetracycline and other antibiotics.

See also VENEREAL DISEASE.

NURSING. See BREAST FEEDING.

NYMPHOMANIA. See HYPERSEXUALITY.

ORAL CONTRACEPTIVE. See PILL, CONTRACEPTIVE.

ORAL SEX is the sexual stimulation of the genitals by the mouth. It is practiced by a large number of adults, both heterosexual and homosexual.

Cunnilingus (from the Latin, meaning "to lick the vulva") is oral stimulation of the female's genitals. Women vary widely in their preferences for types of oral stimulation. Many women enjoy having their genitals kissed or sucked. Some enjoy having the partner's tongue explore their vaginal lips and vaginal opening. Women often find oral stimulation of the clitoral hood especially satisfying. The clitoris itself is more sensitive and may require lighter pressure.

Some women prefer cunnilingus to all other forms of sexual stimulation and regularly reach orgasm in this manner.

Fellatio (from the Latin *fellare,* meaning "to suck") is oral stimulation of the male's genitals. The partner may lick the penis or move the tongue around the head of the penis. Many men find the frenulum— the fold on the lower surface of the head of the penis—particularly sensitive to oral stimulation. Rhythmic sucking of the penis is a mode of oral stimulation preferred by many men. Sometimes, the testicles or perineal area may also be licked or sucked.

Cunnilingus and fellatio simultaneously—also referred to as 69, or in French *soixante-neuf*—refers to oral-genital contact between two people at the same time.

Some couples engage in cunnilingus, fellatio, or both simultaneously, as a prelude to sexual intercourse. For others, oral sex is an alternative form of sexual expression. It is often employed in homosexual relationships.

For people with medical conditions that preclude sexual intercourse, oral sex is often one of the few sexual options left to them. Many such couples report an extremely gratifying sexual relationship through mutual oral sex.

Attitudes toward oral-genital contact vary widely. For some people it is an acceptable and mutually pleasurable form of sexual expression.

Other people consider oral sex perverted and loathsome. For some, it is unacceptable because of its association with homosexuals. Others regard the genitals as "dirty" and "smelly." Some reject oral sex on moral or religious grounds. It is not unusual for people to see the performance of oral sex as an act of submission or degradation.

These cultural taboos and religious prohibitions against oral sex are reflected in our laws. In many states, oral-genital contact, even among people who are married to each other, is illegal and punishable by imprisonment. Such statutes make criminals of a large portion of the population.

The practice of oral sex has increased considerably in the last few decades. When Kinsey did his study in 1948, 45 percent of males said they had performed cunnilingus. By contrast, one recent study shows that of males under 35 with 13 years of formal education, as many as 75 percent say they practice cunnilingus. Of males over 35 with the same education, 66 percent report engaging in the practice. The percentage of males with high school educations who practice cunnilingus has also risen substantially.

Similarly, Kinsey found that 60 percent of married couples had participated in oral sex. Now, a variety of studies show the percentage to be considerably greater. Among young college-educated couples, as many as 90 percent may practice oral sex.

Oral sex can be the focus of sexual conflict in a relationship. One or the other partner may want to impose the practice on the other. Some people have particular preferences or dislikes related to oral sexual practices. It is important for such concerns to be frankly communicated to the sex partner.

It is not unusual, for example, for a woman to enjoy fellatio, but still have an aversion to her partner's ejaculating into her mouth. Although she may permit it, fearing that refusal may upset him, she may nevertheless feel used and resentful. It is important for her to tell her partner about her aversion and assert her wish that he withdraw before ejaculation. (Those who prefer to swallow the semen should be reassured that this practice is safe.)

Oral sex can transmit disease. Some people believe they can avoid venereal disease by engaging in oral sex instead of intercourse. In fact, a number of venereal diseases can be transmitted orally. Gonorrhea and syphilis infections of the throat can be transmitted through fellatio.

Viral diseases, including herpes simplex and cytomegalovirus infections, can be transmitted by cunnilingus. The presence of a cold sore or any sore on the mouth should rule out oral sex.

Pathogens causing gingivitis or a tooth abscess may be passed through cunnilingus, causing vaginal infection. Strep throat or staphylococcal glossitis may give rise to bacterial inflammation of the vagina. Some lesbian women develop inflammations of the vulva as a result of allergies to their sex partners' lipstick or other cosmetics.

There is no danger for a male in performing cunnilingus after the woman has inserted contraceptive cream. Such products are nontoxic even if ingested orally. Some people may find contraceptive jelly—also safe—somewhat more palatable; it is faintly minty.

A small number of couples experiment with flavored creams, sometimes including whipped cream, as part of the orogenital experience. There is likely to be no danger in doing this. But couples should be warned that introducing alcoholic beverages into the vagina can pose a medical hazard. They are rapidly absorbed, damaging the delicate mucous membranes of the vagina.

Cunnilingus can be fatal for a pregnant woman. Extreme care must be taken not to blow any air into the vagina. If the woman is pregnant, this can cause a fatal air embolism. Bubbles of air blown forcefully into the vagina pass through the open cervix into the dilated uterine blood vessels surrounding the fetus. Air in the blood stream can be carried to the lungs or the brain, where it blocks circulation, causing coma and, usually, death.

The practice of blowing air into the vagina should be avoided, particularly if there is the least possibility that a woman could be pregnant.

See also VENEREAL DISEASE.

ORCHIECTOMY. See TESTICLE REMOVAL.

ORGASM is the climax of the sexual response cycle, characterized by release of muscular tensions throughout the body, release of blood from engorged blood vessels, and rhythmic contractions of the genitals. It is a total body response, usually lasting only a few seconds.

From a biological point of view, no matter what part of the body is stimulated before or during orgasm, the same physiological responses occur (i.e., pelvic congestion, muscular contractions). This is true even though not all orgasms feel the same to a woman and may be reached in different ways—through intercourse, oral stimulation, masturbation, breast stimulation, direct clitoral stimulation, etc.

Direct or indirect stimulation of the clitoris usually brings about orgasm in the female. The sole known function of the clitoris is to receive and transmit sexual pleasure. The lower third of the vagina also has extremely sensitive tissue capable of producing orgasm.

The clitoris is richly supplied with nerves. If a woman is not sure where her clitoris is, she can study an anatomical illustration, then explore with a mirror and her hand.

During vaginal intercourse, the thrusting of the penis moves the inner lips (labia minor) down at the entrance of the vagina. These lips come together above the vaginal opening and the urethra to form the hood of the clitoris. This rhythmic motion can stimulate the exquisitely sensitive head of the clitoris.

However—and this is not widely realized—the action of the penis alone frequently is not enough to lead to an orgasm. Additional stimulation, usually with a finger, is very often needed for orgasm.

The cycle of female sexual response can be divided into four parts. The first is the excitement phase, characterized, among other things, by the moistening of the vagina and the erection of the nipples of the breasts.

The plateau phase follows: the rate of breathing increases. Muscle tension is heightened. The tissues around the vagina swell. The clitoris becomes erect and the inner lips change from pink to deep red.

Orgasm is the third phase, consisting of rhythmic muscular contractions of the vagina. In the fourth phase, resolution, the body returns to its preorgasmic condition.

Some women are capable of having multiple orgasms. Masters and Johnson demonstrated that some women experience from 5 to 20 recurrent orgasms, sometimes more, "until physical exhaustion terminates the session."

Multiple orgasms are more apt to occur during masturbation than during intercourse. This is because few men can maintain an erection long enough to provide an opportunity for multiple orgasms in their partners.

Preliminary evidence suggests that women may also be able to experience orgasm through stimulation of the Grafenberg spot (see entry).

In the male sexual response cycle, the excitement phase is characterized by erection of the penis. It increases in size because blood engorges chambers of spongy tissue within it. With the filling of these chambers, the penis both stiffens and rises in its angle of protrusion from the man's body.

Erection comes about from a reflex action. Stimulation of the penis and other genital zones triggers the pudendal nerves. These run to the lower spinal cord, where a nerve center relaxes muscles in the walls of arteries supplying the penis. The arteries expand, causing an increased amount of blood to rush into the spongy tissue. The blood compresses penis veins, sustaining the erection until the artery muscles contract and restrict the blood inflow.

A man also may be sexually aroused by sights or thoughts that stimulate pleasure centers of his brain. These connect to the reflex center in his spinal cord. His erection reflex can be activated by non-sexual stimuli as well: a full bladder, straining during defecation, stress while lifting. An erection can develop in less than 10 seconds.

During sexual arousal, a man also undergoes a tensing and thickening of the skin of his scrotum. The scrotal sac flattens toward his body. His spermatic cords shorten, pulling in his testicles. The nipples of his breasts may become erect because of the contraction of muscle fibers.

In the plateau phase, sexual tension becomes more intensified. The head of the penis may enlarge slightly at its base. A few drops of fluid, from the Cowper's glands, may emerge before ejaculation. This fluid contains live sperm and can cause pregnancy.

Testicles reach an expansion of about 50 percent above their normal size. They are pulled to their maximum into the scrotal sacs. The full elevation of the testicles marks the point of no return—orgasm is imminent.

In the orgasmic phase, the man ejaculates. This takes place in two stages. Before orgasm, fluid containing millions of sperm cells from the man's testicles collects in sacs near his bladder. These structures—the seminal vesicles and the ampullae—contract rhythmically, expelling their contents into the urethra. At the same time, his prostate gland contracts, providing most of the fluid in his semen. A bulb at the base of his penis expands to receive the semen. These changes provide his first sensations of orgasm.

In the second stage, this bulb and his penis contract—projecting his semen out under great pressure.

In the resolution phase, the man's body gradually returns to normal. Then he undergoes a "refractory period," during which he cannot be sexually aroused or have another erection. This period can be extremely short—some young men achieve 3 orgasms in 10 minutes— but it more typically lasts many minutes.

See also FEMALE SEXUAL ANATOMY; GRAFENBERG SPOT; MALE SEXUAL ANATOMY.

ORGASM, SIMULTANEOUS. See SEXUAL DYSFUNCTION.

OSTEOPOROSIS is a gradual decrease in the density and strength of bone tissue. The bones become brittle. It is an extremely common condition of the elderly.

The vast majority of osteoporosis sufferers are over 60 years of age. Women—particularly those who have passed menopause—are especially vulnerable.

Osteoporosis most commonly begins with the bones of the spine. These thinned bones are compressed, or mashed down, by the weight of the body, resulting in low-back pain, a round-back deformity, and loss of height. The person's capacity for physical activity progressively decreases.

Eventually, the bones of the spine collapse. As the disease advances, other bones become thinned, particularly those of the pelvis, arms, and legs. Osteoporosis is responsible for many of the fractures that disable elderly people.

Many people suffer from osteoporosis without being aware of it. The bones are neither painful nor tender until they have become so weak that they break.

Osteoporosis is thought to be due to a combination of factors. In the normal adult, old bone is continually reabsorbed by the body and new bone is produced to replace it. In the osteoporotic, however, the normal breaking up of bone continues, while the regeneration of bone slows.

This is thought to result in part from the aging person's decreasing production of the hormones that help stimulate bone regeneration. Another important factor in osteoporosis seems to be a long-term shortage of calcium. Every adult loses calcium daily, and it must be replaced with new calcium from food and drink. If the amount of calcium in the diet is insufficient, bony strength will lessen.

A third possibility is lack of exercise. A normal degree of activity helps keep bones strong and solid. A person who is inactive suffers from bone loss because of a substantial increase in bone resorption. When younger people are immobilized because of illness or injury, their bone loss is reversible when they resume activity. In older people, bone once lost usually cannot be regained.

Osteoporosis is usually treated with a diet rich in calcium and protein. Adequate doses of vitamin D are needed for normal absorption of calcium.

Hormones may be prescribed to encourage regeneration of bones, and some physical activity is recommended. Such measures may halt or slow the progress of the disorder—but are unlikely to reverse it.

During sexual intercourse, osteoporosis sufferers should take care not to put undue stress on the spine or on arms or legs.

See also AGING; MENOPAUSE.

OSTOMIES are artificial openings (stomas) for the excretion of feces or urine.

Colostomy most often results from surgery for cancer of the colon and rectum. When the surgery is extensive, involving a large portion of the lower colon and the rectum, a surgical opening is made in the abdominal wall to permit elimination of body wastes.

Cancer of the colon and rectum is often called "the cancer nobody talks about." Shame and embarrassment prevent many people from reporting rectal bleeding to their doctors. They may convince themselves that the problem is merely hemorrhoids. Thus, many victims of colon-rectum (or colorectal) cancer treat themselves in privacy with ineffective "pile cures," such as "Preparation H."

Such excessive modesty costs lives. Colorectal cancer strikes some

100,000 Americans each year, more than any type of cancer except skin cancer. Each year there are about 50,000 deaths.

Almost 3 out of 4 patients with colorectal cancer can be saved when the disease is found early and treated promptly. Yet, the actual survival rate is only about 40 percent. The principal reason is that people are not routinely checked for such cancer—nor do they report symptoms to a doctor. An annual physical exam for anyone over 40 should include examination of the rectum with a proctoscope or at the least a digital rectal exam.

The chief symptom of colorectal cancer is bleeding. The cancer obstructs the feces, and bleeding appears as blood in the stool, as streaks, or as actual blood in the toilet bowl. There may be changes in bowel habits—either constipation or diarrhea or both alternately. Intestinal gas may cause varying degrees of abdominal discomfort.

Many bowel cancers begin as tiny hanging pendulums of growing tissue called polyps. They usually begin as benign growths. Late in their development they may start ulcerating and bleeding and become malignant. (Not all polyps become malignant.) If bleeding continues over a long period, the patient may become weak and short of breath, a result of anemia.

Ostomy surgery has varying effects on sexuality. In some men, nerve damage resulting from extensive surgery may cause irreversible sexual impairment. Among men with colostomy for colorectal cancer, some will be impotent, others will suffer from retrograde ejaculation, and many will lose the ability to ejaculate. Most such men are over 50, and may have been suffering from sexual problems because of illness or medications before the surgery.

Ileostomy is performed most frequently because of inflammatory bowel disease. The colon—and usually the rectum—is removed, and the small intestine is fashioned into a stomal opening on the front of the abdomen. The incidence of impotence and ejaculatory problems is considerably less than in colostomy due to cancer.

When colostomy is due to other causes, impotence and ejaculatory problems are also more rare.

An ostomy patient who is impotent after surgery should not assume that the condition is permanent. Some men regain potency several months or even years after the operation.

Little research has been done on the sexual consequences of ostomies among women. Most women seem to retain their interest in sex and their ability to achieve orgasm. Some women report painful intercourse or lack of vaginal sensation.

Colostomy and ileostomy do not usually interfere with a woman's ability to become pregnant or to deliver a healthy child.

The psychological impact of ostomies is enormous—and accounts for far more sexual problems than the physical effects of the surgery. Loss of bowel or bladder control is a terrible insult to self-esteem. Body image is altered by ostomy surgery, and many people feel embarrassment and shame. The sex partner may be revolted and sexually rejecting—or the patient may fear these reactions. There is also the fear of offending a sex partner by odor or unexpected emissions from the stoma. Anxiety about injury to the stoma may also inhibit sexual activity.

When the ostomy results from surgery for cancer, such problems are compounded by anxiety about recurrence. Treatment with radiation therapy or chemotherapy may create health and sexual problems. Depression is common, with consequent diminished sexual interest.

Single ostomates may be particularly concerned about their sexuality. It is common to fear that the surgery will repel a potential sex partner. There is also concern about when—and how—to inform a person who may become sexually intimate.

It is best to tell a potential partner as soon as sexual intimacy becomes a possibility. A simple explanation will usually suffice and might be along the lines of: "I was ill with a disease and needed an operation. Now I have an alternate opening for eliminating waste." The explanation need not be overly detailed. Honest answers should be given clearly and confidently. The emphasis should be on the fact that an ostomy does not interfere with a person's activities or the enjoyment of life.

It is wise for an ostomy patient to join an Ostomy Club before the surgery is performed. The United Ostomy Association (1111 Wilshire Boulevard, Los Angeles, California 90017) can provide information. At such clubs, peer counselors give emotional support and practical guidance in coping with ostomies. A visit prior to surgery can be most reassuring to anxious patients. Some clubs encourage sex partners of ostomy patients to meet with their counterparts. Discussions with a special ostomy nurse may also prove invaluable.

Sexual adjustment with ostomies often depends on the quality of the relationship. A sex partner's responses can do much to promote or decrease an ostomy patient's self-esteem and feelings of sexual desirability. Open communication between sex partners is especially important. It is the cornerstone of effective and satisfying sexual functioning.

Practical considerations can do much to promote positive sexual experiences. A female ostomy patient who is concerned that the stoma will be damaged can have intercourse in the female-superior position.

If an ostomy patient uses a pouch, emptying it just before sexual activity will give a sense of security. (Some ostomates don't use pouches, but learn to irrigate the colon with an enema-type apparatus.) Opaque pouches are preferable to transparent ones. A deodorant can be used in the pouch or on the covering of the stoma for people who irrigate.

For sexual activity, some people may want to tape the pouch onto the body instead of wearing the belt. Others may wish to take if off for the duration and apply a dressing over the stoma. Ostomates often wear scarves or fabric over the stoma or pouch. Some wear panties with the crotch cut out. Each couple has to discover what degree of exposure is comfortable for both partners.

It is wise for ostomates to avoid foods that may cause bowel problems—particularly just before sexual activity is planned. Spicy foods and onions may stimulate bowel activity. Foods such as cabbage, cauliflower, turnips, and onions may increase fecal odor. Such odors may be lessened by eating yogurt or drinking cranberry juice or buttermilk.

For an ostomy patient suffering from irreversible impotence, a penile prosthesis may be a possibility. A couple can also engage in manual or oral stimulation of other erogenous areas. Indeed, for some patients the stoma itself becomes erotic, and stroking it can give a good deal of sexual pleasure.

See also CANCER; CYSTECTOMY; EJACULATION, RETRO-GRADE; PENILE PROSTHESES.

OVARY. See FEMALE SEXUAL ANATOMY.

OVERWEIGHT people commonly suffer social and sexual discrimination.

The slender, youthful, athletic figure is today's standard, while the well-padded figure is deprecated as a sign of gluttony and sloth. This standard of physical acceptability is far more narrowly defined for women than for men. An overweight woman is more likely to suffer social ostracism than an overweight man.

Since most people find overweight—particularly extreme overweight—aesthetically and sexually distasteful, many overweight people have negative sexual self-images. The overweight frequently consider their bodies repulsive. Shame and self-disgust about physical appearance are common.

Very overweight people may have trouble attracting sex partners. They may be loath to make social or sexual advances out of fear of being considered grotesque. When sexual advances are made toward them, they may respond with suspicion. Thus, their opportunities for sexual activity may be severely limited.

For most overweight people, excess weight does not interfere with sexuality. The large majority of overweight people enjoy sex and function normally. In general, the overweight population suffers no more sexual dysfunction than the general population. While the very obese may engage in sexual intercourse somewhat less frequently than people of normal weight, sex is an important source of their pleasure.

But overweight may be associated with a number of medical conditions that increase the risk of sexual problems. Diabetes frequently occurs in overweight people and may result in impotence or orgasmic problems. Hypertension is common among the overweight. Drugs used to control it frequently interfere with sexual functioning.

When people are very overweight, shortness of breath during physical exertion may make sexual intercourse a taxing activity. Chest pain may occur. Such people are advised to engage in very slow intercourse in a passive position: lying on the side or underneath a partner.

Massively obese people—some are several hundred pounds over ideal weight—may experience mechanical difficulties associated with intercourse. Their large abdomens and thighs may make it hard for them to find comfortable intercourse positions. When both partners are grossly obese, the number of sexual positions available to them is extremely limited. Side-by-side may be the only position in which their genitals can come into contact. For many, penile-vaginal penetration is impossible. Such couples may engage in oral sex or mutual masturbation. Sometimes, an obese man may have intercourse between his partner's breasts.

Obesity can alter sex hormones. Obese women have a higher rate of menstrual dysfunction than women of normal weight. Often, gross obesity is associated with hirsutism (hairiness) and lack of menstruation or scanty menstruation. When massively obese women lose significant amounts of weight, menstruation usually returns to normal.

In obese men, testosterone levels are often substantially lower than in normal-weight men.

Some overweight people suffer depression caused by their weight problem. Depression typically results in diminished sexual desire.

A small number of overweight people stay fat to avoid sex. Consciously or unconsciously, they may use overweight to avoid intimate relationships. Obesity may serve as a physical barrier against sexual involvement.

Dieting can put stress on a relationship. In some marriages, the equilibrium is maintained by one partner's being overweight. In such cases, an obese person's spouse may sabotage efforts to diet. A woman may profess to want her very overweight husband to lose weight and may expect to find him more sexually desirable if he does. At the same time, she may fear that if her husband does slim down, he will become dangerously attractive to other women. She may thus undermine his diet by cooking elaborate meals or buying high-calorie desserts.

Similarly, a man may need a justification for extramarital affairs. Keeping his wife fat by sabotaging her diet gives him the excuse he needs.

In fact, both men and women who lose weight are usually so pleased with their new looks—and with other people's appreciation—that they do become more flirtatious than usual, thus feeding the spouse's fears.

What is more, the dynamics of a marriage may change when one partner loses a great deal of weight. The formerly obese person may become more self-confident and assertive. The basis of the marriage may come into question. For people involved in programs aimed at dramatic weight loss, marital counseling is advisable.

Formerly obese people may also require help in adjusting to a changed body image and a new social and sexual status. People who have lost large amounts of weight usually experience an increase in general anxiety. They commonly need reassurance that they are more loved and desirable than when they were obese.

Body image typically does not keep pace with weight loss. A formerly obese person who reaches a normal weight may find the sudden increase in sexual attention alarming. This may be especially true for a young woman who has been obese since childhood. She may need guidance in handling encounters with men.

People who lose a lot of weight may experience increased sexual desire. Some fear that they will be unable to control their sexual impulses. It is also common for people who lose weight to have unrealistic sexual expectations. They may be disappointed if the spouse does not respond to the weight loss with increased sexual attention.

See also DEPRESSION.

OVULATION. See NATURAL FAMILY PLANNING.

PAP TEST. See PELVIC EXAMINATION.

PARASITES. See AMEBIASIS; GIARDIASIS; PINWORMS.

PARALYSIS. See SPINAL-CORD INJURY.

PARKINSON'S DISEASE, a degenerative neurological disease, usually results in sexual impairment. Sufferers often find that its symptoms—arm and leg tremor, muscular rigidity, and slowness of movement—make intercourse difficult. Impotence is common, usually as a result of advanced organic involvement.

Psychological factors may contribute to sexual dysfunction. Victims may be embarrassed by their stooping posture, weak voice, and excessive salivation. Stiff facial musculature can make them seem dull and slow to respond. They may thus tend to withdraw from their spouses, decreasing sexual activity. Some sufferers develop a reactive depression, with reduced sex drive.

Yet it is possible to have a gratifying sexual relationship in spite of neuromuscular symptoms. Parkinson's disease victims should communicate with their sex partners. They should be patient, allowing plenty of time for sexual activity, since responses are bound to be slower.

With levodopa therapy, sufferers are likely to experience improved sexual functioning. Better motor control may make them feel more alert and mildly euphoric. This glow of well-being tends to heat up sexual activity, giving levodopa the unfounded reputation of being an aphrodisiac.

Levodopa may also affect sexual functioning through hormonal changes. Semen may become more copious and viscous. In a postmenopausal woman, the drug may cause increased vaginal secretions (along with uterine bleeding).

Some people are unable to tolerate levodopa. Serious side effects may include psychiatric disturbances, such as severe depression, suicidal tendencies, delerium and hallucinations; heart irregularities; high blood pressure; and phlebitis (inflammation of veins).

PEDICULOSIS PUBIS. See LICE.

PEDOPHILIA literally means "love of children." It describes the need of some adults—usually males—for sexual contact with preadolescent children.

Most victims are girls between the ages of 8 and 11. They may be enticed with favors, gifts, or promises. Some are intimidated or threatened. Rarely is brutality involved.

Often, the pedophile wants merely to look at the child nude. Sometimes the child's genitals are inspected or touched or kissed. In other instances, the child may be required to masturbate the adult or perform fellatio. In a small number of cases, pedophiles have sexual intercourse with their victims.

Most child molesters share a sense of isolation and alienation. They feel inadequate and inept in personal relationships. They experience themselves as helpless victims.

The typical child molester is a married man with marital problems and sexual difficulties. Indeed, his difficulty in sexually functioning with his wife may be a major motivating factor in pedophilia: the man gains a sense of mastery and sexual adequacy through sexual contact with a child. Typically, a pedophile commits the same type of offense over and over again, seeking out children of the same age, sex, and general physical appearance and performing the same acts.

Sometimes, alcohol use is associated with pedophilia. With his inhibitions lowered, the man may be impelled to commit an offense he would be restrained from doing when sober. A small number of pedophiles are retarded or psychotic.

Many types of therapy have been used to treat the pedophile, among them hypnosis, psychotherapy, and behavior modification therapy.

From the child's point of view, molestation is usually upsetting and confusing. But the child is usually far more alarmed when appalled parents overreact to the event.

Parents should take care to deal with the incident so as not to further traumatize the child. This means listening to the story as calmly as possible. It is important not to suggest interpretations, but rather to find out how the child perceived the event. Many children are simply mystified that the adult (sometimes someone they are acquainted with) would want to do so peculiar a thing as, say, smell their panties or touch them in an unexpected place.

Children need reassurance that they are in no way to blame for the incident, that the problem lies with the adult. They should also be absolved of any guilt they may feel for having accepted a treat in return for the sexual favor. The molester can be presented as someone who is mentally sick and in need of help.

See also INCEST.

PEEPING TOM. See VOYEURISM.

PELVIC CONGESTION syndrome can occur when a person repeatedly experiences sexual arousal, but fails to reach orgasm. In men, the condition is colloquially termed "blue balls."

A woman's symptoms are most likely to be pelvic discomfort and backache. She will usually have an increased menstrual flow, with cramps, and a watery vaginal discharge. The heavy aching distress is likely to make her irritable.

While pelvic congestion syndrome is a relatively common condition, people rarely link it to their sexual frustration.

A doctor's examination would find a tender lower abdomen and uterus. The mucous membrane of the vagina may be dark and soft, as if in early pregnancy. The vulva is swollen and sensitive.

Treatment is the release of sexual tension: orgasm by any means. A woman should explore what gives her pleasure—and communicate this information to her partner. But she need not rely on her partner in order to reach orgasm every time she experiences sexual tension. If her partner is unavailable or uninterested, self-stimulation is an option.

See also BACKACHE; EPIDIDYMO-ORCHITIS; MASTURBATION.

PELVIC EXAMINATION is part of a general gynecological examination. It consists of:

1. Observation of the external genitals.
2. Observation of the internal genitals.
3. Bimanual examination of the internal reproductive organs.

For a pelvic examination, a woman lies on her back with her head supported by a pillow and her legs spread apart and supported by stirrups or foot supports—the dorsal lithotomy position.

The pelvic examination should not be uncomfortable if there is no pelvic pathology, if the physician is gentle, and if the woman relaxes her abdominal and pelvic muscles. The doctor's explanations and reassurance also help minimize discomfort—both physical and psychological.

The physician—preferably a board-certified obstetrician-gynecologist—first inspects the woman's external genitals for irritations, signs of infection, or growths.

He or she then inserts an instrument called a vaginal speculum, which lifts the walls of the vagina away from each other, and makes the lateral wall visible. The physician inspects its general character, its color, and the consistency of its mucous membrane.

The cervix (neck of the uterus or womb) is clearly visible, allowing the physician to take a sample of cervical and vaginal cells. These are placed on a slide and inspected for abnormalities. This procedure—called a Pap smear—can detect cervical and uterine cancer and some types of vaginal infection.

For the bimanual examination, the physician removes the speculum and gently inserts the index and middle fingers into the vagina. The doctor's other hand is placed on the woman's lower abdomen. With gentle pressure, the physician checks the uterus, ovaries, Fallopian tubes, and general pelvic area for tumors, cysts, fibroids, or other abnormalities. The physician may also insert one finger into the woman's rectum to examine the area between the rectum and the vagina.

Many physicians find the pelvic examination an excellent opportunity to teach a woman more about her body. Some encourage their patients to feel their ovaries and uterus through the abdominal wall.

If the pelvic examination is part of an annual gynecological checkup, it will also likely include a breast examination. Most physicians also check the thyroid, blood pressure, urine and hemoglobin, and listen to the chest with a stethoscope.

Many women find vaginal examinations an ordeal. The position often makes a woman feel absurd and vulnerable. No matter how many times a woman has been previously examined, she may never get over the feeling of involuntary intrusion. Many women delay an examination for years because of the emotional trauma associated with it.

Some physicians find that warming the speculum aids in making the examination more comfortable. For women who are extremely resistant, or for young girls who are undergoing their first internal examination, it usually helps if the doctor explains just what he is doing and why. Slow, deep breathing will help women relax. Sometimes, the examination may have to be performed over two or more visits. The external genitals can be examined first; at a later time, the bimanual examination can be done. The patient can be shown the warmed speculum and told how it is going to be used before the doctor inserts it.

Occasionally, babies or very young girls require internal examinations. This can best be done with the child resting on her mother's lap and the physician proceeding in a slow, gentle, and reassuring manner.

PELVIC INFLAMMATORY DISEASE (PID, salpingitis) is infection of the Fallopian tubes—although the term is often used to include infection of the cervix, uterus, or ovaries.

PID occurs predominantly in young women who are sexually active. Most often, the cause is gonorrhea, although many other organisms besides gonococcus bacteria may cause PID. Infection may also result after abortion, childbirth, or the insertion of an IUD.

When the infection is gonorrheal, a woman will often have a profuse pus-laden discharge, with malaise and a low-grade fever. There may also be a discharge from the urethra, with frequent, painful urination. Such symptoms may be absent or mild, and tend to subside even without treatment.

PID symptoms are likely to flare up within one to three weeks, frequently just after menstruation. A woman may experience severe lower abdominal pain and tenderness, with fever and a purulent discharge from the vagina.

PID can cause infertility. Blockage of the Fallopian tubes commonly follows infection. Prompt treatment with antibiotics will cure the infection and may avert infertility. Occasionally, PID is life-threatening. An abscess in a Fallopian tube may rupture, causing shock and death within an hour. A ruptured abscess is a surgical emergency.

The sexual contacts of a woman with gonorrheal PID should be examined, since they may harbor asymptomatic gonococcal infection. Untreated, they may cause recurrent infections. Follow-up treatment for women with PID includes repeated pelvic examinations and cultures for gonococcus bacteria.

See also ABORTION; GONORRHEA; INFERTILITY; IUDs.

PENECTOMY. See PENILE CANCER.

PENILE CANCER is rare.

Its usual treatment is surgery. In some cases, only a part of the penis must be removed. This operation—called a subtotal or partial penectomy—usually leaves the prostate, testicles, and lymph nodes intact.

Even if as much as 85 percent of the penis is removed, the remainder of the penis may be capable of erection. The man can still experience orgasm, including ejaculation. Although the glans and frenulum are gone, the bulb of the penis—at the base—can provide extremely pleasurable sensations. With or without erection, the man may enjoy vaginal intromission.

Even when a man retains sexual functioning, he may experience the partial loss of his penis as a mutilation that adversely affects his feelings about himself. A man in this situation may wish to explore whether he is a good candidate for a penile prosthesis.

When the entire penis is surgically amputated and surrounding

225

lymph nodes dissected (total penectomy), a man is left sterile and unable to engage in sexual intercourse. Total penectomy may also be performed on a man suffering from urethral cancer. Such surgery is almost always a profound blow to a man's sense of masculinity and self-esteem. With extensive cancer, a man may also be suffering physical pain, fears about dying, financial problems, and stress in family relationships—all of which may contribute to a sense of helplessness and worthlessness.

For some men with total penectomies, plastic reconstructive surgery is an option. An artificial penis can sometimes be fashioned out of surrounding tissue.

A man with a penectomy should remember that penile-vaginal contact is only one sexual option. He can explore what other forms of sexual activity he enjoys. One penectomy patient found great sexual gratification in realizing the sexual potential of his perineal area. At first he believed that this type of stimulation was a poor substitute for intercourse. But he grew to appreciate it as a valid form of sexual expression in its own right.

See also CANCER; PENILE PROSTHESES.

PENILE PROSTHESES are an option for men who are unable to have erections.

Most candidates for these surgical implants are men who are impotent because of irreversible organic causes. They may suffer from penile trauma or congenital abnormalities; some have neurologic disorders or diabetes; some types of surgery—such as prostate surgery or ostomies—may make erection impossible. Sometimes, penile implants may be recommended for men with psychogenic impotence when psychotherapy and sex therapy have failed. There are two types of devices available:

1. *Semirigid rod devices*—such as the Small-Carrion prosthesis—consist of two sponge-filled silicone rods that are surgically implanted in the penis. The incision is made either in the perineum or on the underside of the penis.

This device has enough length and girth to simulate a normal erection and allow vaginal penetration. It has no movable parts.

The Flexi-Rod prosthesis is a similar device that has a hinged pair of rods that permits the penis to hang down when the man stands.

With the semirigid rod prostheses, the penis remains in a state of semierection. This may be an embarrassment to the man or his partner. On the other hand, the device is relatively easy to implant and inexpensive. Persistent pain and infection are rare.

Brief style (rather than jockey style) underwear is recommended to help disguise the erect penis. The penis can be placed downward in the usual position or flat against the abdomen.

2. *The inflatable penile prosthesis* is a hollow silicone cylinder that is surgically implanted in the penis. A reservoir containing radiopaque solution (which can be seen on X ray) is implanted in the abdomen, and a bulb is implanted in one scrotal sac. The cylinders, reservoir, and bulb are connected by silicone tubes.

When the man squeezes the bulb in the scrotum, the solution flows from the reservoir to the cylinder and causes an erection. A one-way valve keeps the solution in the cylinder. When the man wants the erection to subside, he compresses a release valve in the bulb, and the fluid returns to the reservoir.

Many men find this type of device more psychologically satisfying, since it more closely resembles normal functioning than the rigid device. When not erect, the penis has a normal appearance. On erection, the inflatable implant has greater length and girth than the rod-type implant.

Surgery is more complex and more expensive for inflatable devices. The most common complication is mechanical failure of the device, such as kinks or leaks in the silicone tubing. These mechanical failures are always correctable, but usually require more surgery.

Initial pain may be severe, and mild pain may continue for weeks after surgery. A man with an inflatable prosthesis requires careful instruction in its use. During the first 4 weeks after surgery, he must inflate and deflate the device daily to stretch penile tissue. This is likely to be a very painful procedure the first several times; in the hospital, it is advisable for pain medication to be given about half an hour before the doctor or nurse inflates the bulb.

Choice of the type of device is left to the patient in most cases. But some medical problems make one type or the other more suitable. Men with physical handicaps, for example, may find the inflatable device hard to manage. A young, physically active man should be aware of the possible social embarrassment of participating in athletic activities with a semierect penis. He is probably better suited to the inflatable device. Diabetic men may be predisposed to a higher rate of surgical and postoperative complications than other candidates for prosthesis surgery. Benefits versus risks should be carefully weighed.

Sexual activity can usually begin 4 to 8 weeks after surgery with both types of prostheses. To avoid damage to the penis, the woman's vagina should be sufficiently lubricated before insertion—or an artificial lubricant should be used.

There may be a decrease in the sensitivity of the shaft of the penis, but normal ejaculation and orgasm occur with both types of devices—except if the man's medical condition makes this impossible.

Counseling is recommended to help the man adjust to his implant. Simply adjusting to erection and intercourse can be stressful after months or years of impotence—for both the man and his spouse or sex partner. Men with penile implants commonly fear that the device can be easily dislodged or damaged; they can be reassured that a properly implanted device is made to withstand the rigors of vaginal penetration and thrusting.

See also IMPOTENCE.

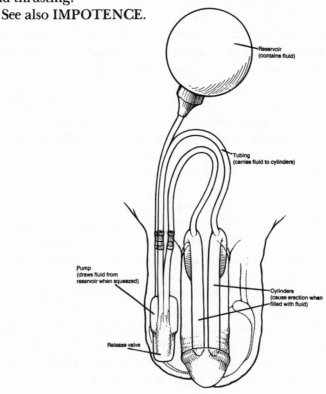

Reservoir
(contains fluid)

Tubing
(carries fluid to cylinders)

Pump
(draws fluid from
reservoir when squeezed)

Cylinders
(cause erection when
filled with fluid)

Release valve

PENIS. See MALE SEXUAL ANATOMY.

PENIS INFLAMMATION almost invariably results in painful sexual intercourse.

Inflammation may involve the head of the penis (balanitis), the foreskin or prepuce (posthitis), or both (balanoposthitis).

Its causes are myriad. Poor hygiene, especially among uncircumcised boys, may cause soreness. A condition called phimosis, in which the foreskin cannot be retracted to uncover the head of the penis, may lead to irritation, redness, and swelling. Circumcision is usually recommended.

One of the commonest causes of sore penis among boys and adolescents is masturbation.

Aggressive masturbation in an adult male may likewise be responsible for penis inflammation. Irritation is especially likely if the penis is rubbed without lubrication. Any water-soluble lubricant (such as K-Y jelly) will minimize irritation during masturbation.

Infectious disease may account for penis inflammation. Venereal diseases such as gonorrhea or herpes may cause inflammation. So may bacterial infections such as E. coli, staphylococcus, and streptococcus. Such vaginal infections as yeast infections and, occasionally, trichomoniasis, may result in penis inflammation.

Skin conditions such as neurodermatitis may appear on the penis. Inflammation may also result from allergy—to contraceptive foam, for example. Rarely, inflammation of the penis is cancerous.

See also CIRCUMCISION; MASTURBATION; VENEREAL DISEASE.

PENIS INJURY ranges in severity from the mild penile numbness bicycle-riders may experience to complete traumatic amputation of the penis.

Anesthesia (loss of sensation) of the penis may occur in bicyclists who ride for long periods without stopping. This occurs because the penis is compressed between the peak of the seat and the pubic bones. Urination, erection, and ejaculation are unaffected. Sensation returns within a few hours.

The condition can be avoided if the cyclist tilts the peak of the seat downward to relieve the pressure. Resting more frequently, or occasionally pedaling with hips raised from the seat, also helps avoid the problem.

Frostbite of the penis occasionally occurs in joggers, walkers, bikers, or outdoor workers in very cold weather. The risk depends not only on the temperature, but also on wind, dampness, and the insulating ability of clothing.

A penis damp from drops of urine or semen, or from wet underwear, is more vulnerable to frostbite since dampness increases heat loss. Men should take care to shake off or wipe the last few drops of urine before venturing outdoors for prolonged periods in cold weather. It is also wise for them to wear multiple layers of light clothing rather than one single item of heavy clothing. Air trapped between layers has an insulating effect. A water-repellent outer layer gives further protection.

For the aching or numbness of mild frostbite, the penis should be immersed in warm water until normal sensation returns. If warm water is not immediately available, the man should warm his penis with his bare hand. Rubbing snow on a frostbitten part is a dangerous myth—it can do permanent damage. Only in very rare cases is penile frostbite so severe that tissue death and ulceration result, with impaired sexual functioning.

Entwining hair or thread around the penis is a common cause of penis injury among children. Most often, the boy is merely playing with the hair or nylon thread and accidentally wraps it too tightly around his penis. In other cases, young boys are thought to be punishing themselves for misdeeds by strangulating their own penises. A few instances of penis strangulation may be child abuse by emotionally disturbed parents. The severity of the injury ranges from mild swelling of the head of the penis to the constriction of the blood supply that results in gangrene and requires surgery.

Entrapment of the penis in a fly zipper is another common penis injury among little boys. The parent can release the penis by cutting the zipper across underneath the caught penis—after first carefully explaining to the child just what is going to be cut. The injury from the zipper is usually slight and can be treated like any other cut or bruise. If there is more than a little bleeding, a physician should determine if the cut requires stitches.

Masturbation sometimes results in penis injury. Inflammation may occur after vigorous rubbing, particularly without lubrication. Some men insert foreign objects into the urethra as a part of masturbating. One physician reports removing mechanical pencils, paper clips, hat pins, and swizzle sticks from men's urethras. Such objects can do irreparable damage to the urethra and the penis. Men who use mechanical suction devices—such as vacuum cleaners—for masturbatory purposes are also liable to cause serious injury to their penises.

In an effort to maintain an erection, a man may try to prevent the escape of blood from his penis by constricting the base with rubber bands, rings, or straps. This is a very dangerous practice. Constricting the blood supply may result in gangrene.

Penis injury occasionally results from sexual intercourse. On rare occasions, the frenulum (the fold on the lower surface of the head of the penis) or the foreskin may be torn, particularly if this is the man's first intercourse. If there is much bleeding, suturing may be necessary.

In some instances, penis injury is self-inflicted. A high percentage of the men who mutilate their penises are psychotic or are under the influence of drugs or alcohol. Physicians have observed gunshot wounds, cuts with sharp instruments, and trauma from blunt instruments.

Amputation is the most severe and life-threatening penis injury. Complete severing of the penis may occur by accident, self-injury, or attack. In one instance, a 20-year-old man's penis was severed with a butcher knife by his girl friend's estranged husband. In another, a psychotic mother cut off her infant's penis. (In cases of penile cancer, part or all of the penis may have to be surgically removed.)

A severed penis can be reimplanted. For best preservation, it should be chilled on ice—but kept from direct contact with the ice. Best results are obtained when the time lapse between the amputation and the surgery is less than 6 hours.

After successful surgery, it is possible for patients to achieve normal urination, erection, and ejaculation. Partial skin sensation may also return.

When the penis cannot be reimplanted, it may be possible for a new penis to be fashioned from neighboring tissues. The reconstructed penis is sufficiently rigid to permit sexual intercourse. The grafts are frequently without nerve supply, thus penis stimulation is not erotic.

But orgasm may be achieved through the caressing of other erogenous areas—nipples, anus, underarms, testicles, etc. Fantasy is also an aid to orgasm in men with reconstructed penises.

See also MASTURBATION; PENILE CANCER; PENILE IN-FLAMMATION; PENILE PROSTHESES.

PENIS MALFORMATION, if uncorrected, is likely to interfere with sexual functioning and reproduction.

Among the more common congenital penis anomalies are:

Hypospadias. This is the most frequent defect of the penis, occurring in approximately 1 in 125 newborn males.

In this condition, the urethral opening is mispositioned on the undersurface of the penis. This causes the male to urinate and ejaculate through this abnormal opening.

In most cases, the defect is minimal, with the urethral opening occurring not far from where it normally should be. Erection, intercourse, and fertility are usually unimpaired by mild hypospadias.

Even so, the condition can cause males to harbor grave doubts about their masculinity. A boy with hypospadias may have to urinate in a sitting position. He may be confused about his sexual identity. Playmates may ridicule him. Adolescents and adults with this defect often avoid sexual situations out of embarrassment.

Further, hypospadias can interfere with a man's chances of conceiving a child if the urethral opening is so near the base of the penis that much of his ejaculate leaks out of the vagina.

Hypospadias can usually be surgically corrected. It is best done at between 2 and 4 years, before the age of memory recall, so that the boy is not troubled with doubts about his sexual adequacy. Surgery is usually not done at infancy because of the great difficulty of repairing such a small penis.

Chordee. The misplaced urethral opening of hypospadias is often associated with chordee, a fibrous band of tissue around the urethra. This results in an abnormal curvature of the penis.

Surgical correction should ideally occur before the boy is of school age. Newborns with a combination of hypospadias and chordee should not be circumcised—since the tissue of the foreskin is used in reconstructive surgery.

Uncorrected chordee may interfere with sexual intercourse. The curvature caused by chordee is accentuated with erection. A pronounced curvature can make vaginal penetration difficult or impossible. Even a relatively slight downward curve may make intercourse uncomfortable for one or both partners.

Sometimes, chordee occurs alone, without urethral anomalies.

Epispadias. In this more rare condition, the opening of the urethra is on the *upper* surface of the penis.

Chordee is often associated with epispadias, making the penis curve upward on erection. Intercourse may be difficult or impossible.

Almost always, a male with an epispadias also suffers from bladder and abdominal wall defects.

Surgery for epispadias is a complicated procedure. The surgery frequently has to correct urinary incontinence, the malpositioned urethra, and the curvature. Often, two or more operations are required for the best functional and cosmetic results. It is usually recommended that the surgery be performed when the boy is roughly 3 to 5 years old.

Even after surgery, sexual functioning may be impaired.

Shortened frenulum. Some men suffer from a taut frenulum—the fold on the lower surface of the head of the penis. This condition predisposes to fissuring or cuts during sexual intercourse.

The head of the penis is likely to be curved slightly downward with erection, thus making vaginal penetration difficult. The man may feel pain during intercourse, which may cause him to lose his erection or to have trouble ejaculating. The problem can usually be surgically corrected.

Rare but severe anomalies include retroscrotal penis, in which a boy's penis or penile tissue occurs beneath his scrotum. He may also suffer defects of the urinary tract. Occasionally, the problem can be surgically corrected, with the penis properly repositioned.

In rare cases, a male baby is born without a penis. Since there is no procedure that can satisfactorily construct a fully functioning penis, parents of such children are usually advised to raise them as girls. The testicles are surgically removed, and an artificial vagina is created. When the child reaches early adolescence, estrogen therapy will bring on female secondary sex characteristics and a female appearance. Reproduction, however, is not possible.

A few other males are afflicted with the opposite problem: two penises. In this rare anomaly (estimated to occur only once in 5.5 million births), it is typical for only one penis to have a fully functional urethra. Before corrective surgery is attempted, a complete urological examination should determine just how the male's genitourinary system functions.

See also PENIS SMALLNESS.

PENIS SMALLNESS is a common concern of normal teenage boys—and of many grown men as well. Adolescent boys frequently worry that their penises are too small to satisfy a woman.

This concern stems from the myth that the larger the man's penis, the more sexual pleasure he gives women. This is simply not true. Many men have an image of the vagina as a vault of a certain size that has to be filled by a sufficiently large penis. A much more accurate image is that of an elastic stocking or an empty sleeve. The vagina expands to accommodate penises of greatly varying sizes.

During sexual arousal, the opening of the vagina narrows as the surrounding tissue becomes congested. At the same time, the inside of the vagina expands, decreasing direct stimulation from penile thrusting and making the exact size of the penis basically irrelevant. Further, the inner two-thirds of the vagina contains few sensory nerve endings—while there is a rich concentration of such nerve endings at the vaginal entrance.

A teenager may begin worrying when he observes that his flaccid penis is smaller than his friends' penises. However, his erect penis is probably roughly the same size as theirs. Smaller flaccid penises usually double in size, while larger flaccid penises may increase only 80 percent. Thus the great variation in sizes of flaccid penises tends to even out when they're erect.

In rare instances, males suffer from micropenis. Their penises are properly formed, but abnormally small. The cause is unknown. In some cases, it may result from a defect in androgen secretion during pregnancy. It has also been observed among some young men whose mothers took the drug DES during pregnancy. The disorder may occur alone, or may be associated with endocrine problems or abnormalities of the testes or chromosomes.

Small boys with micropenis may be treated with testosterone cream for 3 to 6 months, which often produces a small growth in penis size. If not, testosterone injections for 3 months may produce penile growth. The dosage and duration should be carefully controlled, for excessive amounts may prematurely end skeletal bone growth and thus interfere with potential adult height.

PERIOD. See MENSTRUATION.

PEYRONIE'S DISEASE is one of the most common causes of painful intercourse in men. A tender knot develops along the shaft of the penis. This hard scarlike tissue is inelastic. Thus, as the disease progresses, erections are likely to be painful and interfere with intercourse. Moreover, the erection curves at the point of the knot, further impeding sexual activity.

The disease is most likely to affect men over 40. Its cause is uncertain. Some investigators believe that the scar tissue results from an injury or infection. A virus may be implicated. Men who suffer from Peyronie's disease can rest assured that the growth is not cancer, a common fear.

Men with this condition have a very good chance of resuming intercourse. About half of patients recover spontaneously within an average of four years. For the other half, the scarlike region spreads and becomes calcified, making the erect penis bend—usually upward or sideward, occasionally downward—at an angle of up to 90 degrees. Even so, the pain on erection tends to disappear—and there is often enough flexibility to permit penetration.

Early in the disease, the most widely used medical treatment is injecting the knot with steroids. This causes a remission in about 76 percent of the cases. If the deformity becomes permanent, the knot can often be successfully removed by surgery. However, surgery is usually not recommended if the fibrosis extends deep into the penis—because, if too much tissue is removed, the shaft will have a weak point on erection.

See also INTERCOURSE, PAINFUL.

PID. See PELVIC INFLAMMATORY DISEASE.

PILL, CONTRACEPTIVE (oral contraceptive, birth control

pill) is a combination of hormones that prevent conception mainly by suppressing ovulation.

The Pill's major advantage is its high degree of effectiveness. It is more effective than the IUD, although it presents many more potential problems. The Pill is a method appropriate for mature women with established sex lives and regular daily habits.

A woman is a candidate for the Pill only if her menstrual cycle is established and reasonably regular. Most oral contraceptives combine the two kinds of female sex hormones: estrogens and progestogens. They prevent ovulation, the production of the egg cell. They also thicken the mucus in the neck of the uterus, obstructing sperm. Further, they change the lining of the uterus so that it cannot receive a fertilized egg. The combined pill is effective because, if one of the reactions fails to occur, another will do the trick. Combination brands include: Brevicon, Demulen, Enovid, Loestrin. Lo/Ovral, Modicon, Norinyl, Norlestrin, Ortho-Novum, Ovral, Ovulen, Zorane. A "mini-pill" contains progestogen only. It does not stop ovulation, but works by thickening the liquid in the cervical canal so that sperm have more difficulty in reaching the egg. Major mini-pill brands: Micronor, Nor-Q.D., Ovrette.

Before getting a prescription for the Pill, a woman needs a gynecological examination. Her doctor needs to take a careful medical history to find out whether she has a tendency toward any condition that would make it best for her not to take the Pill. He also should take her blood pressure, examine her breasts for lumps, and take a Pap smear to check for cervical cancer.

She starts her first course of pills on the fifth day after her period begins. She should use another method of contraception as well for the first two weeks. Until then, she is not fully protected by the Pill alone.

If she misses even one pill, a woman risks becoming pregnant until her next period. After such a lapse, she should take the pill or pills missed, then continue taking pills daily for the rest of the month—but also use another contraceptive method, such as condoms, spermicidal preparations, or a diaphragm. Contrary to popular belief, there is no medical reason to give her body "a rest" by periodically discontinuing the pills for a month or two. A woman should never use someone else's prescription.

A physician can prescribe an oral contraceptive tailored to a woman's individual needs. Thus, if a woman tends to be hairy, he is likely to prescribe a pill with a low progestogen content. If she develops complications such as vaginal bleeding, he may switch her to a pill with a higher estrogen content.

Many brands of the Pill are available in 21- or 28-day packets. It is a good idea for the doctor to prescribe the 28-day packet, the last seven pills of which are inactive. That way a woman gets used to taking a pill every day. If she goes off the Pill, she needs to start another method of contraception right away. Even if she wants to conceive, miscarriage is more frequent in the first two to three months following stoppage of the Pill. She should use another method of contraception for at least three months.

Before thinking about taking the Pill, a woman needs to face whether its benefits offset its risks. Certainly, she should not consider the Pill if she has intercourse only at great intervals. Its risks are too great for her to take it "just in case." *The Medical Letter* recommends that "the risks in the use of oral contraceptives should be weighed against the psychological effects of fear of pregnancy and the possible physical consequences of pregnancy or abortion." The editors of the publication advise women to use other effective methods of birth control if they can do so.

About 1 in 5 users experience reactions to the Pill. Many of these side effects are similar to the symptoms of early pregnancy, and may disappear after a few months. They may include nausea and vomiting, a bloated feeling, and tender breasts. Many users complain of being perpetually damp from excessive vaginal secretions. Chloasm is darkening of the skin—the "mask of pregnancy," especially common among brunettes and worsened by exposure to the sun. Headache, dizziness, acne, and emotional depression are less common complaints associated with the Pill. Loss of scalp hair is an uncommon side effect.

At unexpected times of the month, a woman may experience some breakthrough vaginal bleeding, marked by staining of her underpants. There is often a tendency to gain weight, probably caused by an increase in appetite and water retention. A change of hormone combination may eliminate or reduce specific side effects. So may a change in dosage or the taking of concurrent drugs, like diuretics to reduce the bloating.

If a woman has a chronic health problem, it may be made worse by an oral contraceptive. Migraine, depression, and asthma are often aggravated by the Pill. Among other contraindications: high blood pressure, diabetes, fibroid tumors in the uterus, and heart, liver, or kidney disease. The Pill may also interfere with the absorption of vitamins and minerals.

Women on the Pill face an increased risk of developing thrombophlebitis—blood clots in the veins possibly leading to loss of limb, paralysis, loss of sight, or death. A woman should contact her doctor immediately if she ever experiences severe headaches, shortness of breath, blurred vision, or pain in the legs or chest. Also, while she is taking the Pill, she should report any unusual swelling and any color changes, such as brownish spotting or yellowish discoloration of the skin or eyes.

Increased risk of stroke, heart attack, and birth defects has also been linked to the Pill. After using the Pill for more than four years, a woman will face almost twice the normal risk of developing malignant melanoma, an often fatal skin cancer—and three to five times the normal risk of getting cancer of the cervix.

See also CERVICAL CANCER; CONTRACEPTION.

"PING-PONG" DISEASE is an infection that is repeatedly passed back and forth between sex partners. Usually, one partner is treated for a genitourinary infection. The other harbors the organisms without any symptoms and thus can reinfect the partner who has undergone treatment.

See also URINARY TRACT INFECTION; VAGINAL INFECTION; VENEREAL DISEASE.

PINWORMS (seatworms, oxyuriasis, threadworms, enterobiasis), like other intestinal parasites, are not usually transmitted sexually.

But it is certainly possible for the worms to be passed from person to person during sexual activity. Transmission is particularly likely if one partner inserts fingers in the infested partner's anus. Anilingus (anus-tongue contact) may also spread the parasite.

Pinworms, unlike other intestinal parasites, do not chiefly infect the rural and the poor. Rather, observes parasitologist Harold W. Brown, these worms are found "even in the seats of the mighty."

An estimated 18 million Americans have this infectious disease.

Pinworms are tiny, delicate, white worms, the largest of them less than half an inch long. Infestation occurs when the microscopic eggs hatch in the small intestine. The young worms then migrate to the large intestine where they attach their heads to the mucous lining, usually in the appendix or nearby.

In about two months, the mature worms emerge, usually at night, at the anus. The females lay eggs by the thousands in the moist folds of skin around the rectal opening.

The most common symptom of pinworm infestation is an itch around the anus. A pinworm sufferer, especially a child, frequently reinfects himself. He scratches and gets the sticky eggs on his hands; later he puts his hand to his mouth or transfers the eggs from his hand to food.

If the anal itching is prolonged, it can lead to sleeplessness and nervousness—a source of the old wives' notion that fidgety children have worms. Infected children sometimes have dark circles under their eyes and are pale, in part from lack of sleep. Restlessness, loss of appetite, loss of weight, and sometimes nausea and vomiting occur. Infected children are apt to be irritable, hard to manage, and inattentive at school.

In women and girls, migrating worms may enter the vulva and vagina, frequently causing vaginal irritation and discharge. After a bowel movement, it is wise to wipe away from the vaginal opening, to lessen the chance of infection. Occasionally pinworms cause intestinal inflammation with symptoms much like appendicitis.

When one member of a household gets pinworms, the others are likely to get infested as well. The eggs may contaminate toilets, night-clothes, bedding, and underwear. They may be carried on air currents and inhaled or swallowed. These parasites can infest pets, especially dogs, which may then infect their owners. Students in classrooms, residents of a dormitory, or institution co-workers may infect each other.

Sometimes worms can be seen on a freshly passed stool or in bed. Giving a shallow enema may bring out worms. Worms may be sighted at night if the sufferer's buttocks are separated and a light is shined on the anus.

If worms cannot be found by these methods, a visit to a physician or public-health laboratory is necessary. In preparation, about 2 inches of cellulose tape, sticky side out, should be wrapped around a tongue depressor or the blade of a blunt knife. First thing in the morning, this swab is pressed firmly on the anal region. Any pinworm eggs will adhere to it and show up under a microscope. Since the worms deposit eggs erratically, it may be necessary to make a swab on 4 or 5 consecutive days before pinworms can be ruled out.

All members of a household should be treated. Even those showing no symptoms may be infested and thus be a possible source of reinfection. The same is true of all sexual contacts of an infected person. Treatment needs to be in the hands of a physician.

Patent medicines should be avoided. They are less effective and possibly more dangerous than pyrantel pamoate (*Antiminth*), pyrvinium pamoate (*Povan*), or piperazine (*Antepar*), the standard medications prescribed for pinworms. Pyrvinium pamoate turns bowel movements bright red.

Physicians often prescribe 5 percent ammoniated mercury ointment around the anal area each night at bedtime for 2 weeks. This furthers destruction of the eggs. Fingernails of small children who may do much rectal scratching should be cut short. They should sleep in tight-fitting pajamas.

Dryness and heat tend to kill the eggs. When people living in crowded conditions are being treated, every morning their underwear, nightclothes, and towels should be boiled or at least heated to 150° F for several minutes. Houses should be dusted frequently.

People being treated for pinworms should pay close attention to personal hygiene. They should bathe daily and scrub the anal region. Hands should be washed thoroughly and frequently in running warm water, especially after the toilet and before handling food.

POSTHITIS. See PENIS INFLAMMATION.

POSTPARTUM PROBLEMS. The period following the delivery of a baby is a time of adjustment not only to infant care, but also to a new life-style.

Extra energy is needed at just the time when it's in most short supply. The infant's schedule during the first 4 to 6 weeks is often very erratic, causing a great deal of strain on the parents. Sleep is at a minimum, adding to the already existing state of exhaustion.

Mood swings or mild depression are common in new mothers. A woman may be irritable and hypersensitive, crying for no apparent reason.

She may experience the feeling of having lost control of her life. All her time may seem taken up with catering to the baby's needs. She may feel exhausted and overwhelmed, and it may seem to her as if life will always be this way. Having to cope with the needs of other young children aggravates these feelings.

Postpartum depression, also called after-baby (or postnatal) blues, usually disappears by itself within a few weeks. The condition is thought to result from a combination of psychological stress and hormonal changes following delivery.

Arranging for time away from the baby at frequent intervals is likely to help a new mother get over the blues. Just a couple of hours of freedom a day may make her feel refreshed and renewed.

It's wise to arrange for assistance with housekeeping, food preparation, and baby care before the baby is born. Such help can come from family members, friends, or, if affordable, professional homemakers or nurses.

After childbirth, it is important for a woman to maintain good nutrition, particularly if she is breast feeding. A diet high in protein is recommended.

If the depression is severe or prolonged, professional psychiatric help is needed. For a few women postpartum depression develops into a serious emotional disturbance.

Vaginal discomfort. Following delivery of a baby, many women experience discomfort in the vaginal area around the episiotomy stitches. (An episiotomy is the incision the doctor makes in the perineum—the area between the vaginal opening and the rectum—during childbirth; it avoids tearing in the area as the baby's head is delivered.) The discomfort after childbirth is due to swelling in the perineal area.

Hot sitz baths several times a day may help. They should be followed by exposing the external genital area to a heat lamp placed a foot away. The physician may also prescribe sprays that anesthetize the area.

Doing vaginal exercises—contracting the vaginal muscles, holding for several seconds, then releasing—may help restore muscle tone and promote healing.

A woman will bleed from the vagina for several weeks after the baby is born. She should wear sanitary napkins, not internal tampons. In the first weeks after delivery, she needs to get as much rest as she can. If she is breastfeeding, her breasts may feel overfull and sore as the milk comes in. Constipation may be a problem—walking soon after the baby is born is thought to prevent a severe case. If any of these problems are more than a little troubling, she should tell her doctor.

Intercourse can be resumed as soon as the episiotomy heals and it is comfortable. Women vary widely in their readiness to resume, both physically and psychologically. Caesarean births will prolong the recovery period because of the added strain of major abdominal surgery.

Some women resume intercourse as early as 3 weeks postpartum; others are not comfortable until many weeks thereafter. What is important is that a couple continue to share warmth and show consideration for each other, for feeling loved is often more important than making love.

Couples are often troubled to find that their sexual desire is low after the baby is born. They can be reassured that, as they feel more rested and become more accustomed to taking care of the baby, their sex drive will return.

The vagina may be dry and thin postpartum because of a decrease in hormones. A water-soluble lubricant such as K-Y jelly will aid penetration. Couples who do not wish to conceive will need to use birth control, even if the mother is breastfeeding.

See also BREASTFEEDING; CONTRACEPTION; PREGNANCY.

PREGNANCY is a normal developmental life crisis. Along with its physiological changes, many psychological and social changes also occur. Familial, societal, religious, and cultural conditioning influence a woman's attitude toward pregnancy.

A woman's attitude about her sexuality also affects the way in which she responds to the changes that occur throughout the pregnancy year (9 months gestation, 3 months postpartum). A woman who values her sexuality and her ability to relate to her partner in a close, intimate manner will often view her pregnancy as a physical manifestation of such closeness. She is likely to greet the changes in her body with curiosity, excitement, and acceptance.

By contrast, for a woman who does not value her sexuality, and who does not relate well to her partner, the pregnancy may stir up negative feelings about herself and/or her partner. She is likely to view the changes in her body as distortion and ugliness. She may complain a lot about the usual discomforts of pregnancy, and be demanding and needy. She may doubt her ability to carry the pregnancy to full term and delivery.

The husband's attitude toward childbearing and rearing also influences the pregnant couple's adjustment to this normal life crisis. Myths and misconceptions about pregnancy may influence his response and his ability to cope with the changes pregnancy brings.

Sex during pregnancy. Any pregnant woman who experiences vaginal or abdominal pain or bleeding during intercourse, or at any other time, should abstain from sex until she has talked with her doctor. Couples should also not engage in intercourse after the membranes have ruptured or if the woman has a history of premature labor. Otherwise, sexual intercourse can ordinarily continue throughout a normal pregnancy.

Throughout pregnancy, it is imperative that no air be blown into a woman's vagina. Deaths to pregnant women have resulted when the forced air passed into the blood vessels of the placenta, causing bubbles that blocked circulation to the heart.

Vaginal bleeding should be reported to the physician. It is typically the first sign of an impending miscarriage (see ABORTION). Other symptoms may include cramps, backache, and nausea.

To lower the risks to herself and her baby, a woman can take the following precautions. She should:

● *Take no drug unless there is a strong medical need for it.* Virtually all drugs pass through the placenta, entering the unborn child's circulation and possibly harming it. *The Medical Letter* recommends that physicians give pregnant women as few drugs as possible. It cautions that "except for urgent indications, all drugs should be withheld during the first trimester (three months)."

Since 1962, when the drug thalidomide was found to cause severe physical abnormalities in the fetus, many other drugs—including some antidepressants, tranquilizers, steroids, anticoagulants, and anticonvulsants—have been implicated in potential birth defects. Iodides, contained in many cough medicines, can cause large goiters and respiratory distress in newborn infants. Progestogen, estrogen, and androgenic hormones can cause masculinized external genitals in the

243

female fetus. Antibiotics containing tetracyclines may inhibit fetal bone growth or produce teeth discoloration.

If the doctor prescribes a drug, the pregnant woman should take it only in the doses and at the times indicated. *She should never take a drug that has been prescribed for someone else.*

● *Rule out VD.* If there is any possibility that a pregnant woman has a venereal disease, she should be tested as soon as possible. During pregnancy VD is not only harmful to the pregnant woman, but it can also injure her infant.

Gonorrhea may cause difficult pregnancies. At University Hospital in Seattle, a study of pregnant women with gonorrhea suggests that they are likely to experience early membrane rupture and premature labor. There is also likely to be bacterial infection of the fetal membranes.

The babies of such women often have gonorrhea bacteria contaminating their uper gastrointestinal and respiratory tracts. The Seattle researchers found that many infants were suffering from fever, jaundice, poor appetite, and weakness. A number had pneumonia. Some died.

Syphilis can be passed to the unborn infant, causing congenital syphilis. Many such babies are stillborn. Others may become deaf, blind, or mentally defective unless they receive immediate treatment.

Yet another common venereal disease—herpes simplex virus infection—can cause grave damage to the fetus as it passes down the birth canal. The infection may start as a skin disease. It usually rapidly involves the liver, adrenal glands, and brain of the baby. Between 75 and 90 percent of the babies die. Of those who survive, an estimated 60 to 80 percent will be left with neurologic damage.

To prevent such a tragedy, a pregnant woman should be on the alert for any suspicious genital lesions. If herpes is caught early in her pregnancy, it can usually be controlled before damage to the baby occurs, and she can deliver her baby normally. But if the infection is discovered only near the end of term, her doctor may deliver the baby by caesarean in order to bypass the infected genital tract. The doctor may also advise keeping the baby isolated from the mother until she is free of infection.

● *Tell her doctor about any swelling.* A woman who experiences swelling of her hands or feet should tell her doctor right away. Edema, the accumulation of fluid in the tissues, is an early sign of toxemia, a severe metabolic disorder marked by the excretion of protein in the urine.

Heavy vomiting and sudden weight gain are other frequent signs of toxemia. In the course of the disease, a victim may experience blurred vision and severe headache. Her blood pressure generally rises abnormally.

If unchecked, toxemia (also called preeclampsia) can progress to eclampsia, a condition of convulsions and coma. Eclampsia is fatal in about half the cases and often results in the death of the fetus.

Nutritional deficiencies, especially lack of protein, may be a cause. Toxemia occurs most often in first pregnancies. It generally appears after the twentieth week of pregnancy. It is most likely to affect women who have diabetes and women carrying more than one fetus.

While it is prudent to bring any swelling to the attention of the physician, most cases of edema have nothing to do with toxemia. Some swelling because of increased water retention is normal during pregnancy. Fingers may be somewhat puffy and stiff, especially in the morning.

Good prenatal care can detect toxemia in its early stages and generally get it under control. A woman who suffers any of the symptoms associated with toxemia will generally be put on a high-protein diet with supplements of folic acid, iron, and vitamin D.

In cases of severe hypertension (high blood pressure), drugs may be prescribed. Bed rest alone, at home or in the hospital, can often control mild or moderate hypertension. If symptoms of toxemia persist after treatment, the physician may recommend inducing labor. Toxemia disappears within a few days after delivery.

• *Cut out all nonprescription drugs.* Except on her doctor's advice, a pregnant woman should not take aspirin, remedies for colds, laxatives, or medicated nose drops. Lotions or ointments containing hormones or other drugs should be avoided.

• *Avoid illicit drugs.* The effect of LSD and marijuana on the fetus is unknown. Heroin, morphine, or methadone addiction in the mother can cause addiction in the newborn—with severe physiological problems or death.

• *Stop smoking.* Women who smoke during pregnancy have a greater than average risk of stillbirths or early infant deaths. The Public

Health Service's report to Congress on cigarette smoking estimates that 4600 stillbirths a year can almost certainly be attributed to the smoking habits of the mothers.

The infant of a smoking mother is more likely to die within its first month. Smoking during pregnancy also tends to reduce the size of the infant.

If a woman gives up smoking by her fourth month of pregnancy, she is likely to eliminate the risk to her baby. The danger to the fetus seems to come from the cumulative toxic effects of the nicotine.

● *Refrain from vaginal douching.* A pregnant woman should douche only if prescribed by the doctor for a medical condition.

● *Stay physically active.* Exercise helps control weight and keep muscles strong. Most doctors urge healthy pregnant women to continue with the kind of exercise they are used to until it becomes uncomfortable to do so. Walking is particularly good.

● *Delay most immunization.* Live virus vaccines (for mumps, measles, polio, and rubella) may be harmful to the fetus. If a pregnant woman is exposed to these or other communicable diseases, she needs to consult her physician about possible preventives.

On the other hand, tetanus toxoid is generally recommended if her immunization has lapsed. The shot will also protect her baby through his first month.

● *Steer clear of X rays.* They can be dangerous to the fetus, particularly during the first three months. All nonessential abdominal X rays should be postponed until after delivery or at least until the fourth month or later. If a woman must have an X ray elsewhere on her body—such as a dental X ray—she should make sure her reproductive organs are protected with a lead apron.

● *Eat sensibly.* A pregnant woman's diet should include milk or milk products (about 4 servings a day). Dairy foods provide protein and calcium essential for the baby's bones and teeth. She should also have daily servings of meat, fish, poultry or eggs, nuts, and beans; vegetables and fruits; breads and cereals. Many doctors prescribe supplementary iron tablets to prevent iron-deficiency anemia.

It is best for a pregnant woman to eat small, frequent meals instead of 2 or 3 large meals every day—since hormonal changes slow down the normal digestive process.

A woman of normal weight should gain roughly 25 to 35 pounds in the course of her pregnancy. Many women fear they will gain too much weight in the wrong places and not be able to lose it afterward. Anxious that this weight gain will make them sexually unattractive to their partners, they restrict their food intake and thus give birth to low-weight babies. These babies tend to have more medical problems than babies of average weight (7.5 pounds).

Most women lose about 12 to 15 pounds after giving birth. With a reasonable amount of exercise and a good diet, normal weight will usually be attained within 12 months.

• *Wear a seat belt low.* It is not necessary to stop wearing a seat belt during pregnancy. Contrary to misbelief, there is no evidence that seat belts pose any threat to the fetus, and in accidents they could save the lives of both the mother and the fetus.

But a pregnant woman should wear the belt low, snugly fastened across the pelvic bones and upper thighs, not across the uterus. For added protection, she should wear a shoulder harness too. She can continue to drive as long as she can fit behind the wheel.

Air travel in a pressurized cabin poses no special hazards. But it is wise for her to avoid long airplane trips during the last weeks of pregnancy because of the possibility of labor or delivery during the flight. Some airlines require a doctor's note to the effect that childbirth en route is unlikely before they will permit an obviously pregnant woman to board.

In late pregnancy, a woman's large abdomen may make some intercourse positions uncomfortable. The male-superior position (face-to-face, man on top) may be particularly awkward.

The female-superior position may be considerably more comfortable. It allows the pregnant woman to control the degree of penile penetration and to accommodate her enlarged abdomen by sitting higher or raising herself with her arms.

A lateral position (partners on their sides) is another alternative. The woman can rest on the man's inner thigh while he places his upper leg between her thighs. This position allows great freedom of movement and makes it relatively easy for the man to accommodate his pelvis to his pregnant partner's abdomen.

Yet another possibility is a rear-entry position, in which the woman lies on her side with her belly supported by the bed. For easier vaginal penetration, her hips may be elevated with a pillow.

247

Throughout pregnancy, it is important for a woman to receive good prenatal care. Optimal health maintenance during pregnancy involves education and counseling as well as medical management.

Childbirth preparation classes are invaluable in reinforcing and amplifying what the pregnant couple learns from the obstetrician. Organizations that provide such classes include Parent-Child, Lamaze, Childbirth Education Association (CEA), ASPO, and Flame.

See also ABORTION; CONTRACEPTION; POSTPARTUM PROBLEMS; VENEREAL DISEASE.

PREGNANCY, ECTOPIC. See ECTOPIC PREGNANCY.

PRIAPISM, a persistent, abnormal erection of the penis, is a medical emergency. It can result in damage to the erectile tissue. Sexual function is rarely recovered unless treatment is prompt and effective.

Most causes of priapism have nothing to do with sexual arousal. Sickle cell anemia, chronic myelogenous leukemia, and polycythemia are among the most common underlying conditions.

Less frequently, the cause may be blood vessel obstruction resulting from spinal cord injury or tumors. Priapism may also be an effect of phimosis, urethral polyps, urethral calculi, or prostatitis.

Occasionally priapism may be the result of trauma to the penis. Blood clotting and swelling from the injury may interfere with blood supply to the penis. A persistent erection may result if less blood can flow out of the vein or if more blood flows through the artery.

Certain drugs—thioridazine, heparin, testosterone, and hyralazine—have occasionally been reported to bring on the condition.

Patients with idiopathic priapism—in which there is no identified cause—often have had transient episodes following intense sexual stimulation. In such cases, a cycle of reflex blood vessel spasm and swelling is thought to obstruct drainage from the tissues of the penis.

The onset of priapism is often associated with vigorous and prolonged intercourse. But it is likely that the intercourse merely exposes the condition, rather than causes it. Indeed, the pathological erection may be what makes the prolonged intercourse possible.

Ice packs are among the many remedies but are rarely adequate alone. The penis is likely to contain thick blood, the consistency of motor oil, in the vein. It may need to be removed through large-bore needles.

Priapism caused by neurological conditions may be relieved by spinal anesthesia. Blood may have to be surgically shunted from the erectile tissue to another blood vessel.

For priapism caused by trauma, there is usually a need for immediate surgery, with drainage of fluid or blood.

See also PROSTATITIS.

PROGESTERONE. See HORMONE DISORDERS.

PROPHYLACTICS. See CONDOMS.

PROSTAGLANDINS. See ABORTION; MENSTRUATION.

PROSTATE CANCER kills more men than any other cancer except lung cancer. It accounts for 15 percent of cancers among white males and 21 percent among black. Prostate cancer is mainly a disease of older men. In men over 65, it accounts for the majority of malignancies. It is extremely rare in men under 40.

The prostate is a small gland about the size of a walnut. It is located under the male's bladder and surrounds his urethra, the tube through which urine passes. The prostate produces most of the fluid of ejaculation.

Men over 40 should have the prostate examined annually. A prostate check is usually part of a rectal examination. The physician feels the prostate through the rectum wall with a gloved, lubricated finger. The examination takes a minute or two. Men can minimize the discomfort by bearing down as if moving their bowels.

Prostate cancer usually progresses slowly and may cause no symptoms. Some men experience frequent, painful urination. There may be a change in the size or force of the urine stream. Sometimes, blood appears in the urine.

There is no known cause of cancer of the prostate. A man is at greater risk of contracting the disease if his father and grandfather had it. If so, he should be checked twice a year.

No relationship has been found between frequency of intercourse and the incidence of prostate cancer. Nor is there a correlation between particular sexual practices—such as masturbation—and the development of the disease.

When the cancer is confined to the prostate, the treatment of choice is usually surgery. Such surgery, called a radical prostatectomy, is much more extensive than the prostatectomy for prostate enlargement (see entry). Since nerve pathways that control erection are damaged, impotence usually results.

Men with this condition may wish to consider penile prostheses. Surgical implants are a possibility for 96 percent of men after radical prostatectomy.

Sexual desire may remain after surgery, and men report varying degrees of sexual gratification. But sensations of orgasm are absent, and there is no ejaculate.

Urinary incontinence is a problem for about 10 percent of men after the operation. It can be surgically corrected in 60 percent of the cases.

In some cases of inoperable prostate cancer, treatment is the removal of both testicles and/or estrogen therapy. With such therapy, sexual desire is usually suppressed and impotence occurs.

See also CANCER; PENILE PROSTHESES; PROSTATE ENLARGEMENT.

PROSTATE ENLARGEMENT (benign prostatic hypertrophy). The prostate gland, a walnut-sized organ wrapped around the male's urethra, produces most of the fluid that helps transport sperm at ejaculation.

By about age 50 or 60, a man's prostate begins to get bigger, sometimes with no symptoms.

Many men with this condition experience difficult passage of urine. There may be related discomforts, such as bedwetting and frequent urination.

The condition should be checked by a physician early. Many of the same symptoms mark cancer of the prostate.

The cause of enlarged prostate is uncertain. A hormonal imbalance is thought to be responsible. It does *not* result from sexual excesses, masturbation, or gonorrhea. Nor is the condition likely to cause sexual problems.

An enlarged prostate puts pressure on the urethra and the bladder, interfering both with the starting of the urine stream and the complete emptying of the bladder. This results in a sensation of irritation and a need to empty the bladder frequently. The stream of urine lacks force and becomes weak and dribbly. Straining to urinate may cause pain and the appearance of blood in the urine.

During the months or years of increasing discomfort, obstruction of urine flow contributes to complications. The muscles of the bladder wall must force urine through the narrowing urethra. These muscles become enlarged from the extra exercise, thickening the bladder wall and reducing the bladder's capacity.

Occasionally the increased muscular effort forces weak spots on the wall of the bladder to become pockets called diverticuli. This can lead to urinary tract infection. Eventually the kidneys may be damaged, preventing the filtering of waste products from the blood. This can be fatal.

No medicine currently available can shrink or dissolve the enlarged glands. In the early stages, prostate massage may be helpful.

Surgery is the recommended treatment when enlargement greatly obstructs the urine flow, or when there is a chronic infection.

There should be no loss in sexual function following surgery. Although the operation is called a prostatectomy (which means removal of the prostate gland), the gland itself is not removed, merely the mass of overgrown urethral glands inside the prostate. The man will be able to have an erection, engage in intercourse, and experience orgasm.

The operation usually causes infertility. After surgery, most men experience retrograde ejaculation: semen is propelled into the bladder instead of being ejaculated through the penis. Since most of the men undergoing such surgery are older, infertility is not a common cercern.

Impotence may follow surgery if a man equates fertility with virility, and feels less a man after surgery. Or he may feel that his sex partner considers him less virile if he can no longer reproduce. If retrograde ejaculation has not been fully explained to him, he may be concerned about this change in sexual functioning, and impotence may result.

Some men become impotent because of fear that intercourse may cause medical complications. Others may get the impression from their physicians that impotence is expected to follow surgery.

An older man may use the surgery as an excuse to stop sexual activity

251

because of declining sexual desire or ability. Some men may suffer from concurrent medical problems—such as diabetes—which may impair sexual functioning following surgery.

Men with psychogenic impotence often respond well to psychotherapy. In cases of organic impotence, a penile prosthesis can be considered.

See also EJACULATION, RETROGRADE; IMPOTENCE; PENILE PROSTHESES; PROSTATE CANCER.

PROSTATITIS is inflammation of the prostate gland. This small organ is located at the base of the bladder in the male. It is wrapped around the urethra, the tube through which urine passes.

The prostate is part of a man's reproductive system. The ducts that carry sperm pass through tunnels in the prostate. At ejaculation, the muscles in the prostate squeeze the embedded glands to discharge a fluid that helps to transport and nourish the sperm.

Pain on ejaculation is a common symptom of prostatitis. There may also be an aching in the groin, testicles, and lower back, pain on urination, and frequent urination.

Often, prostatitis is caused by a bacterial infection. In an acute attack, a man typically experiences fever, chills, rectal and perineal discomfort, and painful, frequent urination. There is often a sense of urinary urgency, and there may be a discharge from the urethra.

Chronic bacterial prostatitis—a more common condition—plagues many men over 50. The infection seems to disappear, only to reappear weeks or months later, a pattern that may continue for many years.

In many men, inflammation of the prostate occurs without any apparent infection. The cause may be bacterial or viral micoorganisms that have not yet been identified.

A marked decrease in sexual activity may result in prostatitis by causing congestion of the prostate. During sexual arousal, fluid in the prostate increases. If the man frequently becomes sexually aroused without ejaculating, the prostate may become congested with fluid. This may cause inflammation.

Prostatitis from this cause is thought to affect many older men, who may have less opportunity for sexual activity.

Congestive prostatitis may also be a sign of a sexual problem in a marriage. With reduced sexual frequency, the prostate may become inflamed.

Less commonly, prostatitis may result from an unusual *increase* in the number of ejaculations in a short period of time. Presumably, the prostate, repeatedly forced to contract during ejaculation, becomes irritated and inflamed. Symptoms usually respond well to warm sitz baths, drinking lots of fluids—and sexual abstinence for several days.

Prostatitis may also be experienced by men who have "feast or famine" sex lives. Such a sexual pattern is common to young men who have periodic intense love affairs or to men who are regularly away from home for several weeks at a time.

Many factors contribute to or aggravate prostatitis. Among these are spicy foods, alcohol, chocolate, caffeine, sitting for long periods of time, riding in bumpy vehicles, and emotional stress.

Sexual problems sometimes result from prostatitis. In acute bacterial prostatitis, some men experience loss of sexual desire. Others, however, find their sexual desire is enhanced—although erection may be painful and ejaculation painful and bloody. Most physicians recommend avoiding sexual stimulation of any sort during acute attacks.

In cases of chronic prostatitis, painful ejaculation may lead to the avoidance of sexual activity and sometimes to impotence. Spasmodic contractions of the prostate during orgasm may cause sharp pain felt in the rectum, testicles, or head of the penis. In some men, the pain is so severe that an aversion to sex develops.

Men with chronic prostatitis may also experience premature ejaculation, bloody ejaculation, and frequent painful nocturnal emissions.

In most cases, there is no reason to abstain from intercourse with prostatitis. But if the cause is bacterial, the ejaculate will usually contain bacteria, and there is a small possibility of causing vaginitis or urinary tract infection in the female. The use of a condom affords protection.

Treatment for prostatitis is a regular pattern of ejaculation— whatever is usual and most comfortable for the man and his sexual partner. This may be once a day for some, once a week for others, once a month for still others. The important factor is not the frequency, but that the man should ejaculate at fairly regular intervals.

If the prostatitis is caused by bacteria, a course of antibiotics is prescribed.

Caffeine-containing products (coffee, tea, cola) are best avoided until symptoms abate. A judicious use of alcohol and spicy foods is also recommended. Sitz baths at least twice a day for 10-20 minutes in very hot water often bring some relief.

Nuts (particularly cashew nuts) increase prostatic fluids, and should be avoided during prostatitis. Some physicians recommend periodic massage of the prostate, usually for older patients. This is done by a physician, who inserts a finger in the rectum. Massage should be avoided during acute bacterial infection.

Symptoms usually respond readily to treatment, and most men quickly resume the level of sexual activity they experienced before the prostatitis. If sexual problems persist after successful treatment, counseling may be appropriate.

See also EJACULATION, BLOODY; EPIDIDYMO-ORCHITIS; PROSTATE CANCER; PROSTATE ENLARGEMENT.

PROSTITUTION is engaging in sexual activity for money. Prostitutes may be male or female, and they may engage in heterosexual or homosexual acts.

Like other people with a large number of sex partners, prostitutes of both sexes are at greater risk of contracting—and spreading—venereal diseases. Male prostitutes are liable to the same medical problems as homosexuals with many contacts—including amebiasis, giardiasis, hepatitis, venereal warts, and problems associated with anal sex.

Female prostitutes may experience pelvic congestion (see entry) if they repeatedly become sexually aroused without experiencing orgasm.

It is not usual for a female prostitute to experience orgasm during intercourse with a client. In a study of nearly 500 prostitutes, one-third reported that they occasionally experienced orgasm while having intercourse with a client. One-fifth sometimes experienced orgasm from cunnilingus performed by a client.

Most had an orgasm once a week or less. Emotionally uninvolved in the sexual activity, many are surprised by their orgasms. Some are embarrassed. Others experience revulsion. To avoid sexual arousal, many prostitutes prefer to provide oral sex rather than intercourse. Prostitutes often relieve sexual tension through masturbation, or through sex with their pimps or male or female lovers.

Generally, prostitutes are young men or women, and their clients are older men. The practice of prostitution is illegal in this country, except for some parts of Nevada.

Studies of female prostitutes reveal that as children they were more likely to have experienced sexual advances from adults than women who are not prostitutes. They were more often involved in incestuous relationships with their fathers. They generally began sexual activity at a younger age, and they experienced a higher incidence of rape. The majority have little education and come from poor families. Many are dependent on drugs.

The typical client of a female prostitute is a middle-aged married man who occasionally goes to prostitutes for sexual acts that his wife will not provide, or that he is reluctant to ask her for. Most often, the practice is fellatio (see ORAL SEX). Some men engage prostitutes to perform sadomasochistic acts, such as whipping or being whipped.

See also AMEBIASIS; ANAL SEX; GIARDIASIS; HEPATITIS; HOMOSEXUALITY; INCEST; ORAL SEX; PELVIC CONGESTION; SADOMASOCHISM; VENEREAL DISEASE.

PUBERTY (from the Latin word *puber*, meaning "adult") is the culmination of the process of sexual maturation: the ability to reproduce.

This process begins when a part of the brain called the hypothalamus triggers a chain of chemical reactions. Researchers do not yet know what signals the hypothalamus to send to the pituitary gland specific hormones, chemical substances secreted directly into the bloodstream. The pituitary, a pea-sized organ on the underside of the brain at eye level, in turn sends hormones that regulate the testes in boys and the ovaries in girls.

Finally the testes and ovaries produce sex hormones—mainly testosterone in boys, estrogen and progesterone in girls. These bring about pubescence, marked by the development of secondary sexual characteristics: breasts, enlarged genitals, pubic, facial, and underarm hair. The physical changes culminate in the adolescents' ability to have children of their own. They are then said to have reached puberty.

There is an enormous variation as to the age when individual children reach sexual maturation. The process may begin at 8 or at 18 or at any time in between. Most boys reach puberty at about 15 or 16; most girls about 2 or 3 years earlier.

But children, and their parents, should be reassured that words like "average," "typical," and "normal" are statistical terms—not the same as "healthy." Sexual development of the human species does not necessarily follow an orderly progression. Stages of a youngster's maturing may be faster or slower or reversed compared to the so-called norms. Most departures from developmental norms are not deficient, but merely different.

Puberty comes unusually early for a small proportion of children. A girl should be checked by a physician if she shows signs of impending puberty before age 8; a boy if he shows pubertal changes before age 9. Some children experience isolated pubertal changes, such as the development of pubic hair or breasts, a condition called incomplete precocious puberty. Others undergo the full range of pubertal changes—complete precocious puberty—including maturation of the reproductive system. If precocious puberty affects a girl, chances are 85 percent it's complete; a boy, 65 percent it's *incomplete*.

Some cases of precocious puberty are so extreme that parents seek immediate medical help. Infant boys 5 months old have had penis development. Five-year-old boys have produced sperm. Menstruation has occurred in babies under a year. The youngest documented pregnancy is that of a 5-year-old Peruvian girl who began menstruating at 3. On May 15, 1939, she gave birth to a 6½-pound boy by caesarean delivery.

If a child shows signs of precocious puberty, chances are nothing is wrong. In most cases, doctors can find no abnormality accounting for the condition and make the diagnosis of idiopathic sexual precocity: the clock of puberty went off too early, but there is no medical cause that can be found. The child will probably be asked to see the physician for periodic checkups, but no medical treatment is required.

In some children, however, there are illnesses causing the precocity. Puberty may be a result of tumors in the genitals or on the adrenal gland. Congenital brain defects, a brain tumor, or an injury to the nervous system similarly may account for precocious puberty. The syndrome is far more likely to be caused by a medical condition in boys than in girls. Sometimes, signs of precocious puberty occur when children accidentally ingest sex hormones, such as birth control pills or medications for menopause.

Children are likely to have a hard time adjusting to their premature development. A girl who is an early developer, for example, may be terribly embarrassed by her breasts, hiding them in layers of loose bulky clothing. Parents should explain to the youngster any medical problems that may be causing the condition. If no medical cause can be found, the child should be told that nothing is medically wrong, and that sometimes the clock that regulates the onset of puberty goes off early. Parents should stress that in a few years, friends will catch up. Then the child will feel more comfortable with pubertal changes. In general, experts feel, it is wisest to treat the child according to chronological age. Make demands and accord privileges suitable to a child of 9—even though the youngster looks 13.

At the other extreme, some youngsters experience delayed puberty. Most girls begin breast development between 9 and 11—usually just after a growth spurt. Puberty should be considered delayed—and a physician consulted—if a girl has no breast buds (slightly protruding nipples) by the time she is 13.

Similarly, most girls begin menstruating between 11 and 13½, although it is not uncommon for a girl to start as early as nine or as late as 18. Most girls get their first periods 2 to 3 years after their breast buds first appear. A girl should see a physician if she still isn't menstruating 4 years after her breast budding.

If a girl is 18 or over and has never menstruated, she requires a physician's attention. Her failure to menstruate, termed primary amenorrhea, may be due to a large number of physiological conditions, many of them genetic. She may have an obstruction of the cervix or vagina. She may have been born with a deformed or missing uterus. Her ovaries may be malfunctioning. She may be suffering from hormonal deficiencies. Psychological stress may also play a part.

In boys, delayed puberty is usually associated with delayed growth. If a boy is much shorter than his classmates and has not begun sexual maturation by about 14 or 15, he may have what is medically termed constitutional delayed growth, a condition that affects 10 times as many boys as girls. It is often an hereditary trait. In some families, for example, males are typically shorter than normal until about 16, then suddenly spurt half a foot.

A typical boy with constitutional delayed growth looks about 3 years younger than he is. He reaches puberty two to four years after his peers. At that time, he will have a growth spurt and catch up to his peers.

Constitutional delayed growth can be confirmed by determining a boy's bone age and correlating it with his height and chronological age. Doctors are able to calculate bone age because the development of bones follows a predictable sequence—although the precise schedule varies from person to person. Developmental standards have been set for specific bones. These averages indicate how far along toward maturity a bone of, say, the wrist typically is at certain ages. By examining a boy's bones by X ray, a physician can relate their degree of maturity to the norms—and thus determine what his bone age is. A 13-year-old boy with a bone age of 13 years is developing according to the average timetable. If his bone age were 14 or more years, he would be considered an early maturer. With a bone age under 13, he would be called a late maturer. If a boy is a slow grower, knowing that his bone maturation is also slow can provide him with a great deal of reassurance that he will reach ordinary height.

Bone age can also help a doctor predict when pubertal development is likely to begin. In general, whatever a boy's chronological age is, he begins sexual maturation when his bone age is around 12.

If a boy is experiencing delayed puberty and growth, the physician will want to rule out any medical conditions that might be responsible. These include chronic conditions such as allergies, malnutrition, diabetes, and glandular disorders. Delayed puberty also can result from sickle cell anemia, problems in digestion, and bone, liver, or kidney disease. Emotional deprivation sometimes accounts for a child's failure to grow.

If a boy is unusually troubled by his small size, professional counseling may be advisable.

Male hormone therapy can trigger a boy's puberty and adolescent growth spurt—but at a cost. Speeding up the growth process may cut one or two inches off his ultimate height. Most physicians advise parents simply to wait. It is only a matter of time before the situation improves without any medical intervention. Most doctors consider hormone therapy for constitutional delayed growth and delayed puberty only when a boy's psychological problems are severe enough to offset his risks in treatment.

See also HORMONE DISORDERS; MENSTRUATION.

PUBIC HAIR REMOVAL. Some people prefer to remove their pubic hair. Or in some cases one sex partner—more commonly the male—may request that the other remove pubic hair. In some cultures, shaving pubic hair is the norm.

Often, such people consider pubic hair "unaesthetic." This feeling may be bound up with the view of sexuality as dirty.

Pubic hair is associated with adult sexuality while a bare pubis is associated with childhood. Thus, a person who removes pubic hair may wish to hark back to an earlier era, a time of sexual innocence. Similarly, a man who wishes his partner to remove her pubic hair may feel safer with a woman who looks more like an immature female. Or perhaps a hairless pubis may impart a necessary incestuous quality to the sexual activity.

Pubic hair has several physiological functions, but none is essential. Adults can safely do without pubic hair. This hair aids in the temperature regulation of the pubic area. By controlling temperature, pubic hair helps maintain the expansion of the blood vessels during sexual excitement. It also acts as a protective cushion, helping absorb the friction of intercourse.

The safest way to remove pubic hair is to shave it. The pubic area should first be washed with hot water. Shaving cream or a thick lather or soap should be applied before the area is shaved with a fresh razor blade. Other methods of hair removal—such as tweezing, electrolysis, or depilatories—are more likely to irritate the delicate tissues of the pubis.

See also HIRSUTISM.

PUBIC LICE. See LICE.

PUBIS. See FEMALE SEXUAL ANATOMY.

RADIATION THERAPY. See CANCER.

RAPE is the fastest rising crime of violence in the United States. While over 50,000 rapes are reported every year, between four and ten times as many are thought to occur. Thus, possibly as many as half a million women are raped each year.

Rape is forcible sexual assault. In many states, it refers only to

259

penile-vaginal penetration, with or without ejaculation. Some states have broadened the definition of rape to include any forced sexual act.

No female is safe. Rapes have been committed on babies of a few months and women in their 90s. But the average age of the rape victim is her late teens; most victims are between 10 and 19 years old.

This age group is particularly vulnerable to rape and its aftermath. Young girls are most easily terrified and shamed into silence. Their schedules are predictable, hence a rapist can easily know when and where school buses stop and what routes girls follow home. Further, teenage girls are most apt to be friendly and trusting.

Rapists are not necessarily strangers. About half are known to their victims. Nor do rapes necessarily take place in back alleys on dark nights. Half of all rapes are committed in homes, often the victim's own.

Virtually all victims experience rape as a psychological trauma. They feel terror, rage, and helplessness at the time. The aftermath may be months or years of fearfulness, psychogenic ailments, confusion about sexuality, and sexual aversion.

The teenage girl may be hardest hit. She is often reluctant to turn to her parents for support, since she is struggling for independence from them. Moreover, during adolescence she is forging a sexual identity, coming to grips with her own sexuality. Thus rape at this time is likely to have a particularly profound impact on her attitudes about herself, about men, about sex.

Added to the trauma of the rape is the shame and guilt she is likely to experience. Experts now understand rape as an assault, an act of violence, that takes a sexual form. The rapist's main goal is not sexual gratification, but rather humiliating his victim, showing his power over her, expressing anger. But popular attitudes are slow to catch up with scientific understanding, and a woman may find that a stigma is attached to being a rape victim.

People may suggest that she somehow enticed the rapist, that perhaps she secretly enjoyed the rape. (In fact, most women report that they were in terror of being killed.) If medical personnel and police are callous and suspicious, the rape trauma is further compounded.

To help protect themselves from rape, women are advised to:
- List only last name and initials on mailboxes and in phone directories if they live alone.
- Keep doors locked.

- Never open a door automatically after a knock. Require the caller to identify himself satisfactorily.
- Never let a strange telephone caller know that they are home alone.
- Never let a child answer the door.
- Keep drapes and shades drawn at night.
- Have the key ready so the door can be opened immediately.
- Don't hitchhike.
- Avoid entering an elevator occupied by a male stranger. If a suspicious-acting man follows you into an elevator, step out.
- When driving, try to travel on well-lighted, populated streets. Keep windows and doors locked. Keep your car in gear when halted at traffic lights.
- If you believe you are being followed by another car, pull over to the curb at a spot where there are people, and let the car pass you. If the car continues to follow you, drive to the nearest place where you can get help—a police station, fire house, gas station.
- While walking alone at night, avoid poorly lit streets, unpopulated areas, vacant lots, alleys.
- If you are walking and believe you are being followed, run. If the man quickens his pace, scream as you run. Some women find that screaming "fire" will bring faster results than "rape" or "help."

If a woman is attacked, should she offer resistance? Considerable controversy exists on this point. If the attacker has a knife or gun, physical resistance may spur him to increased violence. On the other hand, it might frighten him away. In one study of rapists, half said if the woman had resisted, they would have let her go. The other half said they would have become violent, possibly killing the woman.

Some women have found that they could discourage the rapist by claiming to have cancer or a venereal disease. Others have talked their way out of being raped by getting the rapist to see them as real people. Sometimes, speaking in a firm, assertive manner will discourage a rapist, who is seeking a startled, passive woman.

A woman who is attacked may instinctively try to fight off the assailant. If so, she should not shirk from trying to hurt him seriously—clawing at his eyeballs, pushing her thumb into his throat, kicking his shins or genitals, stamping on his feet. At the first opportunity, she should run.

A woman who has been raped is likely to get the most sympathetic

261

and knowledgeable advice if she calls her local rape crisis center. These exist in every large city in the United States and in most smaller cities and towns.

Often staffed by women who have themselves been raped, a rape center will give a woman information about getting medical care, about reporting the rape to the police, about court procedures and the particular state's requirements for proving rape.

If the woman plans to report the rape, she should not wash or douche. If she was raped in her home, she should not clean up. Undergarments and any torn or stained clothing should be given to the police. At the earliest opportunity, the woman should write down everything she can remember about the event.

It is a good idea for a raped woman to have a friend or family member accompany her to the police department and hospital. If no one is available, the rape center may be able to provide a volunteer on request.

Whether or not the woman plans to report the rape, she should have a medical examination. Many physicians recommend preventive treatment for venereal disease, usually an injection of penicillin. If the woman is of childbearing age, was not using contraception, and was possibly ovulating at the time, the physician may also recommend a course of DES (see entry) for the prevention of pregnancy. If the woman chooses not to take DES and misses her next menstruation, she should be tested for pregnancy.

A thorough rape examination includes a great many procedures, among them: repairing any injury that resulted from the attack; doing cultures for venereal disease; taking samples of the vaginal contents for semen typing; taking fingernail cuttings and samples of loose hair or dried blood from the woman's body.

Counseling after rape is one of the important services rape centers provide. It is often of immeasurable help for a raped woman to talk with other women who have had the same experience. Most women can satisfactorily resolve their fear, shame, and anger in a few months to a year.

For some women, however, the aftermath of rape is much more extensive. Years later, they may remain anxious, depressed, or afraid to leave the house. Long-term psychotherapy may be called for.

Sexual disturbances are common after rape. Often, women delay resuming sexual relations afterwards. Some develop an aversion to sex or to certain sexual activities associated with the rape. It is not unusual for a woman to have difficulty experiencing orgasm for some months after being raped. A few women respond to rape with compulsive sexual activity—seeking out one man after another in an attempt to erase the memory of the rape.

Often, a woman's ambivalence about sex after rape is compounded by her sex partner's attitude. A male partner may view the rape as a sexual violation of the woman, rather than as a crime of violence. Feeling that the woman is now somehow sullied, he may be unable to resume sexual relations. This leaves her feeling even more shamed and alienated. Psychological counseling can be invaluable in aiding such couples to resolve their difficulties.

See also DES; INCEST.

RECTAL PAIN following sexual intercourse occasionally occurs among both men and women.

The lower rectum and the genitals are both served by the presacral nerve. The contractions that occur during orgasm include some contractions of the anal sphincters and the bladder neck.

Normally, these contractions are not painful. In some hypersensitive people, however, the sensation of anal contraction is experienced as unpleasant or painful. This is more likely to be true of men than women: ejaculation seems to produce more anorectal contraction than the female orgasm.

Severe rectal pain that occurs after each intercourse requires a physician's evaluation. The problem may be due to a rectal disorder, such as a fissure.

Rectal muscle spasm may be the cause of the pain. Direct rectal stimulation as part of sexual activity might make spasm more likely to occur. In some people, rectal pain after intercourse is thought to be of psychogenic origin.

RECTUM. See FEMALE SEXUAL ANATOMY; MALE SEXUAL ANATOMY.

RENAL FAILURE. See KIDNEY DISEASE.

RESPIRATORY DISEASE

RESPIRATORY DISEASE may significantly impair sexual functioning.

A victim of emphysema and/or chronic bronchitis (often designated as chronic obstructive pulmonary disease, or COPD) may suffer shortness of breath with moderate exertion. Sexual activity may prove difficult because of oxygen deficiency.

COPD is a major cause of disability and death in this country, second only to heart disease as a cause of disability in Social Security statistics. Smoking is a major cause of respiratory disease, and "smoker's cough" may be an early symptom. Other early signs are wheezing, recurrent respiratory infections, and sputum production. Occasionally, first complaints are weakness, weight loss, and decreased sexual interest.

In general, sexual difficulties increase with the severity of the disease. Patients who are short of breath at rest or with only minimal exertion may have significant limitations on their sexual activity. Indeed, sexual exertion may be so taxing that the person with COPD may find it impossible to complete the act. Both men and women may experience loss of libido. Some men become impotent.

Patients with severe disability from COPD are typically anxious about their shortness of breath and fear suffocation. They are thus likely to avoid physical exertion, including sexual activity. Further, as with any chronic debilitating disease, COPD sufferers may become depressed, which contributes to decreased sexual desire and other sexual problems.

In advanced COPD, reduced muscle strength and impaired mental activity resulting from persistent oxygen deprivation further impede sexual activity.

To aid sexual functioning, patients with COPD should experiment with sexual positions that minimize physical exertion—for example, the side-by-side position or the one with the patient supine beneath the partner. It is advisable for COPD patients to rest before sexual activity. Patients are also better off having sex when they feel most well. This may require changing the time of day when sex occurs.

A waterbed may be a good way of easing sexual exertion. Movement by the healthy partner produces a fluid wave that propels the couple without requiring increased oxygen consumption on the patient's part. The use of a bronchodilator before intercourse may also help the patient function better.

Home use of carefully controlled oxygen therapy may both improve the patient's capacity for sexual responsiveness and reduce anxiety.

COPD is irreversible, and therapy does not result in cure. But various medical regimens can provide symptomatic relief and may possibly slow the progression of the disease. Any measure that provides relief may also improve sexual functioning.

RHYTHM. See NATURAL FAMILY PLANNING.

RUBBERS. See CONDOMS.

RUPTURE. See HERNIA.

SADISM. See SADOMASOCHISM.

SADOMASOCHISM. Sadism is sexual pleasure derived from degrading, tormenting, or hurting another person. Masochism is obtaining sexual gratification from being humiliated or hurt by a partner.

The terms are often linked to form one word—sadomasochism— since most people who exhibit such behavior patterns have elements of both sadism and masochism in their personalities and typically switch roles.

Some degree of sadistic or masochistic sexual pleasure is thought to exist in almost all people. Sadomasochistic fantasies are common. For many couples, some elements of hurting or being hurt are part of love play—biting, scratching, pinching, and teasing.

Contrary to popular opinion, sadomasochists are proportionally as common among heterosexuals as among homosexuals.

For the majority of people who engage in sadomasochism, the practice is an elaborate theatrical ritual; often, little or no pain is actually inflicted, merely simulated abuse and suffering. Partners may follow a particular scenario, with props such as whips, chains, and

265

costumes. For most, such play-acting of the fantasy is adequate for sexual release.

Some individuals achieve orgasm at the time of inflicting or receiving pain. For others, the sadomasochistic ritual precedes intercourse. The masochist, who may seem to be the victim at the mercy of the sadist, is often the one who prescribes the amount, type, and duration of the physical and psychic pain he receives.

Much of pornographic literature is devoted to sadomasochism. There are magazines that specialize in sadomasochistic practices; personal advertisements in such magazines often bring people with special requirements together. A wide array of sadomasochistic equipment can be purchased through specialized catalogues. There are even special clubs for sadomasochists.

Various tools are used by sadomasochists, among them knives, ropes, leg irons, handcuffs, whips, paddles, and leather garments and boots.

Most people who engage in sadomasochistic practices do so by mutual consent and inflict on each other no permanent or serious injury or psychological damage.

The practice is likely to be safest when the people involved know and trust each other. Indeed, part of the gratification rests in the security of knowing that the partner can be trusted not to transgress prearranged limits.

Unfortunately, sometimes sadomasochism results in severe injury or death. Whipping, burning, beating, and cutting can obviously cause serious harm.

About 50 deaths in the United States each year result from a practice called "bondage." In this practice, the participants are stimulated not by pain—but by the feeling of helplessness associated with being tied up. Death may result if the person is bound in a full bathtub and slips underwater or if someone is tied or chained and left alone in a fire. In some cases, people employ bondage as a masturbatory activity. It may be fatal if, for example, a man chains himself, then drops the key for the lock and is trapped.

Also sometimes fatal is garroting, in which a masochist hangs himself by the neck as part of a masturbatory ritual. Hanging to accomplish ejaculation—known as sexual asphyxia—is most common in adolescent males. The practice may account for as many as 200 to 400 deaths per year. Usually, the man hangs by his neck for 1 or 2 minutes.

The reduced oxygen to the brain is said to enhance orgasmic sensations. But death can result if the man loses consciousness before he can relieve the pressure on his neck.

SALPINGITIS. See PELVIC INFLAMMATORY DISEASE.

SARCOPTIC ITCH. See SCABIES.

SATYRIASIS. See HYPERSEXUALITY.

SCABIES (sarcoptic itch) is an infestation that may be transmitted through sexual intercourse or other close physical contact.

The condition results when mites, arachnids (close kin of spiders) barely 1/50 of an inch long, burrow under the skin. Reddish zigzag furrows can be observed. The victim usually suffers maddening itching, often with an allergic reaction. Scratching is to little avail and may lead to impetigo, a skin infection marked by pustules.

Mites picked up during sexual intercourse are likely to infest the genital area and buttocks. Scabies also commonly occurs in the webbing between the fingers and around the wrists. Skin folds of the elbows, underarms, breast, and feet are often infested.

Merely sleeping in the same bed may spread the infestation. Mites can also travel from person to person through kissing, hugging, handshaking, and contaminated toilets. The mite thrives where people live in crowded conditions and do not bathe. Scabies often spreads through a family.

It is wise to consult a physician or a hospital clinic when symptoms first appear. Treatment usually entails Eurax cream or Kwell lotion or cream (not shampoo). It is applied from the neck down and left on for a prescribed period before being washed off.

All clothing and bedding that came in contact with the sufferer should be thoroughly cleaned. Fumigating the mattress or the household is not necessary.

See also LICE; VENEREAL DISEASE.

SCROTUM. See MALE SEXUAL ANATOMY.

SEATWORMS. See PINWORMS.

SEDATIVES. See TRANQUILIZERS.

SELF-STIMULATION. See MASTURBATION.

SEMEN. See MALE SEXUAL ANATOMY.

SEMEN ALLERGY. A small number of women experience allergic reactions to semen. They may have stinging, burning, and pain in the vagina, starting during intercourse or immediately after ejaculation. The vagina and vulva become red and swollen, often with bumps (urticaria) on the vulva. These symptoms may persist up to 72 hours.

Some women experience systemic reactions, with sneezing, swelling around the eyes, and a sensation of throat swelling.

In rare cases, the reaction may be life-threatening. Some women have asthma attacks or may go into anaphylactic shock. A few women have had the unfortunate experience of being rushed to the emergency room after their first sexual intercourse.

It is possible for a woman to be allergic to one man's semen, but not to that of others. If allergy is suspected, a specimen of the semen can be used in a scratch test. A small amount is scratched into the woman's forearm. She will have a positive reaction—with redness and swelling—in 20 to 30 minutes. Other tests can confirm the diagnosis.

Use of a condom generally prevents the allergic reaction. Antihistamines may be prescribed to minimize reactions. In some women with milder, localized reactions, desensitization may spontaneously occur following several years of sexual activity. In women with the more severe systemic reactions, attempts at desensitization have not been successful.

See also INFERTILITY.

SEMINAL VESICLE. See MALE SEXUAL ANATOMY.

SEMINIFEROUS TUBULES. See MALE SEXUAL ANATOMY.

SEX THERAPY. It has been estimated that about half of all couples have sexual problems at one time or another. Thus a large number of people are in need of information, advice, counseling, or more extensive therapy for sexual difficulties.

Unless such people choose their sources of help carefully, they're in danger of being victimized.

Beware of charlatans. Quackery is rampant in the field of sex therapy. There are no legal restraints on who can claim to be a sex therapist. Thus a classified ad for "sex therapist" or "sex clinic" can as easily be placed by a high-school student or a prostitute as by a qualified therapist.

Thousands of sex clinics have proliferated in recent years, the vast majority of them staffed by unqualified people. Only a few hundred can be considered legitimate.

Perhaps even worse, some self-styled therapists exploit people with sexual difficulties. The Hippocratic Oath specifically prohibits "lasciviousness" on the part of doctors, and a ban on sexual contact with patients is fundamental to every ethical code. The American Psychiatric Association and the American Psychological Association have recently revised their codes to specifically prohibit sexual contact between therapists and patients. Sex therapists encounter scores of patients who have been seduced as part of their "therapy."

Many people naturally turn to the family physician for help with sexual difficulties. This may be a good choice, for many physicians have become aware of the great need for sex counseling. Most medical schools are responding to a new recognition of this need by providing human sexuality courses. (In 1960, only three medical schools in this country had formal courses in sexuality.)

Indeed, the family physician may be in a unique position to help with sex counseling. A family doctor often knows the total family situation, and presumably has a rapport with the patient. The doctor

269

also knows of medical problems or medications that may be interfering with sexual functioning.

On the other hand, many physicians may fail to help—out of ignorance or prudishness. Even among MDs, sex is often a charged topic. As individuals, doctors are likely to have the same hang-ups as anyone else. Often, a physician's prejudices may interfere with treatment. Further, unless a doctor supplements the basic courses provided by most medical schools, he may not know much more about sex than many of his patients.

It may be a good idea for a patient to ascertain a physician's comfort and experience with sexual counseling by asking such questions as: "Do you feel qualified to give sexual advice?" Or, "Have you studied sexual dysfunction?" The patient can also ask where the physician received training and what affiliations he or she has with academic institutions.

If a doctor is obviously uncomfortable talking about sex, it is wise for a patient to ask for a referral to a qualified sex therapist or clinic.

Many patients with sexual problems require only reassurance that their functioning is normal. Others need to have myths dispelled. Some benefit from physiological explanations of sexual functioning. Many physicians can resolve such difficulties in two or three office visits. If sexual problems persits, a referral for sex therapy may be in order.

Among the most reliable sources of treatment are outpatient clinics in increasing numbers of hospitals across the country. These may be staffed by physicians, nurses, social workers, psychologists, psychotherapists, or others who have been trained in techniques for treating sexual dysfunction.

If there is no such hospital clinic locally, the following organizations can provide names of experienced therapists nearby:

Society for the Study of Sex Therapy and Research (SSTAR)
Medical University of South Carolina
171 Ashley Avenue
Charleston, S.C. 29403

The American Association of Sex Educators,
   Counselors and Therapists
600 Maryland Avenue, S.W., Suite 300 E
Washington, D.C. 20024

The American Association of Marriage and Family Counselors
225 Yale Avenue
Claremont, California 91711

Referrals can also be sought through local medical societies and social service agencies.

Some of the best sex therapy programs are modeled after the pioneering program of William H. Masters and Virginia E. Johnson at the Masters and Johnson Institute in St. Louis. This is an intensive two-week program using a male-female therapy team. There is a one to two year follow-up program.

Both partners undergo therapy, and the focus of the therapy is on improving the couple's intimate relationship, not just its genital aspects—for a couple's sex problems are usually more a symptom than a cause of problems in their relationship.

Further, while one partner may seem to have the sexual problem, the situation is usually much more complex. A woman who enters therapy because she fails to have orgasms may have a husband who ejaculates prematurely, compounding her problem. Similarly, when a woman suffers from vaginismus, her sex partner may develop impotence in frustration.

The focus of the Masters and Johnson approach is on educating the couple and helping them improve their skills at communication. Underlying the therapy is a view of sex as a natural function. Sexual dysfunction is seen not necessarily as a symptom of an underlying personality conflict or a deep-rooted psychological problem. Rather, Masters and Johnson believe, most people suffer from sexual problems as a result of ignorance about physiology, anxiety about sex, and assuming a spectator role in sexual activity—watching themselves, monitoring their responses, judging how well they are succeeding in realizing their goal.

The male-female team helps ensure that each partner has a same-sex listener, who may sometimes act as an advocate. This approach eliminates the possibility that an individual therapist will side with the same-sex partner.

Usually, the male therapist takes a thorough psychosexual history from the male, the female therapist from the female. Then, this process is reversed. The female therapist interviews the male patient, and the male therapist interviews the female patient. This approach helps

271

identify attitudes that may be expressed differently in the presence of one therapist or the other.

A medical examination identifies people whose problem is largely or entirely organic. Others may have medical problems which contribute to the sexual dysfunction, and they are given concurrent medical treatment.

The Masters and Johnson program utilizes a wide range of psychotherapeutic techniques. The focus of the therapy is on the present, rather than the history of behaviors and attitudes.

Central to the therapy in most cases is teaching the couple "sensate focus" techniques or "pleasuring." In the privacy of their hotel room, the couple experience the pleasures of touching and being touched—without the pressure to perform sexually.

Sex therapy usually works best when the sexual problems do not result from a major conflict or mental disorder. In cases where they do, referral to a psychiatrist may be in order.

Some sex therapists use a format of one or two sessions per week for 10 or 12 weeks. This approach allows the couple to live at home during the therapy. It also has the advantage, some therapists feel, of allowing the couple to absorb the therapy slowly.

The therapy is done by either a male-female team or an individual therapist. While most sex therapists prefer to treat sexual difficulties in the context of a relationship, many accept individuals for treatment—for a person with a long-standing or severe sexual problem may not at the time be involved in a relationship. For some people, group therapy has been effective in alleviating sexual difficulties. It has been used successfully for some women with orgasmic problems.

How well does it work? Nobody really knows. Recently even the methods used by Masters and Johnsons for evaluating patients' therapy outcomes have come under attack.

Such controversy stems from the fact that it is unusually hard to ascertain what constitutes success—or failure—in sex therapy. A patient may consider failure what the therapist counts success, and vice versa. There may be relapses; so a couple considered cured may still have unresolved sexual problems. The reverse also happens: initial failures may well yield to success as a couple slowly incorporates knowledge and communication skills. Sometimes, the therapy may help one partner but not the other.

Whatever the success statistics—and they have a wide range, depending on the nature of the complaint and the particular therapist—it is undoubtedly true that hundreds of couples and individuals have benefited from sex therapy over the last 15 years.

See also EJACULATION, PREMATURE; "FRIGIDITY"; IMPOTENCE; MASTURBATION; SEXUAL DYSFUNCTION.

SEXUAL DYSFUNCTION affects about half of all marriages, according to a "guesstimate" by Dr. William H. Masters and Virginia E. Johnson of the Masters and Johnson Institute in St. Louis and authors of the authoritative *Human Sexual Response* and *Human Sexual Inadequacy*.

The most common sex disorders are impotence, premature ejaculation, and orgasmic problems ("frigidity"). Diminished sexual desire is another common problem.

In some people, sexual problems are the result of illness, medications, surgery or other treatments, or congenital malformations of the urogenital system.

Far more people suffer sexual problems because of emotional stress. Frequently, fears about sexual performance lead to sexual problems. Job tensions often play a large part in causing sexual difficulties. Myths about sex contribute to stress.

Sexual dysfunction in a marriage may result from other tensions and difficulties—and vice versa. Marital problems that might easily be solved become aggravated by poor sexual functioning.

But if a husband and wife really want the marriage to work, are willing to try to communicate with each other, and seek competent therapeutic help, they can often resolve their sexual difficulties.

The first step is to break free of sexual myths. These common fallacies are barriers to sexual fulfillment.

● *It is not true* that the larger the penis, the more satisfied the woman. Actually, the vagina is a sleeve of soft tissue, not an empty cavity that must be filled. The flexible vaginal wall will enclose a penis of almost any size with essentially the same sensation for the woman.

● *It is not true* that the larger the clitoris, the greater the woman's orgasm. There is no relationship whatever. Nor is the size of the woman's vagina or breasts important in the production of orgasm.

● *It is not true* that men have greater sexual capacity than women do. Physiological studies show that women in general have a greater potential for sexual responsiveness than men. Women react more intensely and longer to sexual stimulation.

• *It is not true* that the man should always be active, the woman passive. The reverse can be equally satisfying, depending on the couple and how they feel at the moment.

Masters and Johnson make the point that in the past, sex was seen as something the male did *to* the female. Then as more women began to demand sexual fulfillment, the male had the responsibility of doing something *for* the female. Increasingly, sex is coming to be accepted as a mutual undertaking—something the male does *with* the female.

• *It is not true* that simultaneous orgasm should always be the goal. Simultaneous orgasm is difficult to achieve and not necessarily desirable. Each partner may actually gain more pleasure from experiencing the other's pleasure. It is often counterproductive to strive for simultaneous orgasm at the expense of overall enjoyment. Indeed, it is possible for a couple to have extremely satisfying sexual intercourse without orgasm at all—how satisfied they are is what counts.

• *It is not true* that a certain frequency of intercourse is normal. How often intercourse occurs should be as individual as any other aspect of sex—with no special rules to be followed.

People should not rate themselves failures if they have sex less than a given number of times a week, a month, a year. There is no minimum score to be achieved—or a maximum that should not be exceeded.

Sexual frequency is extremely variable from one couple to another and from one week to the next. Activity may decline to zero in periods of busyness or stress and increase accordingly at other times. A problem exists only if one or both partners are dissatisfied.

• *It is not true* that you have to master some specified techniques. Experts agree that the best technique is affection for the sex partner and a wish to give pleasure while receiving it. Instead of concentrating on sexual skills, couples are best off concentrating on having fun, on being caring and involved.

"We don't think sexual technique has any importance at all," compared to "getting across to the general public that sex is a *natural function*," like eating, says Virginia Johnson. "Some people are hungry at different times, some people eat for different reasons, at differing speeds, in different amounts." The same is true of sexual appetites.

Once people learn to accept and express their own sexuality, their own sexual pace and preferences, she believes, 75 to 80 percent of sexual problems will disappear, and "technique will come on the scene automatically."

To increase sexual response, it is important for partners to communicate their sexual preferences. Lovers are not mind readers. Each partner must let the other know what is most pleasurable, without insisting on sexual activities the other feels uncomfortable with.

In this way, each partner takes responsibility for his or her own sexual pleasure. And, far from monitoring the other's performance, each increases his or her own enjoyment.

Experimenting freely can help relieve boredom. Any sort of sexual exploration that is acceptable to both partners is normal.

Many couples get used to sex in the male superior position, with the man on top. This is not necessarily best for either partner. With the female superior, the man can often delay ejaculation longer since he's not so physically active, and the woman gets deeper penile thrusting. A position in which the man and woman both lie on their sides—with the woman's hip resting atop the man's thigh, and his other leg between her legs—allows both partners full use of their hands and arms.

Exploring sexual fantasies can help relieve some sexual problems. Almost all normal people indulge in sex thoughts and fantasies, and these erotic musings can be helpful in arousal during intercourse.

Often sexual daydreams include members of the same sex, or multiple sex partners, or family members. While such fantasies may trouble people, they can be reassured that there is little or no danger of their *acting* on such thoughts. It is best to enjoy them for the harmless flights of fancy that they are.

Some people similarly experience sexual stimulation from works of art, music, pictures, books, or films.

People who remain troubled by sexual disorders should seek competent professional help.

See also EJACULATION, PREMATURE; "FRIGIDITY"; IMPOTENCE; MEDICATIONS; SEX THERAPY.

SEXUAL MOLESTATION. See INCEST; RAPE.

SKIN DISORDERS often make people feel repulsive and sexually undesirable. Shame and self-consciousness may inhibit their sexual response. A sexual partner's revulsion may be perceived or imagined and sexual activity avoided.

Acne Vulgaris is a common skin condition that often causes social insecurity and withdrawal. Adolescents may be plagued by the myth that acne is caused by masturbation. If they feel guilty about masturbating, they may see their acne as a punishment for sin, an outward manifestation of their evil practices.

When acne persists beyond the teens, withdrawal may become more extreme and prevent social or sexual relationships.

Treatment for acne includes oral and topical antibiotics, estrogen therapy, drying and peeling ointments and soaps, and exposure to ultraviolet light. Surgery is available for acne victims with deep scars and pits.

Generalized psoriasis often creates serious sexual difficulties. Not only is the skin's appearance unsightly, but the psoriasis often involves the genital area, so soreness and irritation may follow sexual contact.

Psoriasis is a common chronic and recurrent disease characterized by silvery, scaling sores of various sizes. It is believed to be hereditary. Complete cure is rare, but several treatments have been effective, among them lubricating creams, topical corticosteroids, coal tar, and anthralin. A new and apparently very effective treatment for generalized psoriasis is currently under study. It involves oral methoxsalen followed at a specific interval by long-wave ultraviolet light.

Hair loss in women is a skin disorder that often has sexual repercussions. Hair and femininity are closely associated, and a hairless woman's self-esteem usually plunges. (By contrast, among men baldness is thought by some to be a sign of virility. No research supports this view.)

In women, baldness may be due to poisoning, nervous disorders, X-ray exposure, medications, or thyroid disorder. Other causes are hair dye, teasing the hair, and overuse of hair dryers. Steroids are frequently prescribed to treat hair loss. Psychotherapy may be useful when the problem has emotional origins.

Emotional problems contribute to some skin disorders. Neurodermatitis and atopic dermatitis, for example, are thought to be conditions with a strong psychogenic component. Similarly, itching of the genitals or anus is sometimes thought to be caused by sexual conflicts. Many skin conditions are exacerbated by stressful situations in a person's life, including sexual problems.

Indeed, the relationship between skin problems and sexuality is unusually complex. Sexual problems may be stresses which lead to the worsening of dermatologic symptoms. These symptoms in turn may exacerbate sexual problems, and so on.

In some people, sexual problems and skin disorders may both be part of a depression. People with skin disorders who suffer from decreased libido, impotence, or difficulty in achieving orgasm should suspect clinical depression if they experience such other signs as decreased ability to concentrate, decreased appetite, and sleep disturbances.

Fear of contagion may discourage sexual activity. People may avoid sexual contact because of the fear that their skin conditions may be transmitted. Actually, of all dermatological disorders, only about 10 percent are infectious. Patients should find out from their physicians whether particular skin conditions are transmittable during person-to-person contact.

With counseling or psychotherapy, some people can overcome the feelings of self-consciousness and repulsiveness that detract from sexual satisfaction.

SMOKING commonly impairs sexual functioning.

There has been little systematic or conclusive research on the impact of cigarette smoking on sex drive and capacity. But some evidence suggests that the practive may lower the libido and impair fertility in both sexes.

Smoking during pregnancy is associated with decreased birth weight, increased risk of miscarriage, and greater infant mortality. When a pregnant woman smokes, nicotine constricts the blood vessels in her unborn child, cutting down on fetal blood flow and oxygen supply. With reduced blood and oxygen, the fetus fails to grow as fast as it normally would.

Babies born to smoking mothers average 5 to 8 ounces less than those borne by women who do not smoke during pregnancy. Their babies more often weigh less than 5½ pounds and are exposed to more risk of disease and death. Pregnant women who smoke have a greater number of stillbirths than nonsmoking mothers. Their infants are more likely to die within the first month.

Smoking presents a special hazard to women taking birth control pills, particularly if they are over 40. The total death rate resulting from smoking plus the Pill is greater than from either factor alone. Of

277

100,000 women aged 40 to 44, heart attack kills 11 who use the Pill but do not smoke, 16 who smoke but do not use the Pill—and 62 who both use the Pill and smoke. Recent evidence also indicates an association between smoking and an early onset of menopause.

Smokers tend to have a lower breathing capacity, less ability to provide the body with oxygen in emergencies. Smoking thickens the lining membranes of the air passages and obstructs them with secretions. It contracts the muscles in the air passage walls, which narrows them and further reduces air flow. A single cigarette will markedly reduce the air flow of a smoker. Such reduced breathing capacity may cause discomfort and premature fatigue during sexual exertion.

Smoking is linked with a number of serious medical conditions that often interfere with sexual functioning. Among these are heart disease; respiratory diseases such as emphysema and chronic bronchitis; and cancer of the lung, larynx, esophagus, and mouth.

Conflict may arise when one sex partner is a smoker and the other is not. A nonsmoker may find smoking unesthetic and anti-erotic: smoking leaves an unpleasant odor on the smoker's breath; it yellows the teeth; the smoker may frequently cough and bring up mucus.

See also CANCER; HEART DISEASE; RESPIRATORY DISEASE.

SPECULUM. See PELVIC EXAMINATION.

SPERM. See MALE SEXUAL ANATOMY.

SPERM BANKS. See VASECTOMY.

SPERMICIDES are contraceptive preparations that are inserted into the vagina before intercourse. They can be bought without a prescription. Used properly, they are considered 84-97 percent effective. If spermicides are used in conjunction with condoms, they provide peak protection (99+ percent) with few side effects.

Spermicides destroy sperm cells before the latter pass through the cervix and into the uterus. Some brands contain surface-active agents thought to attach to the sperm, breaking down the cell walls, denying them oxygen, and upsetting their metabolism. Bactericidal agents disrupt the metabolism of the sperm. Acid agents are destructive to sperm, which cannot survive in an environment too acid or too alkaline.

One or more of these chemicals are packaged as foams, creams, jellies, foaming tablets, and suppositories. Some come with applicators to ease insertion.

Vaginal spermicides should be inserted shortly before intercourse. To make it effective, the woman spreads the spermicide evenly and thickly high up in her vagina to form a barrier between the cervix and sperm. She must put more in if she has sex again. If she gets off the bed, she needs to apply additional spermicide, since a large quantity may leak out. If she does not have intercourse within an hour after inserting the spermicide, she needs another application, for by then most spermicides lose their effectiveness. She can urinate but should not douche for at least 6 hours after intercourse. If she or her partner shows an allergy to a spermicide, relief may be found in a type with different ingredients.

Foam. An aerosol like shaving cream, foam is thought to provide generally the best protection of all types of spermicides. Foams (Because, Delfen, Emko, Koromex) disperse and form a physical barrier to the cervix more rapidly than the other spermicides. Foam also has the advantage of being less messy and less easily displaced during intercourse.

A woman needs to shake the can of foam at least twenty times before use in order to activate the bubbles and mix the spermicide. She should insert the foam no more than one-half hour before intercourse because the bubbles go flat. The foam is mostly air, leaving little residue.

Foam should never be inserted directly from the aerosol can into the vagina. Not only can it damage tissues if a woman is pregnant and is not yet aware of it. It can also force a lethal air bubble into the enlarged blood vessels of her uterus. To prevent this from happening, she fills the small plastic applicator that comes with it and uses that to deposit about a teaspoonful of foam into her vagina. Prefilled applicators, which are good for one application and can be carried in a purse, are available. Emko Pre-Fil offers a mixture that can be put into an applicator up to a week before use.

Creams and Jellies. These come in a tube with an applicator. A woman should apply them not more than fifteen minutes before intercourse. These spermicides are not as effective as foam. But, as with foam, when used with the condom their effectiveness is increased.

Reliable creams include Conceptrol, Delfen, Koromex, Ortho-Creme. Major brands of jellies: Koromex, Ortho-Gynol, Ramses.

Vaginal Foaming Tablets and Suppositories. These are generally least effective. The tablets work only when moist, and are not suitable for some women with relatively dry vaginas. The tablets lose their fizz within two weeks after exposure to air.

The suppository melts at body temperature and forms a shield. It does not spread as well as foam, cream, or jelly—indeed, it may not melt at all. For best results one suppository should be inserted within fifteen minutes before intercourse and a second suppository immediately afterward. *The Medical Letter* reports that the Encare Oval, heavily advertised as a "new" type of suppository, "has no established advantage over other typical spermicidal products that have been available for many years."

See also CONDOM; CONTRACEPTION.

SPINAL-CORD INJURY affects mainly teenagers and young adults. Its most frequent victims are males between 15 and 29.

The most common causes are automobile accidents, motorcycle accidents, swimming and diving accidents, gunshot wounds, and falls.

The extent of disability depends on the severity of the injury, and where it occurs on the spinal cord—its "level." People whose injury occurs in the part of the spinal cord called the cervical cord (C1-7 in the accompanying diagram) generally become paralyzed in both arms and legs, a condition called quadriplegia. About 30 percent of all spinal-cord injuries occur in the cervical cord, and many leave their victims with complete loss of sensation from the neck down. Severe injury above C5 is usually fatal.

When the injury occurs in the thoracic cord (T1-12) or the lumbar cord (L1-5), paralysis generally occurs in the legs only—paraplegia. Damage to the sacral nerve roots (S3,4,5) causes complete loss of bladder and bowel control.

Injuries above level L2 are called upper motor neuron lesions; those below L2, lower motor neuron lesions.

Spinal-cord injuries are described as complete or incomplete. In a complete lesion, all nerve fibers are severed or irreversibly damaged. In an incomplete lesion, some connecting fibers remain, and there may be some degree of sensation and ability to function. Sexual functioning is also more likely to be retained when the injury is incomplete. A thorough neurological examination should determine the level of the lesion and its degree of completeness.

Sexual functioning is usually a major concern of people after spinal-cord injury. Once assured they will survive, the second most pressing question for many is "What about sex?" For some patients, regaining sexual functioning is even more important than regaining the ability to walk.

When spinal-cord injury occurs, healthy independent young people are suddenly helpless and dependent. Their sense of self is seriously disrupted by this trauma, and their struggle in the following months is to reestablish a positive self-concept and a sense of independence.

A great improvement in self-concept often results when the spinal-cord injured find that they can continue to be desirable sex partners— and that they can engage in some degree of sexual activity, no matter what the extent of their injury.

Spinal-cord injury has greatly varying effects on sexual functioning. No absolute predictions can be made about the extent of sexual response that will be retained after a particular injury.

Among women, sexual desire is usually retained after injury. But the ability to have orgasms is generally markedly reduced or completely absent after spinal-cord injury, according to the small amount of research in this field. The ability to reach orgasm often depends on the presence of sensation (especially by pin prick) in the clitoris and labia.

On the other hand, many women with spinal-cord injuries seem to experience orgasm based on the recall of past experiences. Vivid sexual dreams accompanied by orgasm are also reported.

Some women experience sexual feeling in unexpected parts of their bodies. The area around or just above the injury on the back sometimes develops erotic sensations.

The breasts often become intensely eroticized in women who retain sensation in the torso. One young woman reported not having enjoyed breast stimulation before her spinal cord was injured in a car accident. Afterward, she was able to experience orgasm through stimulation of her breasts.

Some women do not reach orgasm but nevertheless enjoy intercourse. Many report intense satisfaction at the time of the partner's orgasm.

Some couples find electric vibrators useful in determining where pleasurable sensation exists. A woman who cannot feel sensation below her shoulders might yet enjoy sexual stimulation of her ears, mouth, neck, or any other area where she retains any feeling.

A woman who has no feeling in her genitals should not assume that this lack of sensation is necessarily permanent. After injury, the spinal cord goes into shock, and may require 4 to 6 months to recover. Genital sensation may return even 2 years after the injury.

Sexual intercourse for a spinal-cord injured woman involves some practical considerations. Because the woman's vagina may not lubricate—and because she has little or no vaginal sensation—the use of artificial lubrication such as K-Y jelly may be necessary.

In some women, hip and leg muscle spasms during intercourse may make some intercourse positions difficult. When spasms are severe, medication may be required.

In quadriplegic women, there is a danger of autonomic hyperreflexia during sexual arousal: intense stimulation below the level of the injury can produce a syndrome consisting of high blood pressure, a throbbing headache, stuffed nose, warm flushed moist skin on the face and upper torso, cool dry skin elsewhere, and slowed heart rate or other heartbeat irregularities. The syndrome usually reverses when the sexual activity stops and the woman assumes an upright position. Some women especially prone to this syndrome may require preventive medication.

With spinal-cord injury, bowel and bladder control may be lost, and there is a risk of urinary and bowel incontinence during sexual activity.

To minimize the risk, it is wise for the woman to empty her bladder and to avoid drinking for a few hours before intercourse. A rubber pad under the sheet affords protection in case of accidents.

Women with indwelling catheters usually find it safest to remove them before engaging in intercourse. Some women prefer to tape them to the abdomen or thigh.

Spinal-cord injured women can conceive and deliver normally. After the injury, a woman may experience changes in menstrual patterns, but these rarely persist beyond a year. Fertility is unimpaired unless there is organic damage to the reproductive system.

Such women are capable of carrying a fetus through a normal term and delivering it vaginally. But pregnancy may be complicated by urinary tract infections and anemia. Premature labor is a great likelihood.

As the due date approaches, the woman should be carefully monitored, since she may not feel labor contractions and delivery may be abrupt. Nor is she a good candidate for Lamaze or other natural childbirth techniques, since she is unable to give voluntary assistance in bearing down. Caesarean section is often necessary.

A spinal-cord injured woman who does not wish to conceive should use contraception. The choice of an appropriate method may pose some problems.

Birth control pills should be avoided when the woman has circulatory problems. A paralyzed woman may be at double risk of thrombophlebitis, blood clots in the veins: this is a risk for the spinal-cord injured, and also a potential side effect of oral contraceptives. What is more, such clots may go undetected because of the lack of sensation in arms or legs.

An IUD may similarly be a poor choice since pelvic inflammatory disease or other medical problems—such as uterine perforation—could go undetected because of lack of sensation.

A condom has the advantage of the man taking responsibility for birth control. If he can insert vaginal foam for the woman who is unable to do so, the combination affords maximum protection with virtually no potential side effects. The diaphragm may be a good contraceptive choice for a woman who has the use of her hands.

Surgery for sterilization (vasectomy or tubal sterilization) is a good birth control possibility for couples who are sure they never want to have children.

Among men with spinal-cord injury, sexual desire is usually retained—although it may be diminished by many factors, including depression, anxieties about sexual performance, the absence of feelings in the genitals, and lowered self-worth.

Most men with spinal-cord injuries suffer impaired sexual functioning. The ability to maintain an erection sufficient for intercourse occurs in only about 15 to 25 percent of such men, and their frequency of intercourse is substantially less than before injury.

The ability to ejaculate normally is lost by more than 90 percent of spinal-cord injured men. In general, the ability to ejaculate is more likely among men with incomplete lesions and among those with lesions of the lower motor neurons (injuries below the L2 level).

When men do ejaculate, they may or may not experience the sensation of orgasm.

Some spinal-cord injured men experience what has been referred to as a "phantom orgasm"—a pleasurable orgasmic sensation without the physiological changes characteristically accompanying orgasm. (Conversely, some undergo the biologic changes of arousal and orgasm without any sensation.)

Similarly, some men experience what one researcher has called "a sort of 'para-orgasm'"—an intensely pleasurable feeling at the time their partners achieve orgasm. Some have objected to the terms "phantom" and "para-" orgasm as implying that the experience is somehow less real than a "true" physiological orgasm. Whatever the mechanism, these are perceived as orgasmic experiences and should be accepted and enjoyed as bona fide by the men and their partners.

The great majority of spinal-cord injured men attain erections. Unfortunately, such erections are often insufficient for intercourse.

Many men with high spinal-cord injuries experience reflexogenic erections. These are produced by direct stimulation of the genital area. Reflexogenic erections are controlled by a reflex arc between the genitals and the spinal cord. This arc does not need messages from the brain in order to function; hence it can continue to operate in the portion of the cord below the injury.

Reflexogenic erections are usually extremely brief and are not generally accompanied by any sensation.

Some men experience spontaneous reflexogenic erections—erections occurring without any direct stimulation. Their mechanism is not understood. Such erections may occur at inconvenient times and are usually not attainable when wanted.

Some spinal-cord injured men experience psychogenic erections. These result when messages are passed down the spinal cord from the brain. Stimuli received by the brain through the senses of sight, sound, and smell as well as through fantasy and memory activate these messages.

If the spinal cord is injured between the brain and the area controlling sexual response (T12 to L2 and S2, 3, and 4), the messages are usually short-circuited, and the man is unable to achieve a psychogenic erection.

In some spinal-cord injured men, however, the ability to get psychogenic erections remains. This is more likely in men with lower spinal cord injuries. Such erections are possible because the message from the brain may bypass the injured portion of the spinal cord through the autonomic nervous system.

While psychogenic erections among spinal-cord injured men may not always be complete erections, they usually persist longer than reflexogenic erections and may be sufficient for intercourse. As with reflexogenic erections, there is usually no awareness of the genitals.

It is probably wisest for men to remove indwelling catheters for intercourse. They should be removed and replaced very carefully and slowly. If the bladder is empty, it is usually safe to be without a catheter for 3 to 6 hours. Some men prefer to leave the catheter in place. It can be lubricated with a water-soluble jelly and taped to the penis. The tape should be removed soon after intercourse since the bladder can become distended if the catheter is taped closed for too long.

As with women, men with high spinal-cord injuries may experience autonomic hyperreflexia and spacticity with sexual arousal. If this poses a substantial problem, medication may be required.

When a man cannot maintain an erection and his partner enjoys penile insertion, they can try the "stuffing" technique. The man lies on his back with the woman on her knees above him. She gently stuffs his penis into her vagina and rotates her pelvis. Some women can reach orgasm in this manner. A man whose partner particularly desires penile penetration may consider a penile prosthesis. Many spinal-cord injured men sexually gratify their partners by oral or manual stimulation of the genitals and breasts.

Even with impaired sexual functioning, many spinal-cord injured men experience pleasurable sensations. Physical contact can provide a sense of intimacy and well-being. Sexual functioning may return, sometimes as long as 2 or 3 years after the injury.

Fertility is impaired in most men with spinal-cord injuries. Sperm production and motility are commonly diminished. Erection and ejaculation problems may make fertility impossible even when sperm count and motility could result in conception. Some men suffer from retrograde ejaculation. Attempts to retrieve sperm from spinal-cord injured men and impregnate their wives have thus far been unsuccesful. Some couples may wish to consider adoption.

Spinal-cord injured men and women typically labor under the myth

285

that the disabled are asexual. They have difficulty meeting potential sex partners. Fear of sexual rejection by potential sex partners or spouses is common.

The odds of spinal-cord injured people marrying are less than if they were not disabled. If they do marry, though, their chances of remaining married are about the same as for the general population. Those already married at the time of injury have a greater risk of divorce than the rest of the population.

After spinal-cord injury, it is crucial for couples to work toward developing mutual trust. With open communication of their needs and wishes, couples can discover how they may sexually satisfy each other.

Various sexual positions and options can be explored to see which prove most comfortable and pleasurable.

Many couples find that the use of massage, erotic literature, electric vibrators, and water beds enhances sexual response.

For some couples, it may be advisable to seek outside help for performing bowel and bladder care—from, say, a visiting nurse or a part-time assistant. Sometimes, a spouse who routinely provides bowel and bladder care may have trouble seeing the patient as a sexually desirable partner.

Patience is a prime requisite for people with spinal-cord injury. Sometimes, sexual response and enjoyment improve with time. Many couples come to realize that even without genital function, they can continue to express and receive physical love.

Rehabilitation programs in hospitals that treat spinal-cord injury help individuals become more self-reliant. Many provide individual psychological counseling or group-therapy programs.

Some programs also touch on sexuality. There may, for example, be an opportunity for individual or couple sex-related counseling. Or a lecture or film about the sexual effects of spinal-cord injury may be followed by an opportunity for questions.

A few rehabilitation programs have gone considerably farther and offer much more comprehensive sexual rehabilitation. Such a program might provide, for example, a series of eight weekly meetings at which presentations on sexual topics are made, followed by group discussions. Individual sex counseling is also typically available.

These facilities have special sexuality programs for spinal-cord injured patients:

Craig Hospital
Rocky Mountain Regional Spinal Injury Center
3425 South Clarkson
Englewood, Colorado 80110
303/761-3040

Institute of Rehabilitation Medicine
Spinal Cord Injury Center
400 East 34th St.
New York, New York 10016
212/679-3200

Moss Rehabilitation Hospital
12th and Tabor Road
Philadelphia, Pa. 19141
215/329-5715

Rancho Los Amigos Hospital
7601 East Imperial Highway
Downey, Ca. 90242
213/922-7605

The Texas Institute for Rehabilitation and Research (TIRR)
P.O. Box 20095
Houston, Texas 77025
713/797-1440

Spinal Cord Injury Service
Veterans Administration Hospital
130 West Kingsbridge Rd.
Bronx, N.Y. 10468
212/584-9000

Spinal Cord Injury Service
Veterans Administration Hospital
10701 East Boulevard
Cleveland, Ohio 44106
216/791-3800

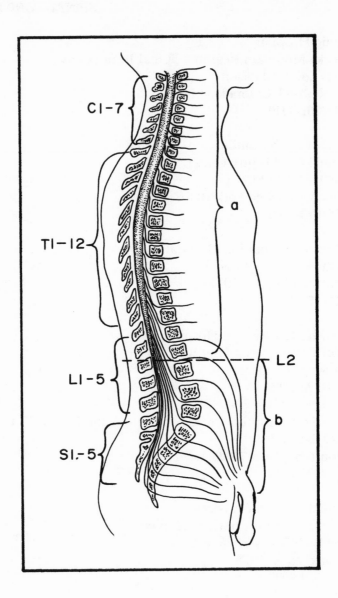

Spinal-cord Injury
a) Injury within this area is referred to as an upper motor neuron lesion.
b) Injury within this area is referred to as a lower motor neuron lesion.

Spinal Cord Injury Center
Veterans Administration Hospital
1400 V.F.W. Parkway
West Roxbury, Mass. 02132
617/323-7700 (ext. 210)

The Rehabilitation Institute of Chicago
345 East Superior St.
Chicago, Ill. 60611
312/649-6179

Santa Clara Valley Medical Center
751 South Bascom
Santa Clara, Ca. 95128
408/279-5116

For more information about spinal-cord injury and sexual functioning, consult the following:

Becker, E. *Female Sexuality Following Spinal Cord Injury.* Bloomington, Illinois: Cheever Publishing, 1978.

Eisenberg, M., Rustad, L. *Sex and the Spinal Cord Injured: Some Questions & Answers.* Washington, D.C.: Superintendent of Documents, 1974.

Mooney, T., Cole, T., and Chilgren, R. *Sexual Options for Paraplegics and Quadriplegics.* Boston: Little, Brown and Co., 1975.

See also CONTRACEPTION; PENILE PROSTHESES; TUBAL STERILIZATION; VASECTOMY.

STERILITY. See INFERTILITY.

STERILIZATION. SEe HYSTERECTOMY; TUBAL STERILIZATION; VASECTOMY.

STEROIDS (corticosteroids) used for up to 10 days will very likely have no effect on sexual functioning.

However, those who must take steroids for long periods may lose their desire for sex. A physician may prescribe long-term use of steroids as replacement therapy, or for such conditions as collagen diseases, blood diseases, chronic allergy, or dermatitis. Loss of sexual appetite can be an early sign of steroid side effects. The physician should be informed if a patient experiences this or any other adverse reaction.

Depression and other mental disturbances can be associated with long-term use of steroids, impairing sexual functioning. Also, steroids over a long term may suppress secretion of sex hormones by interfering with the output of pituitary gonadotropin. In men, large doses of steroids may depress sperm production, causing infertility. Women may suffer menstrual irregularity or may stop menstruating entirely. Steroids also increase the risk of vaginal infection. Prolonged use of steroids—including the use of steroid creams under watertight dressings—can produce stretch marks on the breasts and elsewhere.

These powerful drugs may further have an impact on sexual functioning by causing muscle weakness, vertigo, and headache. Steroids can produce hyperglycemia—and can precipitate latent diabetes, with impotence. Sufferers may feel undesirable—or be sexually rejected—because of changes in appearance from steroid use. Some people develop a moon face, excess body hair, and excess fat.

Conversely, long-term use of steroids sometimes has a positive effect on sexuality. The drug may cause euphoria. The relief of anxiety and depression can enhance sexual functioning.

See also MEDICATIONS.

STROKE (cerebrovascular accident, CVA) is a disorder of the blood vessels of the brain that results in impaired blood supply to the brain. It may be caused by embolism (obstruction), thrombosis (blood clot), or hemorrhage (bleeding). Stroke often follows long-standing untreated hypertension.

Stroke victims who survive sustain greatly varying degrees of neurological impairment. At one extreme are those who are almost completely paralyzed, blind, and unable to speak. At the other extreme are those with very slight residual damage—a somewhat weakened arm, for example.

Most stroke victims have some degree of paralysis on one side of the body. They may have visual and speech problems, memory disorders, and body image disturbances. Changes in tactile sensations, such as numbness or tingling, are common. Some stroke victims lose bladder or bowel control.

Stroke may result in sexual problems. In a small percentage of stroke patients, neurologic damage causes impotence, partial erection, delayed ejaculation, and lack of orgasm. Stroke may diminish sexual desire.

Most often, however, sexual problems after a stroke are due not to neurological problems but rather to a combination of mechanical and emotional factors. A stroke victim may find sexual activity difficult because of weakness, lack of coordination, and paralysis.

The patient's feelings may have an even greater impact on sexuality. Typically, stroke victims feel humiliated at their dependence on others. They may feel overwhelmed and helpless. Their self-esteem is low, and it plummets further if they are treated as stupid or childish because of their speech difficulties. Depression is common after a stroke.

Stroke patients commonly feel great anxiety about sexual failure. Many fear sexual rejection by their partner.

Fear of sex causing another stroke makes many avoid it altogether. Theoretically, the risk of sexual activity precipitating a stroke is highest in patients whose stroke was due to hemorrhage; there is a possibility of elevated blood pressure resulting from sexual arousal causing renewed bleeding. But even in such patients, the risk is thought to be very small.

Sometimes, it is the spouse who avoids sex out of fear of inflicting further stroke damage. The couple should discuss such fears with the physician and ascertain whether there is any realistic risk in engaging in sexual activity.

Sexual rehabilitation after stroke can often be correlated with age and the pattern of sexual activity before the stroke. A small group of younger patients, usually under age 45, experience little if any difficulty with sexual function after the stroke.

Most stroke patients, however, are considerably older—the average age is 70—and many have had sexual difficulties before the stroke as a result of chronic illness, medications, or misconceptions about the effects of aging on sexual functioning.

Drugs that may be required for the treatment of hypertension—commonly seen in stroke patients—may interfere with sexual desire and functioning. These effects may be reversible with a change in drug or dosage.

When stroke patients remain interested in sex, various accommodations can improve sexual enjoyment. If speech problems impede sexual communication, the couple can work out a nonverbal sexual code.

Comfortable sexual positions can be explored. A male stroke victim, for example, may have difficulty in the male-superior position and may prefer lying on his back with the female on top. If poor bladder control is a problem, the stroke patient should urinate just before engaging in sex.

It is important for the couple to insure privacy and to leave ample time for unhurried sexual activity. It is also wise not to set prestroke goals for sexual performance—but rather to enjoy whatever amount of sexual activity ensues. Stroke patients often find that it is a tremendous boost to self-esteem simply to be considered sexually desirable.

See also HYPERTENSION.

SYPHILIS is one of the most severe venereal diseases, ranking as a major killer among infectious diseases. Syphilis typically goes through five stages:

The Primary Stage. This is usually characterized by a sore called a chancre, which appears from ten to ninety days (average: twenty-one days) after exposure. This primary chancre appears on the penis, in the vaginal area, in or around the mouth or anus—wherever the syphilis germ first entered the body. It may look like a pimple, a blister, or an open sore. It often seems hard and punched out. Rarely does it hurt or itch.

The chancre is one of the most contagious forms of syphilis, containing millions of spirochetes (the syphilis bacteria). These germs can be passed to any person whose mucous membrane tissues come in contact with the sore. An untreated person can remain infectious for as long as two years or more.

If a syphilis sore is on the mouth, the disease may be transmitted through kissing. On the other hand, the primary chancre may not appear at all, or it may be so small it is overlooked. In women it may be hidden inside the vulva or vagina.

The chancre can easily be ignored or mistaken for something else. Some people, not realizing they have a syphilis sore, attempt self-treatment with salves or ointments. With or without treatment, the chancre will heal spontaneously within a few weeks. This means only that the spirochetes have moved away from the particular site. The disease has gone underground.

A Symptom-free Period. This stage usually lasts from two to ten weeks, but it may last up to six months. An infected person can still spread the disease to others.

The Secondary Stage. By now the syphilis bacteria have multiplied enough to produce symptoms throughout the body. There may be fever, sore throat, severe headache. Skin reactions are common, ranging from a fine rash to large pox, a measles-type rash or oozing sores. Scalp hair may fall out in patches (alopecia areata). The victim may suffer from sores around the mouth and lips or on the palms or soles.

Secondary symptoms of syphilis may escape notice or be ignored. The rashes do not itch or sting and will usually heal spontaneously. The symptoms of the secondary stage are often mistaken for something else, such as prickly heat or an allergy. Because these symptoms mimic those of so many other diseases, syphilis has been called "The Great Imitator." One clue to a syphilitic rash: it is distributed over the body, but not on the face. Another clue: abnormal patches may appear in the mouth, or on the palms or soles.

Throughout the secondary stage a person remains infectious. Anyone in intimate contact with the syphilitic may contract the disease. This period lasts from six months to two years.

The Latent Stage. This can last a few years or a lifetime. A person may feel perfectly healthy, and can no longer transmit syphilis to others—although it persists internally. Only a blood test can now detect the presence of the disease.

The Late Stage. This is characterized by severe damage to body organs. Roughly 23 percent of people with untreated late syphilis develop crippling or fatal forms of the disease. Most common are heart disease, central nervous system damage, syphilitic insanity (paresis), and blindness.

If a woman is pregnant, she needs to be tested for syphilis as early as possible, for she can infect her unborn child. Many such infants are stillborn. If alive, they may suffer from birth defects. An infant with congenital syphilis may become deaf, blind, or severely mentally handicapped if not treated immediately after birth.

A blood test detects the antibodies the body produces to fight the spirochetes. These are not always found in the first test. A person who has been exposed to syphilis should be retested several times over a three-month period.

Early treatment is important. In later stages, any damage the disease has done to vital organs cannot be repaired. Penicillin or other antibiotics should be administered as soon as possible.

No one should try to treat syphilis at home, as with leftover penicillin tablets. The large doses of penicillin required in the treatment of syphilis must be taken under a doctor's supervision. Covering chancres or rashes with salves and ointments—especially those containing penicillin—will only disguise the symptoms, making diagnosis more difficult. Some salves, especially those containing steroids, may speed up the production of spirochetes.

See also ANAL SEX; GONORRHEA; ORAL SEX; VENEREAL DISEASE.

SYSTEMIC LUPUS ERYTHEMATOSUS (lupus, SLE), a

connective tissue disorder, like any chronic, painful illness, typically alters a patient's body image and decreases self-esteem. Irritability, depression, and apathy are common, and usually reduce libido.

Symptoms of this inflammatory connective tissue disease often interfere with sexual functioning. Fever, weakness, and fatigue may leave a patient disinterested in sex. Facial rash, a frequent symptom, may make an SLE victim feel sexually undesirable.

Joint pains commonly limit movement and make intercourse difficult and painful. A warm bath preceding sexual relations often alleviates discomfort.

A warm bath—and having intercourse in a warm room—will also help reduce discomfort from another common problem of SLE: Raynaud's phenomenon. In this condition, which affects 1 out of 5 SLE patients, decreased blood flow to fingers and toes causes pain, coldness, and a bluish tint. The pain may increase during sexual activity because more blood concentrates in the genital area, further reducing the flow to fingers and toes. The warmth of a bath and a warmed room helps dilate blood vessels and encourage greater blood flow.

It is also important that the patient not support weight on the hands and feet during sexual activity. Such added pressure reduces blood supply. In one safe and common position, the patient lies underneath the partner.

Medications to treat SLE often relieve stiffness and pain during intercourse but may also cause sexual problems of their own. Among the drugs used are cortisone, other steroids, anti-inflammatory agents, and tranquilizers.

Mouth ulcers occur in some SLE patients, making kissing and other oral sexual activities painful. The condition is treated with steroid mouthwashes. Antibiotics are added when there is a bacterial infection.

Some SLE patients experience a dryness of the mucous membranes, including the vagina. Dryness may cause painful intercourse. A water-soluble lubricant such as K-Y often solves the problem.

A small number of SLE patients suffer from vaginal ulcers, which make intercourse painful. Steroid ointments usually relieve the ulcer. In the meantime, intercourse should be avoided, and other forms of sexual activity can be explored.

See also ARTHRITIS; MEDICATIONS; STEROIDS; TRANQUILIZERS.

TB. See TUBERCULOSIS.

TERMINAL ILLNESS. People who are dying need loving concern and physical affection even more than healthy people do.

Sexual needs usually remain even when a person is facing death. Some people wish merely to be held and stroked. Others may have a greater need for sexual intimacy than before their illness.

Among the terminally ill, as among healthy people, sex can be enriching and revitalizing. Further, sex can serve to decrease anxiety and increase self-esteem. It can help the terminally ill temporarily forget the fact of imminent death.

The quality of the love relationship before the illness usually affects the quality of sexual expression afterward. Generally, couples who have had a loving relationship and open sexual communication are also better able to share sex when one partner is terminally ill.

Some factors that may interfere with sexual expression in terminal illness:

Decreased self-esteem. It is common for people to react to terminal illness with shame, guilt, despair, and depression—feelings that typically inhibit sexual desire.

Role changes necessitated by the illness may cause difficulties in family relationships and hence interfere with sexual communication. Thus a man who is dying may not only be suffering from his inability to support his family; he may also feel the burden of his wife's expectation that he will get well. Dealing with her disappointment puts another stress on their relationship.

Guilt about having sexual interest despite the illness can affect either the patient or the partner. Couples may see the giving or receiving of pleasure as grotesque under the circumstances. This feeling may be conveyed by medical personnel. Certainly, sexual expression is rarely encouraged by those who care for the dying. But when doctors, nurses, or social workers fail to even mention the possibility of sex, many patients understandably get the feeling that it must be inappropriate among the terminally ill.

Modes of dealing with stress may have to change when a person is terminally ill. People who have in the past dealt with conflict by engaging in physical activity now find this impossible. If they are unable to learn to handle stress verbally and emotionally, they may become depressed.

Anger. The dying person often feels a rage against fate and may displace this anger onto the sexual partner.

Physical problems associated with the illness may limit sexual functioning. Fatigue, pain, and difficulty in moving may all diminish sexual enjoyment. The disease itself may limit sexual functioning, as in cancer of the genitals. Medication may be blocking sexual desire or functioning.

Feelings of the partner may account for sexual estrangement. It is common for the spouse of a dying person to go through a period of anticipatory grieving, beginning to move away emotionally. Feelings toward a dying partner are commonly a confused mixture of love and hate, closeness and separateness, guilt and blame. This emotional distancing frequently includes sexual separation.

Some partners may fear sexual contact because of an erroneous belief that the illness is catching—or even that death itself is contagious.

Hospital policies may limit the opportunity for sexual expression.

By providing little privacy, hospitals and nursing homes reflect the opinion that the terminally ill are neither interested in sex nor able to function sexually. This frequently becomes a self-fulfilling prophecy.

To help restore sexual intimacy, a couple can discuss feelings that may be interfering with sexual expression, perhaps with the help of a professional psychotherapist.

A terminally ill person can experiment with conditions that may promote a better sexual response. Early in the day, for example, the patient may have more vigor. Some sexual activities may be more comfortable than others when illness limits movement. Dosages and timing of medication can often be adjusted to accommodate sexual experiences at certain times of the day.

Couples can let hospital personnel know that they require more privacy and can even request that a do-not-disturb sign hung outside the door be respected by the staff.

Home or hospice care may be more suitable for the dying person and may also promote more sexual intimacy and loving care.

When a dying person is clinically depressed, medication and psychiatric counseling are usually helpful.

See also DEPRESSION.

TESTES. See MALE SEXUAL ANATOMY.

TESTICLE REMOVAL (orchiectomy). When only one testicle is removed, as in most testicular cancer, potency, ejaculation, and fertility are commonly retained—although some types of treatment may impair ejaculation.

In cases where cancer of the prostate has spread and is inoperable, the usual treatment is removal of both testicles and/or estrogen therapy. Both control symptoms of metastatic spread by reducing testosterone in the blood to low levels.

A majority of men undergoing this regimen experience reduced sexual desire. Some become impotent. Since the testicles produce sperm, men who lose both testicles will be sterile.

After removal of one or both testicles, a man may wish to consider prosthetic testicles. These are surgically inserted into the scrotum.

Usually made of a silicone rubber bag filled with a silicone gel, they have the resilient feel of real testicles and come in several different sizes.

See also PROSTATE CANCER; TESTICULAR CANCER.

TESTICLE, UNDESCENDED (cryptorchidism). In adults,
undescended testicle is linked to infertility and to a higher risk of cancer of the undescended testicle.

In the male fetus, the testicles are normally inside the abdomen. They pass into the scrotum shortly before birth. Sometimes one or both testes fail to descend. The condition occurs in about 3 percent of full-term babies and in about 30 percent of premature infants. It may be due to physiological immaturity or to an obstruction in the inguinal canal (through which the testicles normally descend).

Some testicles will spontaneously descend in the first few years of life. If the testes fail to descend, hormone therapy with human chorionic gonadotropin (HCG) may be recommended. It is successful in 30 to 50 percent of boys with both testes undescended, and less successful when only one is undescended.

If testes do not descend within 3 to 6 months of hormonal therapy, most physicians recommend that surgery be performed before the boy is 5 or 6 years old.

The operation involves opening the inguinal canal, removing any obstructions that may be preventing descent, and placing the testicle in the scrotum.

Boys may become alarmed by the frequent examination of their genitals. By age 4 or 5, most boys have become aware of their genitals, and are conscious of the difference between themselves and other boys. They sense their parents' concern; so they may be particularly troubled when the nature of the problem is kept secret from them.

Child psychiatrists urge parents of a child with undescended testicle to encourage the questions and concerns a young boy inevitably has. The child can be told that the doctor is checking to see if the second testicle has joined the first as it is expected to do. But if it does not, then the doctor can fix it.

A child facing genital surgery is particularly in need of sensitive parental support and open discussions.

A common fear of young boys undergoing genital surgery is that the penis will be removed. Parents should anticipate this anxiety and assure the child that the surgery will involve only his scrotal sac and that his penis will remain exactly the way it was. Most children can handle such information better than their parents expect.

Undescended testicle does not interfere with sexual desire or ejaculation. If both testes are still undescended after puberty, infertility results, since the abdomen is too warm for normal sperm production. If only one testicle is undescended, fertility may be normal. Early hormonal or surgical correction increases the chances of normal fertility.

Treatment also reduces the chance of cancer. While malignant tumors are rare in normal testicles (an annual rate of 2 per 100,000 males), the risk is 30 to 40 times as great in an untreated undescended testicle.

See also INFERTILITY; TESTICLE REMOVAL; TESTICULAR CANCER.

TESTICLES. See MALE SEXUAL ANATOMY.

TESTICULAR CANCER is relatively rare, accounting for only 1.5 percent of male malignancies.

The typical victim of cancer of the testicles—which produce sperm cells and are involved in the production of the hormone testosterone—is in his teens, 20s, or 30s. The cancer often interferes with sexual functioning and fertility.

Men with undescended testicles are more likely to develop testicular cancer—possibly because the body temperature in the abdomen is higher than in the scrotum.

A swelling or mass in the testicle is often the first sign of the disease. Pain in the testicle is not usually an early symptom. It is wise for men to ask their doctors how to self-examine testicles—since early detection gives best treatment results.

Self-examination can be done every six to eight weeks. The best time is after a shower, when the scrotal skin is relaxed and a pea-sized nodule may be felt anywhere in the testis; the cancer may also be signaled by the testicle's becoming harder and larger or by testicular veins becoming slightly enlarged.

Surgical removal of the cancerous testicle is the usual treatment. Radiation therapy may follow. Combination chemotherapy may be used both before and after surgery.

In patients with the type of testicular tumor called seminoma, the survival rate after treatment is very high: 90 percent are still alive 10 years later. Their sexual functioning and fertility are usually unimpaired. Other types have a much lower survival rate.

For some types of testicular cancer, lymph nodes in the abdomen are removed in a surgical procedure called retroperitoneal lymphadenectomy. Many men undergoing this treatment experience ejaculatory problems. Some fail to ejaculate entirely. Others ejaculate very little semen.

Most men will continue to have normal erections and can still experience the sensation of orgasm after the operation.

Decreased sexual desire and impotence afflict some men after treatment for testicular cancer. This may be due to the combined effects of surgery, radiation therapy, and chemotherapy. If blood testosterone levels are very low, testosterone replacement therapy may restore normal functioning. Some types of testicular tumors, however, are accelerated by testosterone, and in these cases the hormone should not be given.

Psychological factors are thought to play a large part in the development of sexual problems following surgery for testicular cancer. Some men equate fertility with virility and feel unmanly if they are no longer able to reproduce. For others, the cancer may be viewed as a punishment for their sexual sins—of, say, masturbation or overindulgence.

To help avert impotence of psychogenic origin, sexual counseling, preferably with the wife or sex partner, is recommended both before and after surgery.

Testicular prostheses are available for men with concern about their appearance.

See also CANCER; TESTICLE REMOVAL; TESTICLE, UNDESCENDED.

TESTICULAR FEMINIZATION SYNDROME. See HORMONE DISORDERS.

TESTICULAR TORSION is the twisting within the scrotum of the spermatic cord—the tube that attaches to the testicle. It is considered a surgical emergency.

Symptoms are sudden severe pain in the testicle, with tenderness and swelling. The testicle retracts to the upper part of the scrotum. Scrotal skin becomes dusky red.

The condition is fairly common, with an annual incidence of one case per 4,000 males below age 25. Most cases occur in boys between 12 and 18.

Torsion is generally caused by an anatomic abnormality of the tunica vaginalis—the membrane covering the testicle and lining the cavity of the scrotum—that predisposes a male to the condition. Torsion rarely occurs, however, until the testicle is enlarged by pubertal growth.

Sometimes the cord spontaneously untwists. Between one-third and one-half of patients with acute torsion describe previous episodes of similar pain that were brief and nearly always on the same side.

But it is unwise to ignore severe testicular pain. Torsion can produce permanent testicular damage within 4 hours. Prompt surgery is thus necessary to preserve functioning of the testicle. Overall, about 50 percent of testicles operated on can be saved. The outlook is generally best if the period of torsion has been only a few hours and the cord has not been twisted through more than 1½ revolutions.

TESTOSTERONE. See HORMONE DISORDERS.

THREADWORMS. See PINWORMS.

TOO-TIGHT FORESKIN. See CIRCUMCISION.

TORSION OF A TESTICLE. See TESTICULAR TORSION.

TOXEMIA. See PREGNANCY.

TOXIC SHOCK SYNDROME. See MENSTRUATION.

TRANQUILIZERS, drugs for treating tension and anxiety, have variable effects on sexual functioning. On the one hand, some users find that their reduced anxiety serves to enhance sexual performance. On the other, the sedative effects of tranquilizers may result in reduced sexual desire and responsiveness in some people.

The two most commonly used tranquilizers in this country are chlordiazepoxide (Librium) and diazepam (Valium).

Both drugs reduce anxiety, relax muscles, and produce some sedation. At high dosage levels or with chronic, prolonged use, a small number of men suffer impotence. These drugs are best avoided during the first trimester of pregnancy since there seems to be an increased risk of birth defects associated with their use.

The drug methaqualone (Quaalude, Sopor, Parest), a nonbarbiturate hypnotic, has recently gained an undeserved reputation in the illicit drug trade as an enhancer of sexual experience. Actually, it is far more likely to impair sexual functioning.

See also BARBITURATES; MEDICATIONS.

TRANSVESTISM (cross-dressing) is the wearing of clothes usually appropriate to the opposite sex. Transvestites are almost always males; they obtain intense sexual gratification when wearing women's clothes. The practice usually begins during adolescence.

Transvestites are not usually homosexual. Most, indeed, are married, employed, have children—and generally dress in male clothes. They are not effeminate—nor, like transsexuals, do they wish to be females.

Their dressing in female clothes is generally an occasional practice. In most cases, it is secretive. Some men will wear merely one or two garments of women's underclothes. Others will be fully dressed in female clothing—including wigs and makeup.

Some transvestites involve tolerant wives in their behavior. They might have intercourse, for example, with the man wearing his wife's slip or bra. Some transvestites are impotent except when wearing some female clothes. For them, women's clothes have a fetishistic quality.

In young children, cross-dressing may be a sign of a disturbance in gender orientation. Parents of a 3- or 4-year-old boy who frequently dresses in girls' clothes should seek psychiatric advice—particularly if the child displays exaggerated female mannerisms.

TRICHOMONIASIS, a vaginal infection, is caused by a one-celled animal (a protozoan) called trichomonas vaginalis. Its main symptoms are a foamy foul-smelling yellow-green discharge and a burning sensation around the vagina. There may be soreness, swelling, and bleeding of the vaginal walls. The urethra and the bladder may also be affected.

Like yeast infection, trichomoniasis is diagnosed by a pelvic examination and a smear or culture of the vaginal discharge.

Trichomoniasis is usually spread through sexual intercourse. Some physicians regard it as a venereal disease. The organism can be carried from the rectum to the vagina by anal intercourse followed by vaginal intercourse or by wiping bowel movements from the rectum toward the vagina—instead of from the vagina toward the rectum.

Because the protozoa can survive outside the body in a warm, moist place, it may also be possible to contract the infection through clothing, toilet seats, towels, washcloths, and other personal articles. Birth control pills may make a woman more susceptible to trichomoniasis.

Men often harbor the organisms in the urethra, prostate gland, or bladder without any symptoms. Thus a woman who has been successfully treated can be repeatedly reinfected by her sex partner.

For this reason, the male partner usually needs to be treated at the same time as the female. It is advisable that the man use condoms during intercourse for several weeks to lessen the possibility of reinfection.

Trichomoniasis is usually treated with the drug metronidazole. In pill form, metronidazole (brand name is *Flagyl*) is usually taken three times a day for 10 days. It should not be taken by a woman who is pregnant or nursing or who has a history of blood diseases or diseases of the central nervous system.

Since *Flagyl* changes the environment of the vagina, it may result in a yeast infection. Other possible side effects include nausea, diarrhea, cramps, dizziness, and dry mouth and vagina. It is best to avoid alcoholic drinks while on this drug since it blocks the metabolism of alcohol and one drink has the impact of several.

Drinking a good amount of water daily will reduce the small chance of dark urine, aftertaste, or furry tongue.

Alternative therapy may include vinegar douches, vaginal suppositories, creams, and jellies. Since trichomonas lives in an environment less acidic than normal, a woman may be able to control the infection at its first signs by douching with a solution of 2 tablespoons of vinegar in a quart of water.

Even with these many methods of treatment, eradicating the organism may prove difficult, and there is a high recurrence rate.

See also ANAL SEX; VAGINAL DOUCHING; VAGINAL INFECTION; VENEREAL DISEASE; YEAST INFECTION.

TUBAL LIGATION. See TUBAL STERILIZATION.

TUBAL PREGNANCY. See ECTOPIC PREGNANCY.

TUBAL STERILIZATION (ligation or coagulation) involves tying off or cauterizing (burning) the Fallopian tubes between the ovaries and the uterus. This prevents the egg from reaching the uterus and the sperm from traveling up the tubes, thus making it a permanent method of contraception. The surgery is performed under general anesthesia in a hospital or ambulatory surgical facility. In rare cases, the severed tubes reunite and a pregnancy occurs.

The most commonly used method is laparoscopy. A long tubelike instrument called a laparoscope is inserted through a small abdominal incision. With the mirrors and lights on the laparoscope, the surgeon locates the tubes and cauterizes, clamps, or cuts them. Cauterizing presents the risk of burning the small or large intestine.

Laparoscopy is sometimes called a "Band-Aid operation" because the umbilical incision is so small that only a Band-Aid is used. It requires at most an overnight stay in the hospital. Many women go home the same day.

In the traditional method of tubal ligation, called laparotomy, a larger incision is made in the abdominal wall. The surgeon cuts each Fallopian tube and ties each separated end. While the operation can be performed at any time, it is often done just after delivery when the uterus is enlarged and the tubes are easily reached.

Laparotomy entails two to six days in the hospital. It is the procedure of choice for women who are 50 pounds or more overweight and for women who suffer severe heart or lung disease or who have had previous pelvic surgery.

Sexual response is not affected by tubal ligation. Menstruation continues; hormones are secreted normally; ovaries, uterus, and vagina are unaffected. An egg is produced and released every month, but when it reaches the cut portion of Fallopian tube, it can go no farther; it disintegrates and is harmlessly absorbed by the body.

Although it is possible to reverse the tubal sterilization, only about half of reversal operations are successful. Thus, it is wise for women to be sterilized only if they are absolutely sure they do not wish to have more children.

A woman also becomes sterile after the removal of her reproductive organs: both Fallopian tubes, both ovaries, or the uterus. These operations are usually performed to remove damaged or diseased tissue. Rarely if ever are they done specifically as sterilization procedures.

See also CONTRACEPTION; HYSTERECTOMY.

TUBERCULOSIS (TB), an infectious bacterial disease, can impair sexual functioning by its general debilitating effect or by its destructive effect on the genitourinary system. Once a common disease, TB has now become increasingly rare.

When TB affects the lungs (pulmonary TB), the patient may experience loss of appetite, fatigue, weight loss, and afternoon fever. Diminished interest in sex is another common symptom of pulmonary TB. In advanced stages, sexual activity may be limited by shortness of breath or exertion.

Sex may be avoided because of fear of contagion. A patient's spouse may be loath to engage in sexual intercourse because of the risk of contracting TB.

Pulmonary TB is transmitted by droplets of liquid containing tubercle bacilli. These small droplets are transmitted when an infectious patient talks, sneezes, laughs, sings, or coughs. The disease is unlikely to be transmitted through contaminated clothes or objects since the bacilli are rapidly inactivated by drying and sunlight.

When one family member is found to have TB, all household members should be tested for the disease. Some physicians recommend preventive therapy for household members at high risk of contracting TB: infants and young children and those who are chronically ill.

Treatment for TB is chemotherapy. Among the drugs used are isoniazid, streptomycin, ethambutol, and rifampin; often they are used in combination.

Patients who are being treated for TB are believed to rapidly decline in infectiousness—even when tubercle bacilli are still present in their sputum. This noninfectious state is believed to occur within 10 days to 2 weeks. Thus patients who are undergoing effective antituberculosis treatment should be able to engage in sexual intercourse without exposing their partners to a substantial risk of infection.

When TB affects the genitourinary system (GUTB), it is likely to have a direct negative effect on sexual functioning. The disease spreads from the lungs through the bloodstream, affecting the kidneys as well as the reproductive organs.

Among women, the Fallopian tubes are involved in 90 to 100 percent with GUTB. The uterus and ovaries are often infected, rarely the cervix. Women with genital TB usually experience infertility, pelvic pain, generalized debility, and menstrual disturbances. Pain is aggravated by sexual intercourse, exercise, and menstruation.

Although it is unlikely that a woman with active GUTB will become pregnant, she should use contraception while she is taking TB medication. If she does become pregnant, the child may suffer from congenital defects caused by the drugs. Amniocentesis is advisable (see entry). If the fetus is found to be suffering from congenital abnormalities, the woman may choose to abort. The child of a woman with tuberculosis will not be born with the disease.

Among men, the disease almost always affects first the kidneys, then the prostate and seminal vesicles. Typical symptoms are difficult and painful urination, urinary frequency and urgency, inflammation of the testicles, and chronic prostatitis. Men with advanced GUTB become sterile.

Even without treatment, it is unlikely for a person with GUTB to transmit it during sexual intercourse. But there is evidence that small children are at risk when family hygiene is lax. Men with untreated GUTB usually have a large number of tubercle bacilli in their urine. Children may contract the illness by being exposed to soiled clothing and sheets contaminated with urine.

As with pulmonary TB, therapy for GUTB is antituberculosis medication. Drugs used to treat tuberculosis are not known to have any negative effect on sexual functioning.

See also PROSTATITIS.

TURNER'S SYNDROME. See HORMONE DISORDERS.

UREMIA. See KIDNEY DISEASE.

URETHRA. See FEMALE SEXUAL ANATOMY; MALE SEXUAL ANATOMY.

URINARY TRACT INFECTION (UTI, urethritis, cystitis)

results from bacteria infecting the bladder, urethra, or other parts of the urinary tract. The most common symptoms are a burning sensation on urinating and frequent, urgent urination. Backache, fever, and pain above the pubic area may accompany the infection. There may be blood in the urine.

Untreated, UTI may pass from the bladder to one or both kidneys, resulting in nephritis. This may ultimately cause uremic poisoning and kidney failure.

About eight times more women than men get UTI. It is common for a woman to develop symptoms after she begins to have intercourse: so-called honeymoon cystitis. It is thought that urethral bacteria are massaged into the bladder, where they may double in number every 20 minutes and cause an active infection of the bladder mucosa. UTI also often occurs when a woman acquires a new sex partner, when her frequency of intercourse greatly increases, or when she resumes intercourse after a long period of abstinence.

During sexual intercourse, a woman's urethra and bladder may become irritated and swollen, particularly in the absence of adequate vaginal lubrication. Infectious organisms in her anogenital region may be introduced into her urethra. UTI may also result if the urethra is contaminated after anal intercourse.

Some vaginal infections make a woman more susceptible to UTI. She is also at higher risk if she has an anal pathology such as anal fistula or prolapsing hemorrhoids.

After menopause, a woman may experience trauma to the urethra—hence a greater likelihood of infection—because of decreased vaginal secretions. In older women, the mucous membrane of the urethra may prolapse through the urethral opening, increasing the likelihood of infection.

Minor anatomical problems cause a small number of women to suffer from recurrent UTI after intercourse. Some women have adhesions between the urethra and the vagina. Others have an incompletely ruptured hymen, which connects the urethral opening to the vaginal opening. On penetration, the penis pulls the urethral opening into the vaginal vault, making contamination likely. A simple surgical procedure corrects the difficulty.

UTI often results from obstructions to the normal flow of urine. Some women are born with an abnormally narrow urethra. In others, tissue damage caused by childbirth may result in some disruption of the normal flow of urine. Tumors in nearby organs may result in an obstruction, as may scar tissue and kidney stones.

When urine stagnates in the bladder, it serves as a culture medium for germs that are usually present in small numbers. The germs multiply rapidly, and infection results. UTI may also be caused by rectal bacteria making their way up the urethra.

Preventing UTI. To protect against urine stagnation, it is wise to drink at least 5 glasses of fluid daily and to urinate often. Women should guard against fecal contamination with E. coli intestinal bacteria after bowel movements by wiping away from the vagina, not toward it (front to back). Anal intercourse requires a condom. The anogenital region should be washed frequently. Irritants like bubble bath, feminine hygiene sprays, and scented douches should be avoided.

It is prudent for women with recurrent UTI to urinate before intercourse, thus reducing pressure on the bladder. Drinking 3 or 4 glasses of water and urinating within 20 minutes after intercourse may expel bacteria before they cause an infection.

If a woman is susceptible to UTI, she may want to refrain from using a diaphragm, since pressure from its ring may irritate her bladder. She should also avoid rear-entry vaginal intercourse, which may cause bladder symptoms.

Treatment of UTI usually consists of at least 10 days of antibiotics. Medication should be continued for the prescribed number of days even though symptoms will probably abate after a day or two.

UTI can be a "Ping-Pong" infection, passed back and forth between partners. One partner may harbor the disease with no symptoms, yet continue to reinfect the treated partner. Thus, it is a good idea for the sex partner of someone with a urinary tract infection to have urine analyzed for signs of UTI.

Analgesics may be prescribed to relieve pain. A sufferer should drink a lot of water or juices (cranberry juice, an American Indian remedy, is often effective)—but avoid coffee, tea, and alcohol, which may irritate the urinary tract.

If UTI is recurrent or difficult to eliminate, a physician may prescribe antibiotics for prolonged periods. When obstruction of the urine flow is responsible for recurrent or chronic UTI, urethral dilatation (stretching with an instrument) and/or surgery is usually recommended.

Pregnancy poses special problems for a woman with urinary tract infection since antibiotics may possibly cause congenital malformation in the fetus during the first three months. Some physicians postpone treatment if the infection is not too serious. Large doses of vitamin C are possibly effective for mild UTI in pregnant women. Chronic, recurrent UTI may be associated with premature childbirth.

See also ANAL SEX; VAGINAL INFECTION.

URINATION during orgasm occasionally occurs among women. Three to 5 percent of women are believed to experience this phenomenon regularly or on occasion.

Involuntary urination may be due to anatomical defects of the urogenital system or to neurological diseases such as multiple sclerosis. Medical problems associated with urinary incontinence, such as diabetes, may account for the problem. Urinary tract infection may cause chronic urgency and loss of bladder control during sexual intercourse.

Women whose incontinence during orgasm is due to underlying disease will most likely experience involuntary urination at other times as well.

Failure to empty the bladder before intercourse is probably the most common cause of urination during orgasm. In some women, the problem may be due to anxiety about sex.

After sexual intercourse, both men and women generally feel the need to urinate. In males, the need arises because of congestion of the prostate, which occurs during intercourse. The prostate is near the bladder, and congestion in the area may produce the urge to void.

In women, the urge may occur because the thrusting of the penis against the urethra and bladder produces the sensation of a full bladder.

See also URINARY TRACT INFECTION.

UTERINE PROLAPSE is the descent of the uterus through the pelvic floor and vaginal outlet. The cause is usually childbirth trauma to the muscles and ligaments that provide support for the uterus. The condition is rare in women who have not given birth.

In first-degree prolapse, the cervix comes down to the vaginal opening but does not protrude. Sexual function is usually not impaired. But if the cervix is in the way, a rear-entry position with the woman on her knees will probably be most comfortable.

In second-degree prolapse, the cervix protrudes through the vaginal opening. The condition is most pronounced when the woman is standing. Intercourse is still possible if the uterus is pushed up to its normal position, but it may be painful.

In third-degree prolapse, also called procidentia, the body of the uterus protrudes through the vaginal opening. The cervix and vaginal walls may become eroded, leading to vaginal discharge and bleeding. Intercourse is all but impossible.

Mild degrees of prolapse can often be corrected by muscle exercises. The majority of more severe cases require corrective surgery.

See also INTERCOURSE, PAINFUL.

UTERUS. See FEMALE SEXUAL ANATOMY.

VAGINA. See FEMALE SEXUAL ANATOMY.

VAGINAL BLEEDING after intercourse may result from a variety of medical problems.

Any woman who experiences vaginal bleeding after sex (or at any other time) should consult a physician—except, of course, if she is menstruating at the time.

Herpes type 2 genital infections may produce changes in the cervix that result in bleeding. Pregnancy and the use of oral contraceptives may similarly cause changes that make the cervix vulnerable and liable to bleed. The cervical changes usually reverse when the woman stops taking the Pill.

Cervical polyps or cancer of the cervix may also result in bleeding after intercourse. Women whose mothers were given DES during their pregnancy may experience vaginal bleeding from a condition called vaginal adenosis. They should have periodic examinations—including examination with an instrument called a colposcope—to check for cervical or vaginal cancer.

Older women may experience relative estrogen deprivation, which makes the vaginal walls thin and prone to bleeding.

Some women experience bleeding from the uterus after intercourse. This bleeding is very likely coincidental—there is usually no cause-and-effect relationship. Some causes of the abnormal bleeding are incomplete abortion; inflammation of the uterine lining after abortion; or abnormal pregnancy, such as a pregnancy that occurs in the Fallopian tubes.

See also CERVICAL CANCER; CERVICAL EROSION; DES; MENOPAUSE; PILL, CONTRACEPTIVE; VAGINAL INFECTION; YEAST INFECTION.

VAGINAL CANCER is relatively rare—although other cancers may extend or spread to the vagina.

Early symptoms include vaginal bleeding or discharge. In late stages of the disease, pain on intercourse is a typical symptom. Persistent, intractable itching is also a common symptom.

Extensive pelvic surgery is usually the treatment of choice. Most often, intercourse is physically impossible after such surgery. But couples may engage in manual or oral sexual activity.

Plastic reconstructive surgery of the vagina is a possibility for some women. Daily dilation of the vagina is necessary to prevent constriction. Frequent intercourse is helpful. Antibiotic and hormone-containing creams may also be needed.

For a few women, the anatomy of the vagina after surgery allows for intercourse. An artificial lubricant is usually necessary since vaginal lubrication is often impaired as a result of scarring and changes in blood-flow patterns to the remainder of the vagina.

See also CANCER.

VAGINAL DOUCHING is irrigating and cleansing the vagina with a solution of vinegar and water or another douche preparation. It is usually done with either a fountain syringe or a disposable syringe.

Douching should be done only when prescribed by a physician for a medical condition. In a healthy woman, the vagina is self-cleaning. Some clear vaginal discharge is perfectly normal.

A woman who is troubled with excessive foul-smelling or greenish-yellowish discharge should consult her doctor. She may have a vaginal infection or other illness.

Hazards of douching. Strong chemicals in the douche solution can injure cells in the lining of the vagina. Further, the normal secretions of the vagina contain protective bacteria that tend to prevent infections of the vaginal tract. By habitually flushing the vagina, a woman invites the very germs she hopes to avoid by douching.

Douching should not be used as a means of birth control. It is an extremely unreliable method. Nor should a woman douche during pregnancy.

Doctors often recommend douching in the treatment of certain vaginal infections or some other conditions. In such cases, the doctor will usually prescribe the powder or liquid to be used. Many doctors recommend a douche solution consisting of one tablespoon of white vinegar to each quart of water. This helps maintain the normal acid medium of the vagina.

Over-the-counter douching solutions and products can be dangerous. Perfumed brands can provoke allergic reactions.

Many women have permanently damaged their vaginal membranes

by using strong douching formulas passed on from mothers and grandmothers—such as phenol household disinfectants, bichloride of mercury, and potassium permanganate. Other douche solutions may contain harmless, but useless, ingredients—such as borax and soda or table salt.

Tips for safety. In cases where douching is prescribed, some women injure themselves by improperly using the douche. Here are some tips for successful douching:

● A woman should always read the directions on the douching preparation. It is particularly important not to use too much of the chemical.

● Water should be put in the douche bag before the chemical. Otherwise, the concentrated chemical at the bottom of the bag reaches the vagina first, possibly injuring the delicate tissues.

● Only mild pressure should be used so that the solution will not be forced into the uterus or the peritoneal cavity. The douche bag should be no higher than two feet above the woman's hips. Syringe-type douches can be hazardous. One safe way to douche is for a woman to hang the douche bag on the edge of a bathtub, and insert the nozzle while lying on her back in an empty tub. The douche bag should never be connected directly to a faucet.

● The douche bag should be kept hygienic. It should be thoroughly washed and dried after every use, then stored in a clean place.

See also VAGINAL INFECTION; VAGINAL ODOR.

VAGINAL DRYNESS during intercourse usually results from insufficient sexual arousal, anxiety, fatigue, or lack of involvement.

One of the first physiological signs of female response to sexual stimulation is vaginal lubrication. In premenopausal women, sexual stimulation causes vaginal lubrication in 10 to 30 seconds.

Lubrication results from congestion of the blood vessels in and around the vagina causing seepage of fluid through the tissue of the vaginal walls to the inside of the vagina. This process is often referred to as the "sweating" reaction.

In most cases, a woman more easily reaches orgasm if she first passes through this earlier phase of her sexual response cycle.

Moisture eases the insertion of the penis into the vagina. However, when the vagina is insufficiently lubricated, insertion may be difficult,

313

and both partners may find intercourse uncomfortable or painful, with burning, itching, or aching.

Besides insufficient arousal, other conditions may account for vaginal dryness. Just after childbirth and during breastfeeding, vaginal lubrication is likely to be scanty because of a relative lack of estrogen. After menopause, it takes a longer period of stimulation for a woman to produce lubrication, and the amount of lubrication may be decreased.

Some medications interfere with a woman's ability to lubricate. These include certain drugs used in treating peptic ulcers, some tranquilizers, narcotics, sedatives, and antihistamines.

A variety of illnesses may cause vaginal dryness. In advanced diabetes, the capacity to lubricate may be decreased. Multiple sclerosis may cause decreased lubrication. A woman with spinal-cord injury experiences little or no lubrication. Vaginal surgery or X-ray therapy may interfere with the ability to lubricate. Hormone problems may result in decreased estrogen, which interferes with vaginal lubrication.

Some oral contraceptives may decrease the ability of the vagina to lubricate. This is especially likely with a birth control pill that is extremely low in estrogen. A switch to a different type will correct this problem.

Lack of sexual interest is common cause of vaginal dryness in a healthy woman with normal hormone levels. A woman may feel uninterested in sex on a particular occasion or may feel negative toward her sex partner. Fear of pain during intercourse can produce a marked decrease in vaginal lubrication. A woman who is tense about intercourse and anxious about her sexual performance may similarly fail to lubricate adequately. Such a woman may benefit from psychotherapy or sex therapy.

Sometimes, women produce sufficient lubrication for easy penetration, but find that intercourse later becomes dry and irritating. This most often happens when intercourse is prolonged. While vaginal lubrication increases during the early excitation phase of sexual response, it decreases during the advanced, or plateau, levels. Therefore, a woman who remains in the plateau level for a long time may experience a decrease in lubrication with resulting irritation.

When additional lubrication is needed, saliva is often sufficient. Water-soluble contraceptive or surgical jellies are very effective. The lubricant can be put on the penis, or at the vaginal opening, or both.

It is unwise to use cold cream as a lubricant. Many creams are mixed with oils and may contain perfumes that can cause allergic reactions in either the man or the woman. Petroleum jelly (such as Vaseline) is also a poor lubricant for sexual intercourse. It obstructs the seepage of the woman's own vaginal fluid and can also impede the vagina's self-cleansing mechanism. If the man wears a condom, the petroleum jelly may damage the thin rubber.

Some women complain of the opposite problem: *excessive* vaginal lubrication. This should be distinguished from vaginal discharge resulting from infection or venereal diseases.

Women vary greatly in the amount of normal lubrication they produce. An excessively fastidious woman may find a normal amount of lubrication bothersome or embarrassing. Women typically produce more lubrication during pregnancy because of increased blood flow to the pelvis.

Prolonged sexual stimulation may sometimes produce an over-abundance of lubrication. Some women are extremely susceptible to sexual excitation and are frequently lubricating in response to it.

A few women report a gush of fluid from the vagina at the moment of orgasm and wonder if they are ejaculating. This may be a squeezing of lubricating fluid from the vagina as a result of vaginal contraction at orgasm. Preliminary research suggests, however, that some women may ejaculate from the urethra a fluid similar to prostatic fluid (see GRAFENBERG SPOT).

A woman who believes she is experiencing over abundant lubrication should consult her gynecologist. In a few cases, it may be due to medical problems.

See also AGING; MENOPAUSE.

VAGINAL EXAMINATION. See PELVIC EXAMINATION.

VAGINAL EXERCISE is the tensing and relaxing of the muscles surrounding the vagina and rectum.

The pubococcygeal muscle, which incorporates the vaginal area, is rich in nerve endings. Toning up the muscle with the Kegel exercise increases its sensitivity during intercourse. A stronger muscle also enables the woman to grip her partner's penis tightly and squeeze rhythmically if desired.

To start practicing the exercise, a woman can stop the flow as she is urinating two or three times for about three seconds each time—providing the same effect as if she were bearing down on a penis. There is nothing harmful in interrupting the flow of urine.

Once a woman becomes more aware of her vaginal muscles, the exercise can be done anywhere at any time—doing the dishes, riding a subway, or talking on the phone.

This exercise is extremely valuable for postpartum patients. Not only does it tighten the muscle for sexual pleasure, but it also, by improving circulation, reduces the pain and edema resulting from the episiotomy. Women can start doing the exercise soon after delivery—indeed, in the delivery room if possible. Vaginal exercise also decreases the amount of stretching of pelvic muscles that may come with aging.

See also POSTPARTUM PROBLEMS.

VAGINAL INFECTION constitutes the most common women's disease. It may be caused by bacteria, trichomonas, fungi, or other microorganisms. A woman can have more than one type of vaginal infection simultaneously (mixed vaginitis).

The most common symptoms of vaginal infections are vaginal itching, a heavy discharge, an unpleasant vaginal odor, and possibly a burning sensation when urinating. Sexual intercourse is likely to be painful.

Form-fitting panty hose and girdles—particularly those made of nylon or other synthetics—have increased the incidence of all types of vaginal infections. These garments raise body temperature and keep moisture from evaporating. The organisms that cause vaginal infections flourish in such a moist, warm environment. Women who have recurrent infections should dispense with tight nylon undergarments. Regular stockings can be substituted for panty hose, cotton underpants for nylon.

Besides yeast infection, gonorrhea, and trichomoniasis, the most common vaginal infection is *nonspecific vaginitis.* This infection is caused by potentially harmful bacteria that normally inhabit the vagina, such as streptococci, staphylocci, colon bacteria, chlamydia, or haemophilis vaginalis.

Changes in the vaginal environment can allow bacteria to cause infections. The acid/alkaline balance of the vagina changes during ovulation, menstruation, and pregnancy, enabling infection to develop. Vaginal douching likewise can change the vagina's chemical environment.

Another infection in the body can also set the stage for a vaginal infection as can exhaustion and poor diet. So too can aggressive intercourse that causes inflammation of the cervix or the vaginal walls. Some women taking the birth control pill seem more prone to vaginal infections. If a woman is taking antibiotics for an infectious disease, yeast in her vagina may flourish unchecked, causing monilial vaginitis. Some types of vaginal infection may be transmitted during sexual intercourse. Although vaginal infections are of course diseases of females, if a woman has a steady sex partner, he should be checked for the organism and treated simultaneously if he proves infected. He may harbor the organisms in his prostate, urethra, and bladder without any symptoms and thus can reinfect the woman after she has undergone treatment.

Infection may also be acquired if a woman has anal intercourse, then vaginal. The contaminated penis may transfer rectal bacteria (E. coli) to the vagina. It is advisable for the man to wear a condom for the anal intercourse, then dispose of it before entering the vagina. At the least, he should wash his penis after anal penetration.

Women who wear very tight jeans are also at greater risk of contracting vaginal infection from E. coli organisms. After bowel movements, any organisms remaining around the anal region or on underwear may migrate to the vagina with the constricting rubbing action of the skin-tight jeans.

One preventive is to wear looser-fitting pants. Another is to cleanse the perineal region after each bowel movement. For times when soap and water are not at hand, as in public rest rooms, a woman can carry a package of foil-wrapped towelettes.

Symptoms of nonspecific vaginitis include a pussy yellow or white discharge, possibly streaked with blood. The walls of the vagina are cloudy, puffy with fluid, and covered by a thick accumulation of pus. One of the early symptoms of the infection may be frequent and burning urination since the infection may quickly spread to the urethra.

The infection can also spread into the uterus and Fallopian tubes. Chronic infections can cause the cells of the cervix to grow abnormally and make a woman more susceptible to cancer of the cervix. The engorgement of blood that occurs during sexual excitement and orgasm may cause the organisms to reach the circulation and thereby spread to other parts of the body.

Other symptoms of nonspecific vaginitis may be lower back pain, cramps, and swollen glands in the abdomen and thighs.

To diagnose nonspecific vaginitis, the physician examines the cervix and vagina. (The woman should not douche for at least 24 hours before her appointment.) The discharge examined under a microscope will show a large number of bacteria and white blood cells.

Vaginal infections are almost always curable. Treatment usually involves some combination of prescribed tablets and salves, vaginal suppositories, and medicated douches.

Physicians often advise abstaining from sexual intercourse for at least two weeks. If suppositories are prescribed, they should be inserted at bedtime with clean fingers, not a plastic gadget that can retain organisms. All the medication prescribed should be finished. The infected area should be washed frequently and gently patted dry with a soft towel.

Treatment may be complicated by a secondary infection. As one type of organism in the vagina is killed off during treatment, others may increase to cause a renewed problem. Thus antibiotics used against haemophilus vaginalis may destroy bacteria that have been keeping yeast in check—giving rise to a case of yeast infection.

See also ANAL SEX; HAEMOPHILUS VAGINALIS; TRICHO-MONIASIS; YEAST INFECTION.

VAGINAL ODOR—like perspiration odor—is caused by bacteria acting on the perspiration, mucus, and oil that accumulate on skin, hair, and clothing. This is a special problem on body areas that are normally warm and moist like the vagina and vulva.

To combat normal vaginal odor, a woman should wash daily with soap and water and wear fairly loose-fitting cotton underwear. Close-fitting nylon underwear, panty girdles, and panty hose delay the evaporation of perspiration and may thus accentuate the odor.

A woman with an abnormally strong and persistent odor should consult a physician, for she may be suffering from a vaginal infection or other pathological conditions, including a forgotten tampon. She should not attempt frequent vaginal douching to eliminate vaginal odor.

Danger of vaginal deodorants. Such products are unnecessary and potentially harmful. This is particularly true of genital deodorants in spray cans.

Feminine deodorant sprays are aerosols for application to a woman's external genital area. Most consist of oils and perfumes of the type used in cosmetics, antibacterial agents, and a propellant. They act much as underarm deodorants do to inhibit bacterial growth and reduce the possibility of offensive odor.

Many women have allergic reactions to the sprays. Many more develop skin conditions. The Food and Drug Administration has received scores of complaints from women irritated by genital deodorant sprays. The most common complaint involves burning sensations. There are many cases of rashes, blisters, itching, or irritations, Other reactions include a feeling of urinary urgency with pain, swelling, or open sores.

In a lawsuit filed against one spray manufacturer, a woman who used the spray while pregnant claims that she developed huge painful swellings. She had difficulty walking and had to be hospitalized. Her doctor diagnosed the condition as a severe reaction to the spray.

Part of the problem may stem from confusing advertising that leads some women to believe the spray is intended for use *in* the vagina. Actually, it is meant to be applied to the *external* genital area only since it can easily injure the delicate mucous membranes of the vagina. Worse yet, widespread advertising of genital sprays may persuade many women with vaginal infections or an unsuspected tumor to put off seeking medical advice while using the sprays instead.

There are also strong objections to the implications of the advertising for deodorant sprays: that women will be offensive to men unless they are completely deodorized.

Reducing hazards. A woman who feels she must use vaginal deodorant spray can reduce the hazards by:

● Spraying it only on the external genital area, not into the vagina.

● Not spraying onto a tampon, which would bring the deodorant in contact with vaginal tissue.

● Not using a spray just before sexual intercourse. It can cause genital irritation for men as well as women.

319

● Not using an underarm antiperspirant spray on the genital area. It may contain aluminum salts, which can be extremely irritating to the mucous membranes of the genitals.

● Spraying at least eight inches from the skin.

● Using the spray sparingly, and not more than once a day.

● Not using the spray on broken, irritated, or itching skin. A woman who develops any such disorder in her vaginal area should see a family doctor or a gynecologist.

See also VAGINAL DOUCHING; VAGINAL INFECTION.

VAGINAL SOUNDS during intercourse occur among many women, and are frequently a source of great embarrassment.

A likely cause for the vaginal sounds is that the woman is assuming coital positions in which her pelvis is elevated—with her hips on a pillow or in any supine position where her knees are close to her chest. Her uterus and posterior vaginal wall fall backward'from gravity, causing a vacuum that sucks in air through the vaginal opening. Changing position can make the uterus and vaginal wall move, forcing air out. Similar flatulentlike sounds are often heard in female exercise and yoga classes.

Penile thrusting may introduce air into the vagina; the pistonlike motion may also force air out, contributing to the sounds.

These sounds are perfectly normal. There is no reason for a couple to try to avoid vaginal sounds by abandoning positions they enjoy; an elevated pelvis tends to permit deep penile penetration and thus is gratifying to many couples. Rather, the couple should try to accept such sounds as an aspect of lovemaking.

VAGINAL SPASM (vaginismus) is an involuntary spasm of the muscles of the outer third of the vagina and the vaginal opening.

Such spasms usually occur whenever there is an attempt to introduce an object into the vagina. Penile penetration of the vagina is usually impossible, and attempts are likely to be very painful.

Women suffering from vaginismus may be sexually responsive and experience orgasm through clitoral stimulation or other sex play. Usually, however, vaginal lubrication and sexual desire are impaired. Typically, women with vaginismus are distressed by their inability to engage in sexual intercourse.

In less severe forms of vaginal spasm, it may be possible to insert a finger or a tampon into the vagina, even to use a speculum for vaginal examination. Only the penis may be prevented from entering the vagina. In some cases, penetration may be possible despite the spasm—but very painful for the women.

Psychological causes are most common. Many women with vaginal spasm have had a strict upbringing in which sex was considered dirty or taboo. Some have had traumatic early experiences with sex—rape, childhood molestation, incest, or painful first intercourse.

In a few cases, the cause is a first pelvic examination by a doctor who is insensitive and rough. Phobias about pregnancy, venereal disease, or cancer may also be causes. In others, vaginal abnormalities or pelvic pathology may result in pain on penetration. The vagina reacts by developing a spasm.

In primary vaginismus, a woman has never been able to have successful intercourse. Sometimes, marriages remain unconsummated for many years because of this problem. In some such marriages, the husband may suffer from erectile difficulties. Both may have come from backgrounds in which premarital sex is viewed as sinful. They may have trouble making the transition to viewing sex as acceptable after marriage.

In other relationships in which the woman has vaginal spasm, her sex partner may develop a pattern of premature ejaculation because he anticipates anxiety and frustration if he attempts penetration. Problems with erection may develop after a while because of repeated failure—further compounding the couple's sexual problems.

In secondary vaginismus, the woman has had satisfactory intercourse in the past. Vaginal spasm may develop because of sexual aversion or trauma or because intercourse becomes painful for any of a wide variety of reasons. The muscles react by involuntarily protecting the vaginal opening.

Vaginal spasm is usually curable. Most sex therapists and physicians use the approach developed by Masters and Johnson, or a variation of it.

Therapy is aimed at showing both partners that the vaginal spasm is real. Illustrations are used to explain vaginismus physiologically. Some couples do not realize what it is that prevents penetration.

The physician explains to the couple that the spasm is not under the woman's voluntary control. This explanation may lift a great burden of guilt from the woman. The physician may demonstrate the spasm by

321

attempting to insert a finger into the woman's vagina: involuntary spasm closes the outlet. The husband is present during the medical examination and sees what is happening.

The woman can be taught to help reverse this reflex by voluntarily tightening her vaginal muscles as hard as she can, then letting go. This results in some lessening of the spasm.

A thorough pelvic examination should identify and correct any medical problems that may be contributing to vaginal spasm.

For home practice, the woman is given plastic vaginal dilators ("Young" dilators)—beginning with one about the size of a tampon and continuing with others of gradually increasing size. She is instructed to slowly and gently insert the lubricated dilator about 4 times a day and to leave it in place for 10 or 15 minutes. She may also be encouraged to try to fall asleep with it inside her. Her sex partner may be encouraged to participate in inserting the dilators.

Therapy is also directed at solving emotional difficulties or problems in the relationship that may have contributed to vaginal spasm.

When the woman can comfortably insert a dilator about the size of a penis, intercourse can be attempted.

See also INTERCOURSE, PAINFUL.

VAGINAL STRETCHING commonly occurs after months or years of sexual intercourse, after childbirth, and sometimes as part of the normal aging process. This slight stretching of the vaginal opening rarely interferes with the enjoyment of intercourse.

Sometimes, however, a woman or her sex partner complains that the vagina is too loose for satisfactory intercourse.

In many cases, such complaints are due to misinformation or unrealistic expectations. Sometimes, problems in the relationship focus on this complaint.

Some women believe that it is necessary to have a tight vaginal opening to please men sexually. Actually, for most men vaginal tightness is only a minor element of sexual pleasure. Further, as men become older their erections may become too weak to penetrate a relatively narrow vaginal opening.

Some middle-aged women erroneously believe that to keep their husbands from straying they ought to have their vaginas surgically tightened. This is very rarely necessary.

For many couples, the problem is not so much that the woman's vagina is stretched—but that its muscles are unexercised and weak. Vaginal exercise can improve gripping of the penis and increase enjoyment for both partners. This involves squeezing and relaxing pelvic muscles as if starting and stopping the flow of urine. Once a woman becomes aware of these muscles, she can further practice by contracting and relaxing with her finger or her partner's in the vagina.

A loose feeling inside the vagina has a lot to do with the woman's stage of sexual arousal. During the excitement stage, the inner two-thirds of the vagina begins to expand. If the penis enters the vagina during this phase, the woman may experience the feeling that the penis is lost in her vagina. The man may likewise complain of little feeling of containment.

As the woman becomes more sexually aroused—during the plateau stage—the outer third of her vagina contracts (the orgasmic platform), gripping the penis. For both partners, the loose feeling may now disappear. Thus, simply making sure the woman has become sufficiently aroused may "solve" the whole problem of vaginal stretching.

A husband who complains his wife's vagina is overstretched may actually be experiencing sexual changes of his own. In middle age, his erections may be less firm, and he may ejaculate more slowly, or sometimes not at all. During intercourse, he may partly lose his erection. These and other normal changes may make him anxious about his sexual adequacy. His less-firm erections may make him feel that his wife's vagina is too loose. In an attempt to deny his own sexual concerns, he may blame his wife's stretched vagina for these alterations in their sexual activity.

From the woman's point of view, the tightness or looseness of her vagina may have some effect on her sexual enjoyment. While a stretched vagina may not impair a woman's ability to reach orgasm, it may affect the amount of stimulation she feels with thrusting. This may be remedied by vaginal exercise.

Some intercourse positions increase penile *friction* and give a feeling of tightness when the vaginal opening is stretched. In one such, the woman lies on her back with her legs together. The man lies on top with his legs apart or with one leg pressed between her legs. Couples should experiment with different positions to find those which produce the desired sensation.

In rare cases, vaginal stretching may be due to congenital defects, trauma resulting from childbirth, scarring from vaginal surgery, or poor episiotomy repair. Corrective surgery may be used to tighten the vagina. Special care should be taken not to make the vaginal opening too tight, particularly if the woman's sex partner is over 50 and may not have erections firm enough to penetrate a very narrow opening.

See also VAGINAL EXERCISE.

VAGINISMUS. See VAGINAL SPASM.

VAS DEFERENS. See MALE SEXUAL ANATOMY.

VASECTOMY is an operation in which the vas deferens is severed, hence sperm is prevented from mixing with the semen. It is an increasingly common form of birth control. An estimated one million men a year are vasectomized.

Vasectomy generally leaves sexual performance unimpaired. The testicles, which manufacture semen, are not affected by the operation. A man can continue to have intercourse, ejaculate normally, and enjoy orgasm as before. The vasectomy has no effect on the production of the male sex hormones or on the appearance of the genitals.

The sole physical effect of vasectomy: no sperm in the semen, hence no possibility of pregnancy. The sperm cells—still produced by the testicles but now having no outlet—dissolve and are absorbed into the bloodstream. Although some controversy exists about the side effects of vasectomy, they are usually considered minimal to nonexistent.

What it entails. The vasectomy involves removing a small segment and tying the ends of the vas deferens, the tubes that carry sperm cells from the testicles. To do this, the surgeon—preferably a urologist—makes in the scrotum two incisions, each about half an inch long. The operation is usually performed in the office under local anesthesia and takes about 20 minutes. Some doctors prefer to do vasectomies in the hospital under a short-acting general anesthesia.

Vasectomy clinics often charge no more than the patient can afford to pay. Many medical and hospitalization plans now cover the cost of vasectomy.

A man who undergoes a vasectomy may be able to return to work and resume normal activities the day after the operation. He is likely to experience discomfort and swelling for several days. To get relief, he can apply ice packs the first day, pain-killers thereafter.

In extremely rare cases, healing may be delayed by infections and other complications, including painful inflammations and internal bleeding. No deaths have been reported from vasectomies.

Sperm may remain in the seminal tract (the path the sperm follow) for weeks or months, depending on how frequently the man ejaculates. Some 10 to 15 ejaculations are generally necessary before all the sperm are gone. It may be wise for a man to have intercourse or masturbate frequently just before the vasectomy so that the seminal tract empties faster. Monthly examinations of semen for several months after a vasectomy are advised.

In perhaps 6 in 1,000 vasectomies, the severed ends of the vas deferens grow together and fertility is accidentally restored. So, until the surgeon has verified that a man's semen is free of sperm, he should use other methods of birth control. Semen analysis is recommended every other year for six years.

A man may have intercourse as soon as he desires after the vasectomy. Many men find sex is comfortable after 10 to 14 days. Some are able to resume much sooner. Couples often report that they enjoy sex more since they feel confident there will not be a pregnancy.

Psychological consequences. About two-thirds of vasectomized men report an increase in sexual pleasure during intercourse.

On the other hand, for some men vasectomy triggers emotional problems. A man may believe his virility depends on his ability to produce a child. He may regard his sterility as a loss of masculinity. Feeling less like a real man, he may suffer impotence.

Some men react to vasectomy with greatly increased, sometimes compulsive, sexual activity. For example, a husband may want sexual relations 1 to 3 times a day, considerably more than was usual for him. This may persist for some time after the operation. A man also may refuse to do "women's jobs" like washing dishes and helping with the children.

Such men are evidently overcompensating for unexpressed concerns about their masculinity. In addition, a husband who has consented to vasectomy to resolve the couple's contraceptive problem might feel that he should be rewarded by continual sexual access to his wife, rather than sexual activity by mutual inclination.

Psychological disturbances over vasectomy usually occur in men who already had doubts about their sexual adequacy or who have serious conflicts with their sex partners. Some men unrealistically hope a vasectomy will solve sexual and marital problems. Psychological shock waves may also result when a man resentfully submits to the operation under pressure from his wife or when he has a vasectomy against his wife's wishes. Until such conflicts are resolved, a man is generally better off with other methods of contraception.

Vasectomy should be regarded as irreversible. The procedure should be considered only if a man is certain he will never want to father a child afterward. An estimated 1 out of every 2,000 men who have vasectomies seek reversal of the procedure.

Attempts to reverse the vasectomy are only 28 to 40 percent successful. Unlike the vasectomy, reversal is a risky, lengthy, and expensive operation. Even when the operation (termed a reanastomosis) is successful and sperm are once more ejaculated, there is a strong possibility that the sperm will not be able to fertilize the egg. Despite a technically successful operation, the ability to conceive may be reduced by perhaps 50 percent. The longer the surgery is delayed, the less chance there is of successful reversal.

Bank sperm? Before vasectomy some men have quantities of their sperm frozen in sperm banks. Their hope is that, in the event that they change their minds about having more children, their defrosted sperm would be capable of impregnating their wives by artificial insemination. Thawed sperm has produced hundreds of pregnancies and healthy babies, including two after more than 10 years.

Frozen sperm, however, declines in fertility. One study found a nearly 50 percent reduction in the movement of thawed sperm. The longer the sperm is frozen, the less likely it will be able to cause pregnancy.

Further, artificial insemination has no higher pregnancy rate than natural coitus. Couples trying to conceive often must engage in intercourse many times before succeeding. The supply of fertile sperm may be exhausted before the woman can become pregnant.

Artificial insemination by frozen sperm is more likely to result in pregnancy than attempts at surgical reversal. Even so, in its present state of development it cannot be counted on as "fatherhood insurance."

See also CONTRACEPTION; IMPOTENCE.

VENEREAL DISEASE.

VENEREAL DISEASE. The United States is in the grip of a VD epidemic of unparalleled proportions—one that affects all strata of society.

Increasingly, VD is an affliction of the educated middle- and upper-classes. Investigators for the Oakland County, Michigan, Health Department have their hands full tracking down gonorrhea and syphilis in the affluent Detroit suburbs of Bloomfield Hills, Birmingham, and Southfield. In Prince George's County, Maryland, a suburb of Washington, D.C., the gonorrhea rate has increased fivefold in the last decade.

VD is particularly on the increase among young people. One person in five with gonorrhea is under 20. The rate of infection among 15-to-19-year-olds is rising faster than in any other age group. More than 55 percent of all reported cases of VD occur in persons under 25.

The reservoir from which a person might be infected is enormous. As contagious diseases, syphilis and gonorrhea are outranked in incidence only by the common cold. VD is now first among reportable communicable diseases. The number of cases each year exceeds those of strep throat, scarlet fever, measles, mumps, hepatitis, and tuberculosis *combined.*

Each year, over 600,000 new cases of gonorrhea are reported. An estimated four cases occur for every one reported, so the real figure is more than 2 million. In Atlanta, 1 person in 40 has gonorrhea; in San Francisco, 1 in 50.

For syphilis the figures are similarly disturbing. There are half a million Americans with untreated syphilis today. This year their ranks will be joined by 85,000 new cases.

At any given time, an estimated 14 million Americans have syphilis or gonorrhea or both.

There are over a dozen venereal diseases besides gonorrhea and syphilis. These include herpes, hepatitis, vaginal infections, lice, and a number of others of growing concern. They are "venereal" in the true sense of the word's derivation—from Venus, the Roman goddess of love (venereus is Latin for "sexual desire"). These conditions are also termed STD—sexually transmitted (transmissible) diseases.

The great spread of VD is largely due to increased exposure to sources of infection. More people have multiple sex partners. Unaware—or unconvinced—of the widespread occurrence and severe health hazards of venereal diseases, they take no measures to protect themselves.

The switch from condoms to other methods of birth control has also contributed to the VD epidemic. Formerly, condoms were the most popular form of birth control for the young. Since they prevent direct penis-vagina contact, condoms provide a measure of protection against VD, especially gonorrhea. Now, the widespread use of oral contraceptives and other birth control methods among young people virtually eliminates condoms as a preventive measure.

In recent years, there has been a large increase in the number of infected women. This has grave epidemiological effects. It is the female who is, as a rule, the carrier of these diseases—unwittingly so because in women most cases of infection have no symptoms. In spreading VD, the sexually active woman is increasingly a Typhoid Mary.

If a woman is promiscuous, she is that much more of a carrier. Center for Disease Control epidemiologists tell of Truck Stop Annie, a California waitress, who gave syphilis to 311 men.

A promiscuous carrier can infect men indefinitely, each of whom is likely to give the infection to someone else. If she seeks a cure, she is likely to be reinfected by one of her many sexual contacts. Such reinfection is extremely common.

At the first suspicion of VD, a physician or clinic should be consulted immediately. Medical personnel are trained to treat VD nonjudgmentally, as an infectious illness like any other.

To ward off "Ping-Pong" reinfection, a steady sex partner should go for treatment at the same time. The partner may harbor the disease asymptomatically, and thus may pass it on anew. It is also important to cooperate in giving VD inspectors the names of any casual sexual contacts. Health officials are combating the VD epidemic by tracking down contacts of known cases.

All VD records are confidential. Sexual contacts are not identified to one another or to anyone else.

In one case, an 18-year-old West Virginian was found to have syphilis during a preemployment physical examination. In a confidential interview, the young man volunteered the names of 6 recent sexual contacts, 2 of whom were found to have the disease. From interviews with these 2 people, 41 more contacts were examined. Eleven of them were diagnosed as having syphilis. In all, 137 persons were examined, and 18 new cases of syphilis were identified. Both heterosexual and homosexual behavior played a part. One case of a baby born with syphilis is directly related to this outbreak.

See also CHANCROID; GONORRHEA; HERPES GENITALIS; HEPATITIS; LICE; LYMPHOGRANULOMA VENEREUM; SCABIES; SYPHILIS; VAGINAL INFECTION.

VIBRATORS are sometimes applied to the genitals during masturbation, or as an alternative form of sexual stimulation with a partner.

Usually made of plastic or rubber, vibrators are either electric or battery-operated. Some are phallus-shaped. Others come with a variety of parts for various types of stimulation or massage.

Stimulation of the clitoral area with a vibrator is sometimes used as part of treatment for women who have never experienced orgasm.

Used with care, vibrators generally give pleasure without harm. Some cautions:

• Vibrators may be allergenic. Some people are sensitive to a vibrator's rubber, plastic, or metal parts. They should be especially wary if they are subject to contact dermatitis from nickel jewelry or rubber gloves. Use of the device should be stopped at the first sign of reddening, swelling, itching, or blistering. Warm-water baths and douches may relieve the inflammation. If not, an estrogen cream may be prescribed to promote vaginal healing. Persistent irritation requires a vaginal examination.

• Inserting a vibrator into the vagina or rectum may be hazardous, possibly causing bruising, tearing, or inflammation of delicate tissues. Before being inserted, a vibrator should be lubricated, then introduced slowly. While it is inside, the sex partner's weight should not press on it.

• To prevent infection, vibrators should be washed frequently with soap and hot water. If a vibrator is inserted into the rectum, it should be thoroughly washed before being applied to the genitals or inserted into the vagina.

• Frequent or prolonged use of vibrators can cause numbness of the genital area. This is usually temporary.

See also "FRIGIDITY"; MASTURBATION; SEX THERAPY.

VOYEURISM. A voyeur (or Peeping Tom) obtains sexual gratification by observing others undressing or engaging in sexual activity.

To a certain extent, almost all people are voyeurs. It is almost universal for people to be interested in what other people's bodies look like. It is similarly common to be curious about others' sexual activity. There is a voyeuristic quality to viewing sexual activity in movies, reading about it in books, and even observing one's own sexual activity in a mirror.

During childhood and adolescence, occasional peeping is frequent. The practice is more common among males, who may peep in small groups.

When an adult voyeur has a compulsion to peep—and when it is his only means of sexual gratification—his behavior is considered deviant, and he is thought to be in need of therapy.

Voyeurs will rarely observe women they know. It is also rare for them to approach the women they view. Some voyeurs masturbate while peeping. The typical adult voyeur is a man who is very shy with women. He is generally passive, socially inhibited, and fearful. He has less heterosexual experience than usual and strong feelings of inferiority. He may have sexual difficulties in heterosexual relationships.

VULVA. See FEMALE SEXUAL ANATOMY.

VULVITIS is inflammation of the vulva, the female's external genitals. Itching, swelling, pain, and burning are common symptoms. Intercourse may be painful.

Vulvitis may result from a wide variety of causes. Among them are venereal diseases, vaginal infections, venereal warts, and parasitic diseases such as pubic lice or scabies.

Inflammation may also result from skin conditions such as psoriasis, or from allergic reactions to clothing, detergents, or drugs. Scratching or chafing may also cause inflammation. Sometimes the condition is cancerous. Persistent vulvitis may require biopsy and/or colposcopy (examination with a special instrument).

To treat vulvitis, the underlying cause must be determined, and appropriate therapy administered.

Oral antihistamines and cortisone creams are usually prescribed to control itching and irritation. The sedative effect of the antihistamines helps women whose sleep is disturbed by itching.

WARTS, VENEREAL (condylomata acuminata). Generally sexually transmitted, these warts are caused by a virus. They appear on the genitals or around the anus.

Anal warts are a common problem among women who engage in anal intercourse and homosexual men who are anal-receptors. In others, warts around the anus may have spread from genital warts.

Venereal warts may be pink, white or brown-gray. If neglected, the warts may grow together to become large cauliflowerlike structures.

In women, the growth of warts on the genitals is likely to be stimulated by pregnancy or irritating vaginal discharge.

Anal warts may be mistaken for hemorrhoids. Despite the high frequency of anal warts, most people are ignorant of this condition. They often assume that these painless, sometimes itchy, lumps are hemorrhoids. Like hemorrhoids, anal warts may bleed, especially after bowel movements or anal intercourse. Embarrassment and shame are common reactions to the diagnosis of anal warts. Patients with anal warts are advised to avoid anal-receptive intercourse until the warts are treated. Patients with genital warts should similarly refrain from intercourse as long as warts are present.

Treatment is as for other types of warts: with caustic chemicals like podophyllin, surgical excision, electrical burning, or cryotherapy (freezing). Internal anal warts may be treated with trichloroacetic acid.

Follow-up examinations are recommended since venereal warts tend to recur after treatment.

See also ANAL SEX; VENEREAL DISEASE.

WET DREAM. See NOCTURNAL EMISSION.

WHIPPING. See SADOMASOCHISM.

WITHDRAWAL (coitus interruptus) is probably the oldest form of birth control. It requires the man to withdraw his penis from the woman's vagina just before he ejaculates. While better than no method of birth control at all, withdrawal is woefully subject to failure.

In theory this common method costs nothing and is always available. But it can make the woman pregnant if the man is slow in withdrawing and deposits even a drop of semen in her vagina. Preseminal fluid may also leak into her vagina long before he ejaculates. It contains live, active sperm, which may cause pregnancy. If he ejaculates near her vagina, some sperm may get inside and swim up into her uterus.

Withdrawal makes great demands on the man's self-control. The split-second timing required can interfere with a couple's enjoyment of sex. The stress connected with the frequent use of withdrawal may lead to sexual and psychological problems. The woman is often anxious over whether the man got out in time. He may not know if he did and so may be plagued by worry and guilt.

See also CONTRACEPTION.

WOMB. See FEMALE SEXUAL ANATOMY.

YEAST INFECTION (moniliasis, candidiasis, fungus infection) is a vaginal infection caused by the fungus candida albicans. It is characterized by itching in and around the vagina, and a thick cottage-cheesy discharge with white patches. The vagina and outer genital area may be reddened, raw, and irritated. Intercourse may be painful. Some sufferers feel a need for frequent urination, sometimes with a burning sensation.

Yeast infection is caused by yeast spores which usually inhabit the rectum and vagina, causing no harm. But when the normal balance of bacteria, fungi, and other organisms in the vagina is disturbed, the yeast may cause symptoms. Women often develop yeast infections while taking antibiotics for infectious disease. The antibiotics also kill the normal bacteria in the vagina, allowing yeast to grow unchecked.

Women in pregnancy and women with diabetes are more susceptible to yeast infections because their balance of organisms is changed. Taking birth control pills may promote yeast infections since the pills lessen the acidity of the vagina. Vaginal douching, or bathing in bubble baths or very soapy water, can also change the normal acid/alkaline balance of the vagina, resulting in infection.

A woman is also more susceptible to yeast infections when her resistance is low from another infection (even another vaginal infection, which changes the content of the vagina), poor diet, insufficient sleep, or drug taking.

The infection is sometimes transmitted through sexual intercourse. Many men who have yeast infections show no symptoms. But they can pass the infection to women during intercourse. A woman who seems to have a chronic yeast infection may actually be recurrently reinfected by her mate.

If a woman is suffering from a yeast infection when her baby is born, the baby may acquire the fungus as it passes through the birth canal. The infection affects the baby's mouth and is called thrush.

Physicians diagnose yeast infection by noting the characteristic discharge and redness in the vagina. A vaginal smear examined under a microscope confirms the diagnosis.

A number of remedies have been used successfully, but yeast infections tend to recur. Sometimes, the infection seems to be gone, only to flare up after the next menstrual period alters the environment of the vagina.

For treatment, a woman may first need to reduce the inflammation by means of soda bicarbonate sitz baths and wet compresses, avoiding soap. Antihistamines such as Periactin may be prescribed.

Many doctors advise their patients to stop using oral contraceptives when they have yeast infections. Physicians may also advise against having sexual intercourse while a woman is infected. Some physicians recommend using condoms.

An effective traditional treatment is the use of aqueous solution gentian violet. The physician paints it on the vagina, cervix, and outer genitals. Then the patient can use gentian violet gels, creams, or tampons daily. Among these are Gentia Jel, Gentersal Cream, Genepax Tampons, and Hyva Vaginal Suppositories. The major drawback of gentian violet is its messiness. Everything it touches is stained purple, so it is a good idea to wear a sanitary napkin for the duration of the treatment.

Many doctors prefer to prescribe miconazole (Monistat) vaginal cream or nystatin (Mycostatin) or candicidin (Vanobid) vaginal suppositories, one or two daily. The treatment is usually continued for 10 to 15 days, and may have to be repeated. If the suppositories alone are not effective, oral tablets 3 times daily may be prescribed concurrently. This may control a possible intestinal source of the yeast infection. Since the symptoms may disappear even though the infection remains, a woman should be checked 4 to 6 weeks after treatment is discontinued.

To help prevent yeast infections it is wise to wear cotton instead of nylon underwear. The vaginal area should be kept clean and dry, and the labia should be spread apart when bathing. Women should be sure to wipe themselves from the vagina toward the rectum, so that organisms from the rectum will not get into the vagina.

Panties, bathing suits, and tub surfaces should be thoroughly washed. A woman who uses a diaphragm should wash it particularly thoroughly with soap and water. If she has had recurring and persistent yeast infections, it may be best to throw the diaphragm away.

At the first sign of an infection, a woman can try to restore the normal acid/alkaline balance of her vagina by douching with 2 tablespoons of vinegar in a quart of water. This may possibly stop the infection. So may a douche of 2 tablespoons of active culture yogurt in a quart of water. Douching should be avoided during pregnancy.

See also VAGINAL DOUCHING; VAGINAL INFECTION; VENEREAL DISEASE.

INDEX

Eyes
  and amyl nitrate, 17
  circles under, 239
  infection, 207
  pain, 203
  protrusion, 129
  swelling, 268
  venereal disease and, 108, 118, 120, 202

Face, 127, 134, 220, 255
  See also, Hirsutism
Fainting, 17, 90, 175, 199
Fallopian tubes
  blockage of, 157
  and ectopic pregnancy, 75
  infection of, 107, 157, 224-25, 317
  and IUDs, 161
  and pregnancy, 155
  and sterilization, 304-5
  See also, Female sexual anatomy
Family physician, 269-70
Fantasy
  aid to orgasm, 68, 105, 178, 232, 275
  and clitoral swelling, 59
  and fetishism, 95
  oral impregnation, 22
  sadomasochistic, 265-66
  sharing of, 79
Fatigue
  and depression, 67
  from hormonal disorders, 128-29
  and illness, 72, 118, 296, 305
  after intercourse, 116
  with "male climacteric syndrome," 167
  and sexual dysfunction, 102, 142
  with SLE, 294
  and vaginal problems, 313, 317
Fear
  aftermath of rape, 260, 262
  of contagion, 277, 305, 321
  of debilitation, 203
  of dying, 46-48, 52, 226
  of fatherhood, 82

of hurting, 43, 52, 81
of loss of control, 48, 81, 90, 102
of pain, 29, 314
of pregnancy, 81, 100, 155, 321
of rejection, 172-73, 291
and severe menstrual pain, 199
of sexual failure, 142-43, 150, 273
of sexuality, 76
of suffocation, 264
of women, 90
Feces, contaminated, 13, 18, 106
Fellatio, 208-10, 221, 255
Female sexual anatomy, 91-95
Female Sexuality Following Spinal Cord Injury, 289
Feminine hygiene sprays, 136, 160, 308, 319-20
Femininity, loss of, 172-74, 276
Feminization, 64
Feminizing interstitial-cell testicular tumors, 152
Fenfluramine, 181
Fertility. *See* Infertility; Pregnancy
Fertilization, 155, 161, 197, 204
Fertility clinics, 155
Fetishism, 95, 137, 302
Fever
  after abortion, 5-6
  after circumcision, 56
  with hernia, 119
  in infants, 244
  with infection, 13, 19, 252, 307
  with pelvic inflammatory disease, 225
  with pulmonary tuberculosis, 305
  with SLE, 294
  with venereal disease, 107-9, 118, 121, 293
Fever blisters. *See* Cold sores
Fibrocystic breast disease, 34, 44
Fissures, anal, 18
Flagyl, 13, 106, 303
Flame, 248
Flashing. *See* Exhibitionism
Flatulence, 13, 18

Infectious disease, 238-40, 244, 292-94, 305

See also Venereal disease

Inferiority, 87, 136-37

Infertility, 155-58

and aphrodisiacs, 22-23

and endometriosis, 84-85

and genital tuberculosis, 306

and heroin, 120

and hormone disorders, 127, 128, 132, 134

and IUDs, 163

and Kidney disease, 163-64

and mental retardation, 201

and pelvic inflammatory disease, 162, 225

and smoking, 277

with spinal-cord injury, 282, 285

after surgery, 251, 299-300

treatment for, 190

and undescended testicles, 298-99

of the airways, 26

of the cervix, 317

and excessive menstruation, 200

of the eye, 207

of the intestines, 239

pelvic, 162

of the penis, 56, 159, 229

of the prostate, 252-54

of the testicles, 86, 133, 159, 306

of the vagina, 210, 317

of veins, 221

of the vulva, 210, 330

See also Pelvic inflammatory disease; Prostate, inflammation

Ingestion of female hormones, 152

Inguinal hernia, 119

Inhibited ejaculation, 81-83

Injury

clitoral, 57-58

head, 87

nervous system, 256

pelvic, 83

penile, 149, 159, 229-32

rectal, 17, 85, 125

spinal, 83, 101, 133, 248, 280-89

vaginal, 312

See also Nerve injury

Insanity, syphilitic, 293

Insecurity, 27, 276

Insemination, 83, 158, 326

Insomnia, 67, 116, 126, 144, 185, 194, 205, 239

Institute for Sex Research, 101

Institute of Rehabilitation Medicine, 287

Institutions, 8, 50, 201, 202, 297

Insulin, 128

See also Diabetes

Intercourse

affected by disability, 15-16, 25, 27, 47-49, 164, 214, 282

anal, 17-19

with animals, 20

conditions aggravated by, 51, 114, 248, 263, 307

and the elderly, 8-11

as exercise, 29-30

among family members, 153-55

frequency of, 68-69, 96-101, 136-37, 143, 156, 164, 172, 312

and heart disease, 114-17

impossible, 136, 311-12, 320-22

during menstruation, 197

possibly dangerous, 119, 138

during pregnancy, 243, 247-48

and reconstructed penis, 231

resumption of, 242, 325

and sexual dysfunction, 76-80, 81-82, 102-5

techniques for conception, 156

and vaginal problems, 6, 311, 322-24, 317

See also Venereal disease

with aging, 9

with cancer, 52, 311

after childbirth, 38

from endometriosis, 84-85

and hymen problems, 136

and ostomies, 216